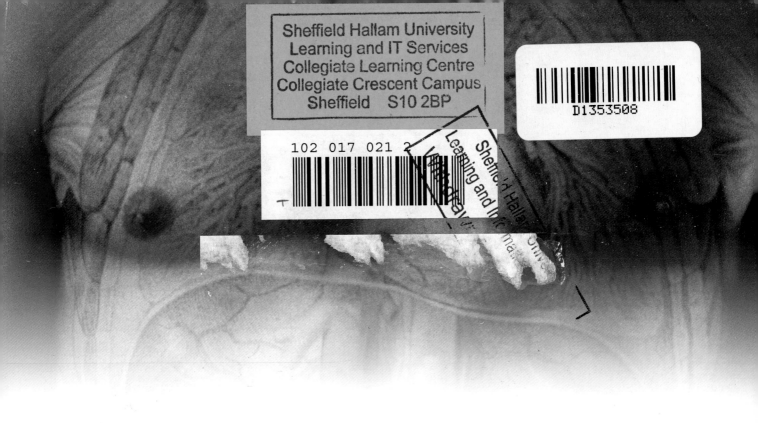

MCMINN & ABRAHAMS'

CLINICAL ATLAS OF
HUMAN ANATOMY

SEVENTH EDITION

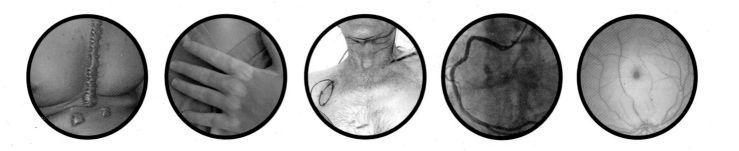

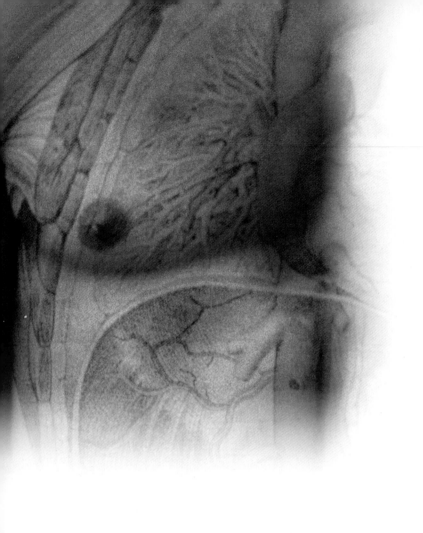

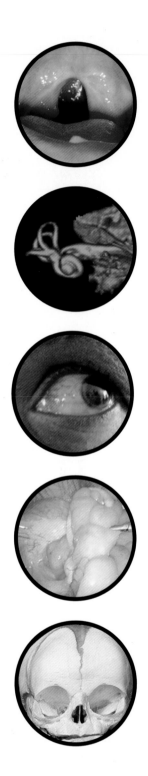

Content Strategist: **Madelene Hyde**

Content Development Specialists: **Rachael Harrison, Sharon Nash**

Publishing Services Manager: **Patricia Tannian**

Senior Project Manager: **Sarah Wunderly**

Design: **Russell Purdy**

Illustration Manager: **Jennifer Rose**

Illustrator: **Oxford Designers & Illustrators**

McMinn & Abrahams'

CLINICAL ATLAS OF
HUMAN
ANATOMY

SEVENTH EDITION

Peter H. Abrahams, MB BS, FRCS (Ed), FRCR, DO (Hon) FHEA
Professor of Clinical Anatomy, Warwick Medical School, UK
Professor of Clinical Anatomy, St. George's University, Grenada, W.I.
National Teaching Fellow 2011, UK
Life Fellow, Girton College, Cambridge, UK
Examiner, MRCS, Royal Colleges of Surgeons (UK)
Family Practitioner, Brent, London, UK

Jonathan D. Spratt, MA (Cantab), FRCS (Eng), FRCS (Glasg), FRCR
Consultant Clinical Radiologist, University Hospital of North Durham, UK
Examiner in Anatomy, Royal College of Radiologists, UK
Visiting Fellow in Radiological Anatomy, University of Northumbria, UK
Visiting Professor of Anatomy, St. George's Medical School, Grenada, W.I.

Marios Loukas, MD, PhD
Professor and Chair, Department of Anatomical Sciences
Dean of Research, School of Medicine
St. George's University, Grenada, W.I.

Albert-Neels van Schoor, BSc MedSci, BSc (Hons), MSc, PhD
Senior Lecturer, Department of Anatomy, School of Medicine, Faculty of Health Sciences
University of Pretoria, Pretoria, Gauteng, South Africa

For additional online content visit studentconsult.com

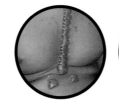
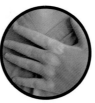
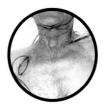
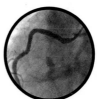
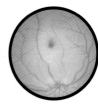

ELSEVIER
MOSBY

ELSEVIER
MOSBY

© 2013, Elsevier Limited. All rights reserved.

First edition 1977 by Wolfe Publishing
Second edition 1988 by Wolfe Publishing
Third edition 1993 by Mosby-Wolfe, an imprint of Times Mirror International Publishers Ltd
Fourth edition 1998 by Mosby, an imprint of Mosby International Ltd
Fifth edition 2003 by Elsevier Science Ltd
Sixth edition 2008 by Elsevier Ltd

British Library Cataloguing in Publication Data
A catalogue record for this book is available from the British Library

ISBN: 978-0723-43697-3
International edition: 978-0723-43698-0

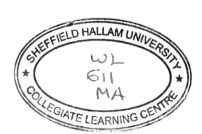

Printed in China

Last digit is the print number: 9 8 7 6 5 4 3 2 1

Dedication and Preface

"To all our long-suffering spouses and children who rarely see us enough and to our international students who see us too much!"

As with most academic literature, there is a large element of truth to the often misquoted "If I have seen further it is by standing on ye sholders of Giants" as written by Sir Isaac Newton to Robert Hooke in 1676. In our case it is not only the giants of our own discipline of anatomy and especially its clinical branch; this atlas has also benefited from a real contribution from our students, colleagues, teachers and mentors.

This new seventh edition of McMinn and Abrahams' *Clinical Atlas of Human Anatomy* is the culmination of 40 years' work by a huge team. The first three editions of this seminal colour atlas were authored by Professor Bob McMinn, Ralph Hutchings and Bari Logan, and the last four editions have been the results of a combined academic endeavour of the now departed "giants" Professors John Pegington (University College London), Sandy Marks (University of Massachusetts, USA) and Hanno Boon (Pretoria, South Africa) working with myself (PHA). For previous dedications see the sixth edition dedication online (www.studentconsult.com).

In the autumn of 2012 we heard the sad news of Bob McMinn's passing at the age of 88. Following in his father's footsteps Bob, graduated from Glasgow University in medicine in 1947. His main academic career was in London, first as Professor at Kings College, London and then as the William Collins Professor at the Royal College of Surgeons of England. Along the way Bob not only gained an MD but a PhD as well in the field of wound healing and tissue repair. However, it is for this revolutionary *McMinn's Colour Atlas of Human Anatomy,* first produced in 1977, that Bob's name is known worldwide. Not only will this seventh edition bring sales to over 2 million in some 30 languages, including Latin, Korean, Chinese, Japanese and most European languages, but this book is also very popular with the art world – something of which he was most proud.

As a founding member of the British Association of Clinical Anatomists and past secretary of the Anatomical Society of Great Britain, Bob was one of my mentors (PHA) and a truly kind, warm-hearted and generous gentleman, whose invitation to work with him on the third edition in 1989 changed my own academic direction and pointed me to the "light" of clinical anatomy. I shall always remember the BACA/AACA

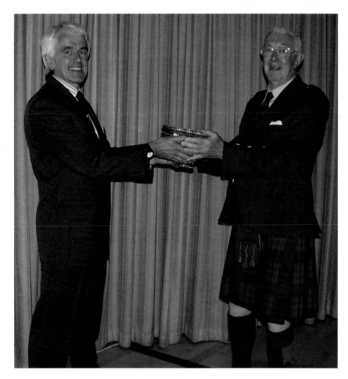

Cambridge meeting in 2000 when Bob, the true Scot, arrived for his presentation as only a Scot can!

This new edition is authored by PHA and Jonathan Spratt, a Director of Radiology at Durham who worked on the sixth edition, and to replace the lost multi-talented giants of clinical anatomy we have transfused some new young anatomical blood.

First we have Professor Marios Loukas MD, PhD, Chair of Department of Anatomical Sciences and Dean of Research, at St. George's University, Grenada, West Indies, who for the last decade has made anatomical waves with his amazing energy and prolific academic output. PHA has known Marios since he was a first-year medical student in Poland and noted his potential even 15 years ago. He is now an internationally recognised and published author and brings to this new edition his wide European education in Greece, Poland and

Germany, as well as his postgraduate experience in Harvard and the Caribbean.

To add to this truly global academic input we also welcome Dr. Albert Van Schoor, anatomist from Pretoria and Honorary Secretary of the Anatomical Society of Southern Africa (ASSA), who is truly following in the footsteps of his own mentor, Professor Hanno Boon. Albert's passion for both teaching and clinically applied research – his PhD was on clinical anatomy of practical procedures in children – was instilled in him by Professor Boon. His African experience and connections with physicians have brought us illustrations from the developing world that often are unavailable in Western culture. Gross pathologies seen in the tropics are vividly illustrated on our web pages.

We, all the authors both old and new, have essentially followed the pattern of Bob McMinn's original work to produce an atlas of the human body aimed at health professionals but have moved the emphasis to correlating the "real" human body dissections directly with clinical practice such as radiology, endoscopy or clinical problems, both in the atlas itself and especially in the clinical vignettes on the website. To this end we have included and done the following:

- Added 100+ new dissections including lymphatics
- Added 100+ radiological images (MR and CT) correlated with dissections
- Added 300+ radiological images for the clinical vignettes on the web
- Increased the clinical anatomy case vignettes to nearly 500 – all now on the web with full download ability as jpeg files onto any student's notes.
- Increased the images on the web to 2000+ which include clinical cases operative images, radiological techniques, endoscopy, etc.

- Added a new video section of 200+ 3D rotations and video loops (mainly 64-slice CT scan reconstructions and angiography) to help students appreciate the anatomical three-dimensional relationships (thanks especially to Dr. Richard Wellings, University Hospitals Coventry and Warwickshire, for most of this collection).

We hope that teachers, especially those in less developed parts of the world, will now be stimulated to give presentations with the latest technology to help their students learn anatomy in all its 3D glory. These video loops are marked by the video icon shown in the key below on the relevant page in the atlas and are all to be found in the 3D files on the web filed under anatomical structures (e.g., arteries, veins, brain, thorax). We hope this latest technology will excite all students in their study of the human body.

For additional electronic content look out for the below icons:

 Go online to view 200+ 3D rotations and video loops

 Go online to view 2000+ clinical cases

PHA
JS
ML
AVS

Acknowledgements

Dissections

Heartfelt thanks to all our **donors and their families** for their ultimate donation for the benefit of mankind and future generations of medical knowledge. This supreme gift to mankind educates and enriches the human experience for generations to come, for today's medical students are tomorrow's clinicians and professors.

The production of this atlas and accompanying web site has been a huge team effort over 5 years and has involved prosectors and professors, teachers and students from four continents but especially from England, South Africa, the United States and the West Indies. We, the four authors, would like to thank all those who worked with us to deliver this new exciting clinical atlas and accompanying web site.

Prosection preparation

Daniële Cavanagh, Franci Dorfling, Heinrich Hesse, Professor Greg Lebona , Lané Prigge, Soné du Plessis, all from the University of Limpopo, Medunsa Campus, South Africa

Nkhensani Mogale, University of Johannesburg, South Africa

Rene Human-Baron, Elsabè Smit, University of Pretoria, South Africa

Theofanis Kollias, Elizabeth Hogan, Mohammed Irfan Ali and faculty Drs. Kathleen Bubb , Deon Forester, and Ewarld Marshall, Department of Anatomical Sciences, St. George's University School of Medicine, Grenada, West Indies.

Many of the new dissections were carried out at the second Hanno Boon Masterclass in Grenada in July of 2011. Those contributing their skills and in honouring the international memory of Professor Hanno Boon (R.I.P.) were Vicky Cottrell, Paul Danse, Maira du Plessis, Alison Tucker, Richard Tunstall, George Salter, Shane Tubbs and the following Warwick University Medical students in the UK—Ross Bannon, Matthew Boissaud-Cooke, Michael Brown, Edward Dawton, Sarah Diaper, Zara Eagle, Elizabeth Jane Harris, Morag Harris, Daniel Lin, Riwa Meshaka, Rob Neave, Charlotte Oakley, Chris Parry, Alison Rangedara, Farah Sadrudin, Jon Senior, Catherine Tart, Adam Walsh, Melanie Whitehead, John Williams, Katie Wooding, Dr. James Chambers.

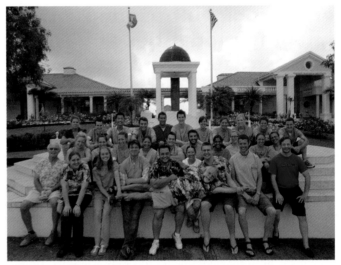

The second Hanno Boon memorial dissection masterclass participants, Grenada, 2011.

Photographic, technical and research

Laura Jane van Schoor (Laura Jane Photography, South Africa) and Joanna Loukas (Department of Anatomical Sciences, St. George's University) for their photographic skills.

Marius Loots, Gert Lewis, and Samuel Ngobeni (Department of Anatomy, University of Pretoria, South Africa) for technical assistance.

Carslon Dominique, Rodon Marast, Christopher Belgrave, Ryan Jacobs, Nadica Thomas-Dominique, Jacqueline Hope, Salisha Thomas and Yvonne James of the Department of Anatomical Sciences at St. Georges University, for their technical and lab assistance.

The following research fellows of the Department of Anatomical Sciences at St. Georges University for their contribution—Drs. Asma Mian, Irfan Chaudhry, Philip Veith, Amit Sharma, Edward Sorenson, Matthew Prekupec and Christa Blaak.

All the mistakes, though hopefully very few, are ours but the following individuals have kept the errors to a minimum with their proof reading skills and expert knowledge: Eng-Tat Ang, PT, PhD; James Chambers, MBChB, BSc(Hons); Sundeep Singh Deol MSc, PhD, MD; Petrut Gogalniceanu, BSc, Med, MRCS; Ruth Joplin, PhD; David A. Magezi MA(Cantab), BM BCh (Oxon), PhD (Notts); David Metcalfe, BSc(Hons), LLB(Hons), MRCS; Barry S Mitchell, BSc, PhD, MSc, FSB, FHEA; Tom Paterson BSc(Hons)Anatomy, MBChB Glasgow; Jamie Roebuck BSc, MBChB, FHEA; R. Subbu, MBChB, MRCS, BSci(HONS); Kapil Sugand, BSc, MBBS; Richard Tunstall, BMedSci, PhD, PGCLTHE, FHEA; Tom Turmezei, MA, MPhil, BMBCh, FRCR; Anne Waddingham, BSc, LCGI.

Clinical, operative, endoscopic, ultrasound, other imaging modalities and videos cases (see also the sixth edition clinical cases acknowledgements on the web page).

Drs. Elias Abdulah MD, Chrystal Antoine MD, Nicole Avril MD, Prof. Danny Burns MD, PhD, Melissa Brandford MD, Katusha Cornwall MD, Adegberno Fakoya MD, Nicole George MD, Prof. Robbie Hage MD, PhD, DLO, MBA, ENT Surgeon, Kennard Philip MD, and Kazzara Raeburn MD, Department of Anatomical Sciences, St. George's University, Grenada, West Indies; Prof. Kitt Shaffer MD, PhD, Department of Radiology, Boston University, Boston Massachusetts, United States; Dr. Robert Ward MD, Department of Radiology, Tufts University, Boston, Massachusetts, United States; Dr. MA Strydom, Steve Biko Academic Hospital, Pretoria, South Africa; Drs. MJ Heystek, M Maharaj, E Poulet, and E Raju, Department of Family Medicine, Tshwane District Hospital, University of Pretoria, South Africa; Dr. PS Levay and Prof. D van Zyl, Department of Internal Medicine, Kalafong Hospital, University of Pretoria, South Africa; Dr. AK Mynhardt, University of Pretoria, South Africa; Dr. MY Gamieldien, Oral & Dental Hospital, University of Pretoria, South Africa; Members of the Department of Plastic and Reconstructive Surgery, University of Limpopo (Medunsa campus), South Africa; Dr. Richard Wellings, Consultant Radiologist and Hon Associate Professor, UHCW Trust and Warwick Medical School, United Kingdom; Ms.Kavita Singh and Mr. Janos Balega, Consultant Gynaecological Oncologists, Sandwell and West Birmingham Hospitals Trust, Pan-Birmingham Gynaecology Cancer Centre Birmingham, United Kingdom; Dr. Adam Iqbal, UHCW Trust and Warwick Medical School; Mr. Michael Brown and Mr. Mark Mobley, Warwick Medical School, University of Warwick, Coventry, United Kingdom; Ms. Nadia Boujo and Mr. Alfred Boujo, London; Dr. Vibart Yaw, Consultant Oral and Maxillofacial Surgeon, General Hospital, St. George's, Grenada, West Indies; Dr. Ankur Gulati, Cardiology Specialist Registrar, The London Chest Hospital, UK

User Guide

This book is arranged in the general order 'head to toe'. The Head and Neck section (including the brain) is followed by the Vertebral column and spinal cord, then Upper limb, Thorax, Abdomen and pelvis, Lower limb and finally Lymphatics. In each section, skeletal elements are shown first followed by dissections, with surface views included for orientation. All structures are labelled by numbers, and these are identified in lists beside each image. An arrowhead at the end of a leader indicates that the structure labelled is just out of view beyond the tip of the arrow. Text has been limited to that needed to understand how the preparation was made, and is not intended to be comprehensive.

Contents

Abdomen and pelvis   5

Lower Limb   6

Lymphatics   7

Orientation

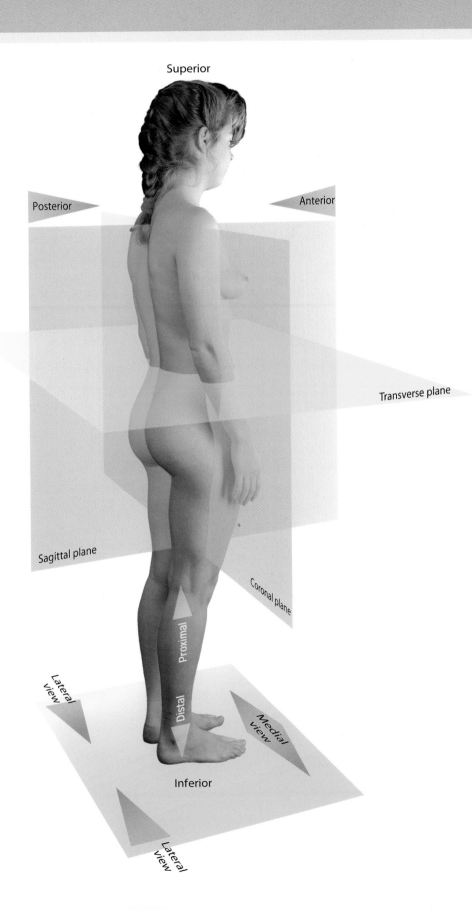

Superior

Posterior

Anterior

Transverse plane

Sagittal plane

Coronal plane

Proximal

Distal

Lateral view

Medial view

Inferior

Lateral view

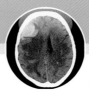
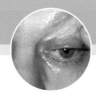
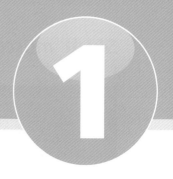
Skull *from the front*

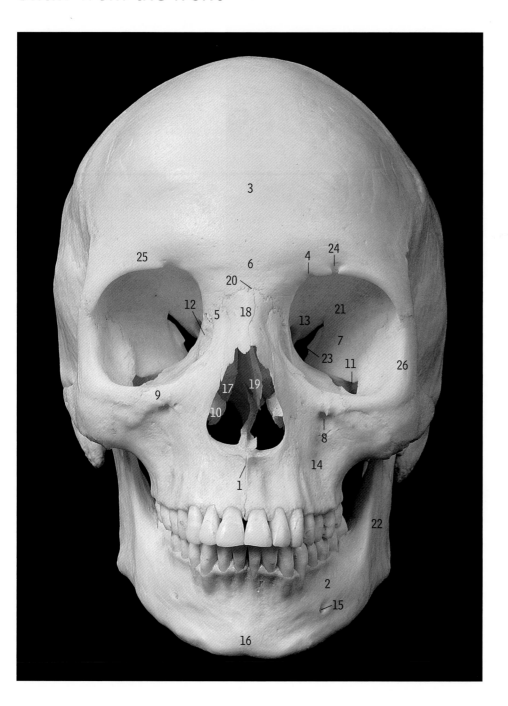

1 Anterior nasal spine
2 Body of mandible
3 Frontal bone
4 Frontal notch
5 Frontal process of maxilla
6 Glabella
7 Greater wing of sphenoid bone
8 Infra-orbital foramen
9 Infra-orbital margin
10 Inferior nasal concha
11 Inferior orbital fissure
12 Lacrimal bone
13 Lesser wing of sphenoid bone
14 Maxilla
15 Mental foramen
16 Mental protuberance
17 Middle nasal concha
18 Nasal bone
19 Nasal septum
20 Nasion
21 Orbit (orbital cavity)
22 Ramus of mandible
23 Superior orbital fissure
24 Supra-orbital foramen
25 Supra-orbital margin
26 Zygomatic bone

The term 'skull' includes the mandible, and 'cranium' refers to the skull without the mandible.

The calvarium is the vault of the skull (cranial vault or skull-cap) and is the upper part of the cranium that encloses the brain.

The front part of the skull forms the facial skeleton.

The supra-orbital, infra-orbital and mental foramina (24, 8 and 15) lie in approximately the same vertical plane.

Details of individual skull bones are given on pages 18–27, of the bones of the orbit and nose on page 12, and of the teeth on pages 13–19.

Tripod fracture, see pages 80–82.

Skull *muscle attachments, from the front*

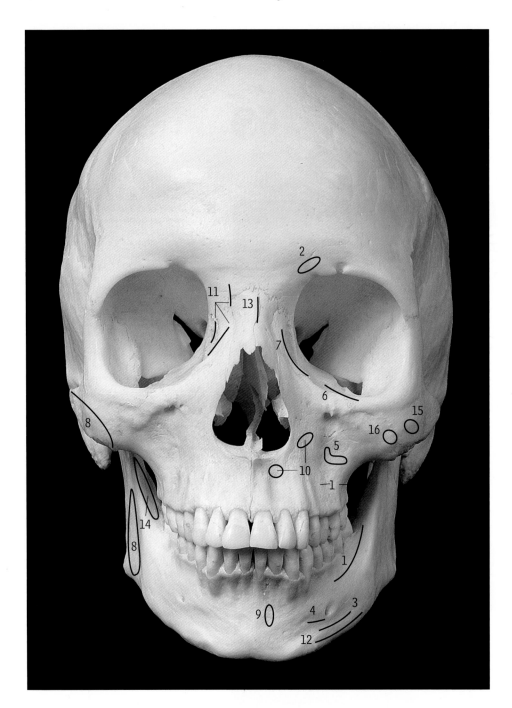

1 Buccinator
2 Corrugator supercilii
3 Depressor anguli oris
4 Depressor labii inferioris
5 Levator anguli oris
6 Levator labii superioris
7 Levator labii superioris alaeque
   nasi
8 Masseter
9 Mentalis
10 Nasalis
11 Orbicularis oculi
12 Platysma
13 Procerus
14 Temporalis
15 Zygomaticus major
16 Zygomaticus minor

Skull *radiograph, occipitofrontal 15° projection*

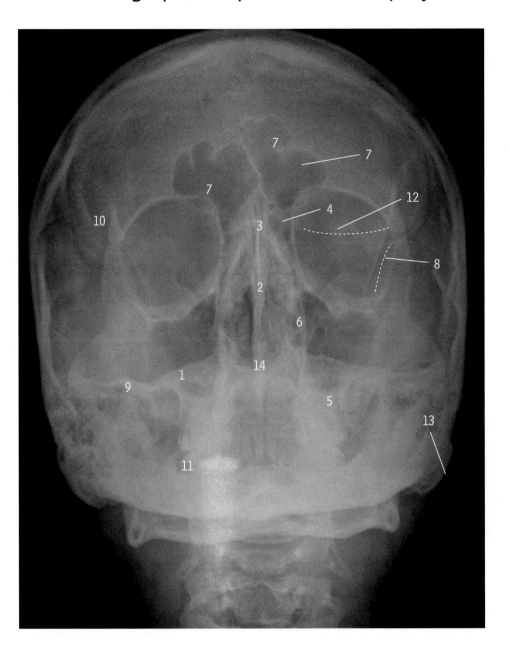

1 Basi-occiput
2 Body of sphenoid
3 Crista galli
4 Ethmoidal air cells
5 Floor of maxillary sinus (antrum)
6 Foramen rotundum
7 Frontal sinus
8 Greater wing of sphenoid
9 Internal acoustic meatus
10 Lambdoid suture
11 Lateral mass of atlas (first cervical vertebra)
12 Lesser wing of sphenoid
13 Mastoid process
14 Nasal septum

Skull *from the right*

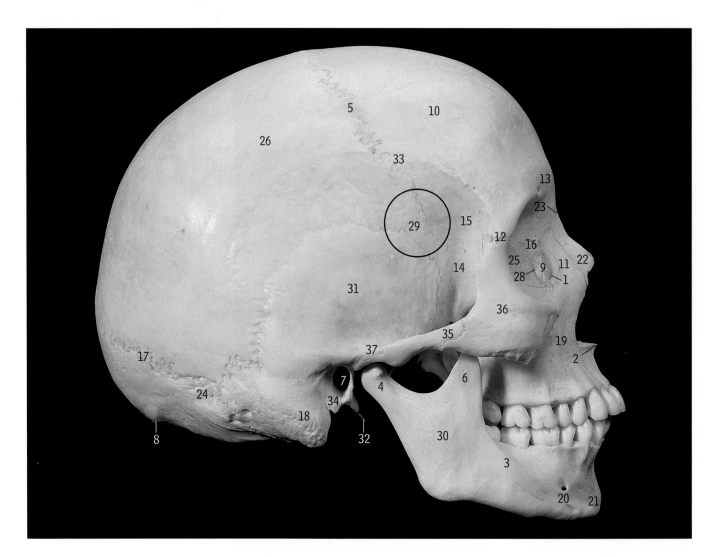

1 Anterior lacrimal crest	**10** Frontal bone	**20** Mental foramen	**30** Ramus of mandible
2 Anterior nasal spine	**11** Frontal process of maxilla	**21** Mental protuberance	**31** Squamous part of temporal
3 Body of mandible	**12** Frontozygomatic suture	**22** Nasal bone	bone
4 Condylar process of the	**13** Glabella	**23** Nasion	**32** Styloid process of temporal
mandible	**14** Greater wing of sphenoid	**24** Occipital bone	bone
5 Coronal suture	bone	**25** Orbital plate of ethmoid	**33** Superior temporal line
6 Coronoid process of mandible	**15** Inferior temporal line	bone	**34** Tympanic part of temporal
7 External acoustic meatus of	**16** Lacrimal bone	**26** Parietal bone	bone
temporal bone	**17** Lambdoid suture	**27** Pituitary fossa (sella turcica)	**35** Zygomatic arch
8 External occipital	**18** Mastoid process of temporal	(see Figure A on page 5)	**36** Zygomatic bone
protuberance (inion)	bone	**28** Posterior lacrimal crest	**37** Zygomatic process of
9 Fossa for lacrimal sac	**19** Maxilla	**29** Pterion (encircled)	temporal bone

Pterion (29) is not a single point but an area where the frontal (10), parietal (26), squamous part of the temporal (31) and greater wing of the sphenoid bone (14) adjoin one another.

It is an important landmark for the anterior branch of the middle meningeal artery, which underlies this area on the inside of the skull (page 17).

  Extradural haemorrhage, see pages 80–82.

Skull

A radiograph, lateral projection

C coloured bones

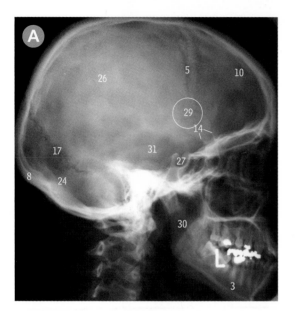

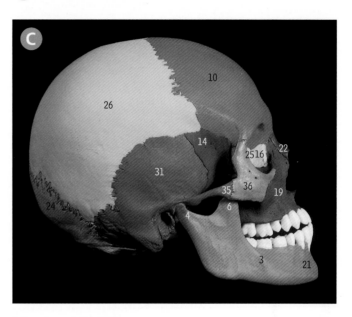

See label list on page 4 for A and C labels

B scalp dissection

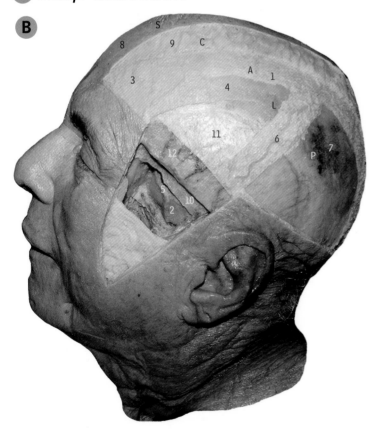

Scalp layers

S, skin; **C**, connective tissue; **A**, aponeurosis of occipitofrontalis; **L**, loose areolar tissue; **P**, periosteum.

1 Aponeurosis of occipitofrontalis
2 Dura mater
3 Frontalis muscle (covered by loose areolar tissue)
4 Loose areolar tissue
5 Middle meningeal artery impression on dura mater
6 Parietal branch of the superficial temporal artery
7 Periosteum
8 Skin
9 Subcutaneous tissue
10 Temporal bone
11 Temporal fascia
12 Temporalis muscle

Skull *muscle attachments, from the right*

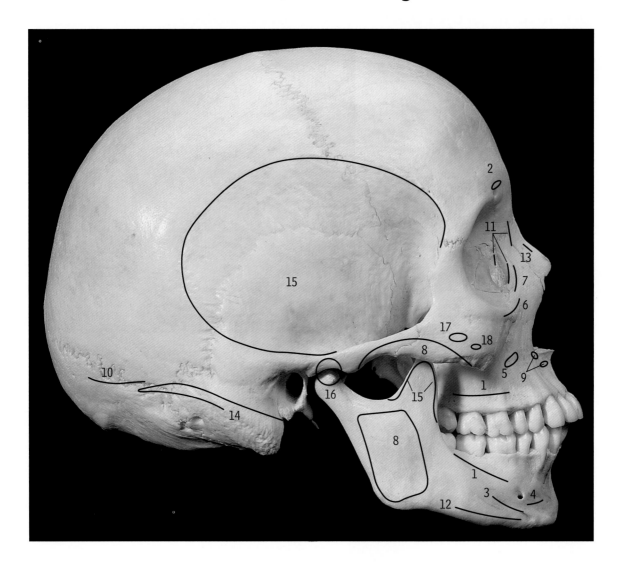

1 Buccinator
2 Corrugator supercilii
3 Depressor anguli oris
4 Depressor labii inferioris
5 Levator anguli oris
6 Levator labii superioris
7 Levator labii superioris alaeque nasi
8 Masseter
9 Nasalis
10 Occipital part of occipitofrontalis
11 Orbicularis oculi
12 Platysma
13 Procerus
14 Sternocleidomastoid
15 Temporalis
16 Temporomandibular joint
17 Zygomaticus major
18 Zygomaticus minor

The bony attachments of the buccinator muscle (1) are to the upper and lower jaws (maxilla and mandible) opposite the three molar teeth. (The teeth are identified on pages 13–19.)

The upper attachment of temporalis (upper 15) occupies the temporal fossa (the narrow space above the zygomatic arch at the side of the skull). The lower attachment of temporalis (lower 15) extends from the lowest part of the mandibular notch of the mandible, over the coronoid process and down the front of the ramus almost as far as the last molar tooth.

Masseter (8) extends from the zygomatic arch to the lateral side of the ramus of the mandible.

Temporomandibular joint (TMJ) dislocation, see pages 80–82.

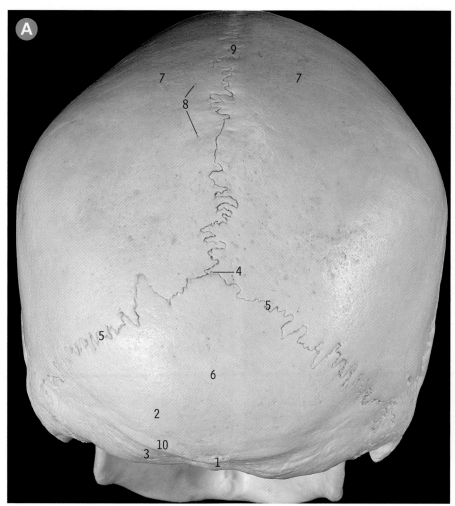

A Skull *from behind*

1 External occipital protuberance (inion)
2 Highest nuchal line
3 Inferior nuchal line
4 Lambda
5 Lambdoid suture
6 Occipital bone
7 Parietal bone
8 Parietal foramina
9 Sagittal suture
10 Superior nuchal line

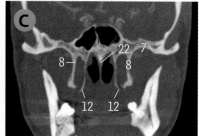

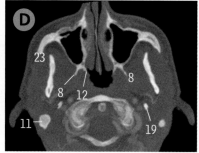

See label list below for C and D.

B Skull *right infratemporal region, obliquely from below*

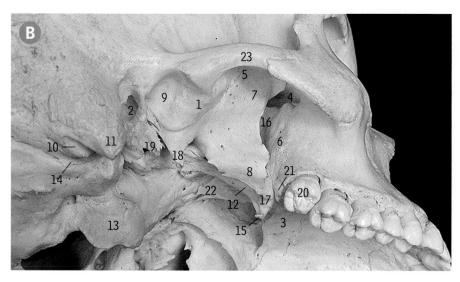

1 Articular tubercle
2 External acoustic meatus
3 Horizontal plate of palatine bone
4 Inferior orbital fissure
5 Infratemporal crest
6 Infratemporal (posterior) surface of maxilla
7 Infratemporal surface of greater wing of sphenoid bone
8 Lateral pterygoid plate
9 Mandibular fossa
10 Mastoid notch
11 Mastoid process
12 Medial pterygoid plate
13 Occipital condyle
14 Occipital groove
15 Pterygoid hamulus
16 Pterygomaxillary fissure and pterygopalatine fossa
17 Pyramidal process of palatine bone
18 Spine of sphenoid bone
19 Styloid process and sheath
20 Third maxillary molar tooth
21 Tuberosity of maxilla
22 Vomer
23 Zygomatic arch

A Skull *from above*

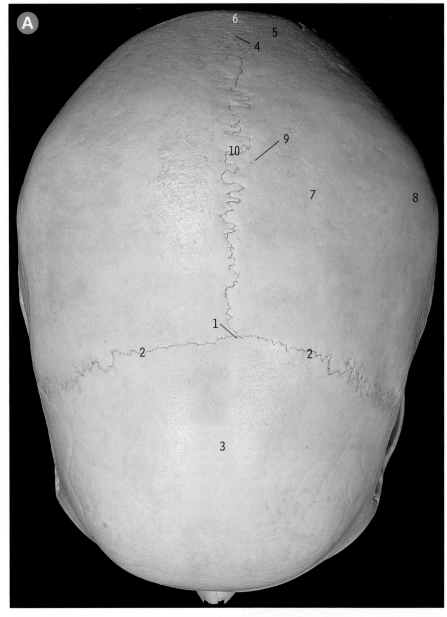

B Skull *internal surface of the cranial vault, central part*

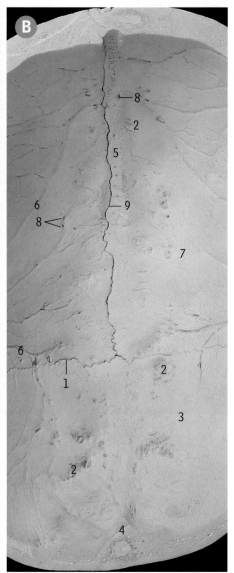

1 Bregma	
2 Coronal suture	
3 Frontal bone	
4 Lambda	
5 Lambdoid suture	
6 Occipital bone	
7 Parietal bone	
8 Parietal eminence	
9 Parietal foramen	
10 Sagittal suture	

In this skull, the parietal eminences are prominent (A8).

The point where the sagittal suture (A10) meets the coronal suture (A2) is the bregma (A1). At birth, the unossified parts of the frontal and parietal bones in this region form the membranous anterior fontanelle (page 14, D1).

The point where the sagittal suture (A10) meets the lambdoid suture (A5) is the lambda (A4). At birth, the unossified parts of the parietal and occipital bones in this region form the membranous posterior fontanelle (page 14, C13).

The label A3 in the centre of the frontal bone indicates the line of the frontal suture in the fetal skull (page 14, A5). The suture may persist in the adult skull and is sometimes known as the metopic suture.

The arachnoid granulations (page 62, B1), through which cerebrospinal fluid drains into the superior sagittal sinus, cause the irregular depressions (B2) on the parts of the frontal and parietal bones (B3 and 7) that overlie the sinus.

1 Coronal suture
2 Depressions for arachnoid granulations
3 Frontal bone
4 Frontal crest
5 Groove for superior sagittal sinus
6 Grooves for middle meningeal vessels
7 Parietal bone
8 Parietal foramina
9 Sagittal suture

Pepperpot skull, see pages 80–82.

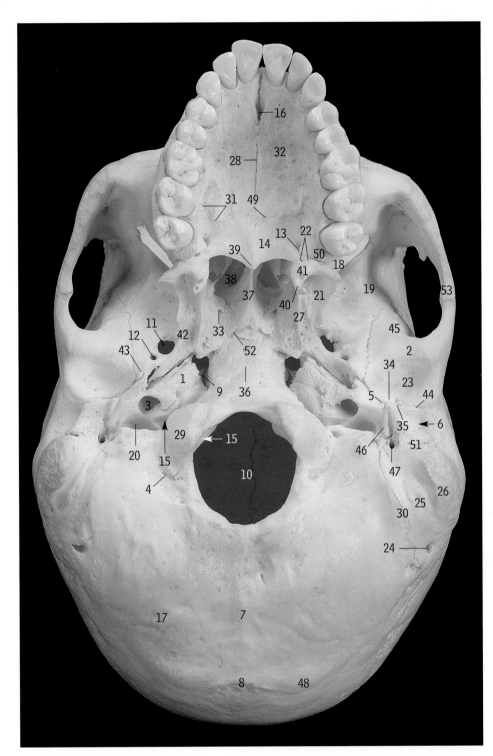

Skull
external surface of the base

1 Apex of petrous part of temporal bone
2 Articular tubercle
3 Carotid canal
4 Condylar canal (posterior)
5 Edge of tegmen tympani
6 External acoustic meatus
7 External occipital crest
8 External occipital protuberance
9 Foramen lacerum
10 Foramen magnum
11 Foramen ovale
12 Foramen spinosum
13 Greater palatine foramen
14 Horizontal plate of palatine bone
15 Hypoglossal canal
16 Incisive fossa
17 Inferior nuchal line
18 Inferior orbital fissure
19 Infratemporal crest of greater wing of sphenoid bone
20 Jugular foramen
21 Lateral pterygoid plate
22 Lesser palatine foramina
23 Mandibular fossa
24 Mastoid foramen
25 Mastoid notch
26 Mastoid process
27 Medial pterygoid plate
28 Median palatine (intermaxillary) suture
29 Occipital condyle
30 Occipital groove
31 Palatine grooves and spines
32 Palatine process of maxilla
33 Pharyngeal canal
34 Petrosquamous fissure
35 Petrotympanic fissure
36 Pharyngeal tubercle
37 Posterior border of vomer
38 Posterior nasal aperture (choana)
39 Posterior nasal spine
40 Pterygoid hamulus
41 Pyramidal process of palatine bone
42 Scaphoid fossa
43 Spine of sphenoid bone
44 Squamotympanic fissure
45 Squamous part of temporal bone
46 Styloid process
47 Stylomastoid foramen
48 Superior nuchal line
49 Transverse palatine (palatomaxillary) suture
50 Tuberosity of maxilla
51 Tympanic part of temporal bone
52 Vomerovaginal canal
53 Zygomatic arch

The palatine processes of the maxilla (32) and the horizontal plate of the palatine bone (14) form the hard palate (roof of the mouth and floor of the nasal cavity).

The carotid canal (3), recognized by its round shape on the inferior surface of the petrous part of the temporal bone, does not pass straight upwards to open into the inside of the skull but takes a right-angled turn forwards and medially within the petrous temporal to open into the back of the foramen lacerum (9).

Intracranial spread of infection, skull fracture, see pages 80–82.

Skull *muscle attachments, external surface of the base*

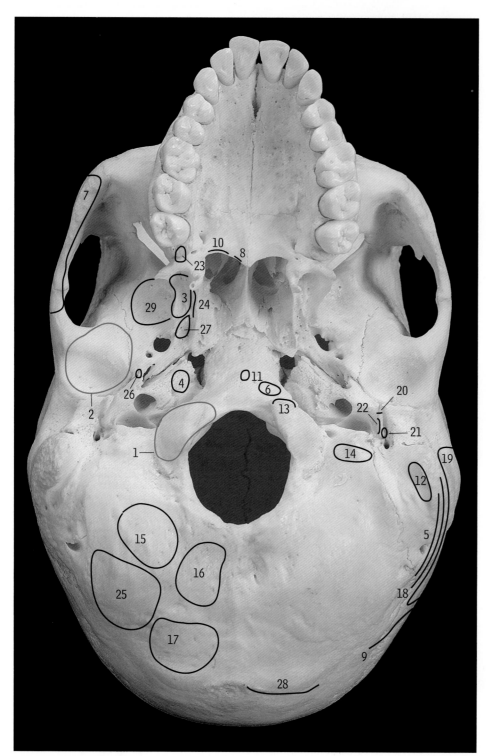

**Green line = capsule attachments
of atlanto-occipital and
temporomandibular joints**

 1 Capsule attachment of atlanto-
    occipital joint
 2 Capsule attachment of
    temporomandibular joint
 3 Deep head of medial pterygoid
 4 Levator veli palatini
 5 Longissimus capitis
 6 Longus capitis
 7 Masseter
 8 Musculus uvulae
 9 Occipital part of occipitofrontalis
10 Palatopharyngeus
11 Pharyngeal raphe
12 Posterior belly of digastric
13 Rectus capitis anterior
14 Rectus capitis lateralis
15 Rectus capitis posterior major
16 Rectus capitis posterior minor
17 Semispinalis capitis
18 Splenius capitis
19 Sternocleidomastoid
20 Styloglossus
21 Stylohyoid
22 Stylopharyngeus
23 Superficial head of medial pterygoid
24 Superior constrictor
25 Superior oblique
26 Tensor tympani
27 Tensor veli palatini
28 Trapezius
29 Upper head of lateral pterygoid

The medial pterygoid plate has no
pterygoid muscles attached to it. It
passes straight backwards, giving
origin at its lower end to part of the
superior constrictor of the pharynx
(24).

The lateral pterygoid plate has both
pterygoid muscles attached to it:
medial and lateral muscles from the
medial and lateral surfaces,
respectively (3 and 29). The plate
becomes twisted slightly laterally
because of the constant pull of these
muscles which pass backwards and
laterally to their attachments to the
mandible (pages 18–19).

Skull fractures, see pages 80–82.

Skull *internal surface of the base (cranial fossae)*

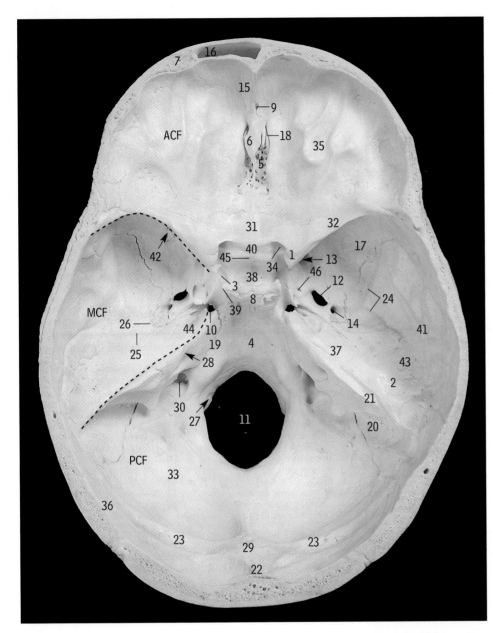

1 Anterior clinoid process
2 Arcuate eminence
3 Carotid groove
4 Clivus
5 Cribriform plate of ethmoid bone
6 Crista galli
7 Diploë
8 Dorsum sellae
9 Foramen caecum
10 Foramen lacerum
11 Foramen magnum
12 Foramen ovale
13 Foramen rotundum
14 Foramen spinosum
15 Frontal crest
16 Frontal sinus
17 Greater wing of sphenoid bone
18 Groove for anterior ethmoidal nerve
   and vessels
19 Groove for inferior petrosal sinus
20 Groove for sigmoid sinus
21 Groove for superior petrosal sinus
22 Groove for superior sagittal sinus
23 Groove for transverse sinus
24 Grooves for middle meningeal vessels
25 Hiatus and groove for greater
   petrosal nerve
26 Hiatus and groove for lesser petrosal
   nerve
27 Hypoglossal canal
28 Internal acoustic meatus
29 Internal occipital protuberance
30 Jugular foramen
31 Jugum of sphenoid bone
32 Lesser wing of sphenoid bone
33 Occipital bone (cerebellar fossa)
34 Optic canal
35 Orbital part of frontal bone
36 Parietal bone (postero-inferior angle
   only)
37 Petrous part of temporal bone
38 Pituitary fossa (sella turcica)
39 Posterior clinoid process
40 Prechiasmatic groove
41 Squamous part of temporal bone
42 Superior orbital fissure
43 Tegmen tympani
44 Trigeminal impression
45 Tuberculum sellae
46 Venous (emissary) foramen

The anterior cranial fossa (ACF) is limited posteriorly on each side by the free margin of the lesser wing of the sphenoid (32) with its anterior clinoid process (1), and centrally by the anterior margin of the prechiasmatic groove (40).

The middle cranial fossa (MCF) is butterfly-shaped and consists of a central or median part and right and left lateral parts. The central part includes the pituitary fossa (38) on the upper surface of the body of the sphenoid, with the prechiasmatic groove (40) in front and the dorsum sellae (8) with its posterior clinoid processes (39) behind. Each lateral part extends from the posterior border of the lesser wing of the sphenoid (32) to the groove for the superior petrosal sinus (21) on the upper edge of the petrous part of the temporal bone.

The posterior cranial fossa (PCF), whose most obvious feature is the foramen magnum (11), is behind the dorsum sellae (8) and the grooves for the superior petrosal sinuses (21).

For cranial dural attachments and reflections, see pages 51–53 and 62.

Anosmia, skull base fracture, see pages 80–82.

Ⓐ Skull *bones of the left orbit*

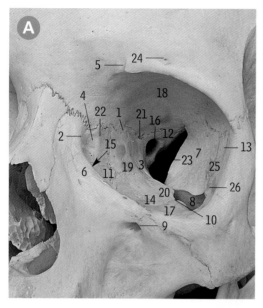

Ⓒ Nasal cavity *lateral wall*

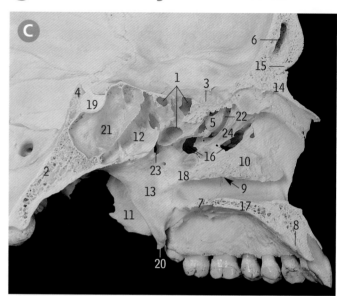

1 Anterior ethmoidal foramen
2 Anterior lacrimal crest
3 Body of sphenoid bone, forming medial wall
4 Fossa for lacrimal sac
5 Frontal notch
6 Frontal process of maxilla, forming medial wall
7 Greater wing of sphenoid bone, forming lateral wall
8 Inferior orbital fissure
9 Infra-orbital foramen
10 Infra-orbital groove
11 Lacrimal bone, forming medial wall
12 Lesser wing of sphenoid bone, forming roof
13 Marginal tubercle

14 Maxilla, forming floor
15 Nasolacrimal canal
16 Optic canal
17 Orbital border of zygomatic bone, forming floor
18 Orbital part of frontal bone, forming roof
19 Orbital plate of ethmoid bone, forming medial wall
20 Orbital process of palatine bone, forming floor
21 Posterior ethmoidal foramen
22 Posterior lacrimal crest
23 Superior orbital fissure
24 Supra-orbital foramen
25 Zygomatic bone forming lateral wall
26 Zygomatico-orbital foramen

In this midline sagittal section of the skull, with the nasal septum removed, the superior and middle nasal conchae have been dissected away to reveal the air cells of the ethmoidal sinus, in particular the ethmoidal bulla (5).

1 Air cells of ethmoidal sinus
2 Clivus
3 Cribriform plate of ethmoid bone
4 Dorsum sellae
5 Ethmoidal bulla
6 Frontal sinus
7 Horizontal plate of palatine bone
8 Incisive canal
9 Inferior meatus
10 Inferior nasal concha
11 Lateral pterygoid plate
12 Left sphenoidal sinus

13 Medial pterygoid plate
14 Nasal bone
15 Nasal spine of frontal bone
16 Opening of maxillary sinus
17 Palatine process of maxilla
18 Perpendicular plate of palatine bone
19 Pituitary fossa (sella turcica)
20 Pterygoid hamulus
21 Right sphenoidal sinus
22 Semilunar hiatus
23 Sphenopalatine foramen
24 Uncinate process of ethmoid bone

The roof of the nasal cavity consists mainly of the cribriform plate of the ethmoid bone (C3) with the body of the sphenoid containing the sphenoidal sinuses (C21 and 12) behind, and the nasal bone (C14) and the nasal spine of the frontal bone (C15) at the front.

The floor of the cavity consists of the palatine process of the maxilla (C17) and the horizontal plate of the palatine bone (C7).

The medial wall is the nasal septum which is formed mainly by two bones – the perpendicular plate of the ethmoid and the vomer – and the septal cartilage.

The lateral wall consists of the medial surface of the maxilla with its large opening (C16), overlapped from above by parts of the ethmoid (C1, 5 and 24) and lacrimal bones, from behind by the perpendicular plate of the palatine (C18), and below by the inferior concha (C10).

Ⓑ Skull *Left orbit, individual bones*

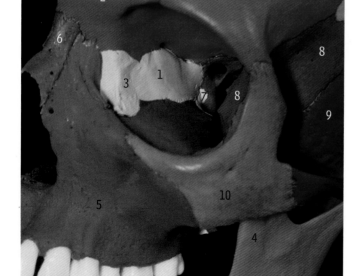

1 Ethmoid
2 Frontal
3 Lacrimal
4 Mandible
5 Maxilla

6 Nasal
7 Palatine
8 Sphenoid
9 Temporal
10 Zygomatic

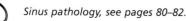

Sinus pathology, see pages 80–82.

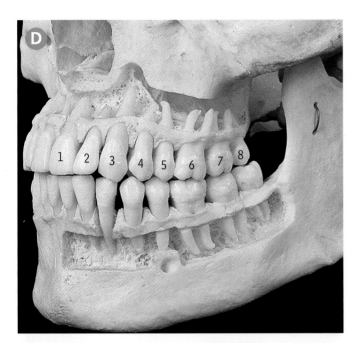

D Permanent teeth
from the left and in front

1 First (central) incisor
2 Second (lateral) incisor
3 Canine
4 First premolar
5 Second premolar
6 First molar
7 Second molar
8 Third molar

The corresponding teeth of the upper and lower jaws have similar names. In clinical dentistry, the teeth are usually identified by the numbers 1–8 (as listed here) rather than by name.

The third molar is sometimes called the wisdom tooth.

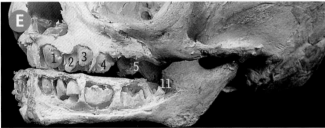

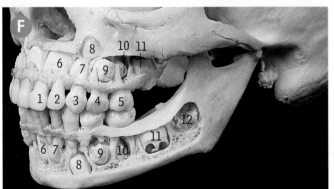

Upper and lower jaws
from the left and in front

E in the newborn with unerupted deciduous teeth

F in a 4-year-old child with erupted deciduous teeth and unerupted permanent teeth

1 First (central) incisor of deciduous dentition
2 Second (lateral) incisor of deciduous dentition
3 Canine of deciduous dentition
4 First molar of deciduous dentition
5 Second molar of deciduous dentition
6 First (central) incisor of permanent dentition
7 Second (lateral) incisor of permanent dentition
8 Canine of permanent dentition
9 First premolar of permanent dentition
10 Second premolar of permanent dentition
11 First molar of permanent dentition
12 Second molar of permanent dentition

The deciduous molars occupy the positions of the premolars of the permanent dentition.

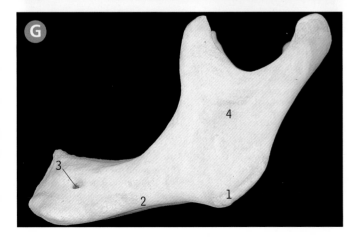

G Edentulous mandible
in old age, from the left

1 Angle
2 Body
3 Mental foramen
4 Ramus

With the loss of teeth, the alveolar bone becomes resorbed, so that the mental foramen (3) and mandibular canal lie near the upper margin of the bone.

The angle (1) between the ramus (4) and body (2) becomes more obtuse, resembling the infantile angle (as in E and F, above).

Skull of a full-term fetus

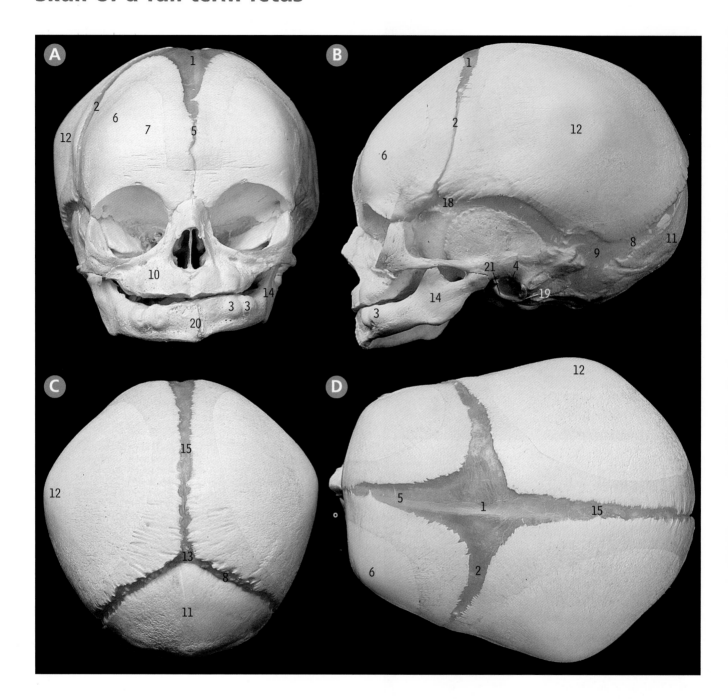

Cleft lip and palate, see pages 80–82.

A **from the front**

B **from the left and slightly below**

C **from behind**

D **from above**

1	Anterior fontanelle	**11**	Occipital bone
2	Coronal suture	**12**	Parietal tuberosity
3	Elevations over deciduous teeth in body of mandible	**13**	Posterior fontanelle
		14	Ramus of mandible
4	External acoustic meatus	**15**	Sagittal suture
5	Frontal suture	**16**	Sella turcica
6	Frontal tuberosity	**17**	Semicircular canals, superior
7	Half of frontal bone	**18**	Sphenoidal fontanelle
8	Lambdoid suture	**19**	Stylomastoid foramen
9	Mastoid fontanelle	**20**	Symphysis menti
10	Maxilla	**21**	Tympanic ring

Fetal skull radiographs **E** *frontal projection* **F** *lateral projection*

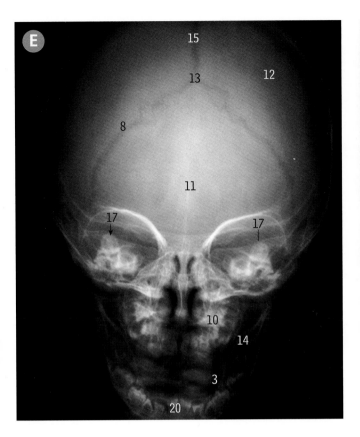

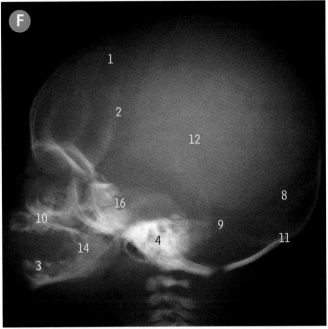

The face at birth forms a relatively smaller proportion of the cranium than in the adult (about one-eighth compared with one-half) because of the small size of the nasal cavity and maxillary sinuses and the lack of erupted teeth.

The posterior fontanelle (C13, E13) closes about 2 months after birth, the anterior fontanelle (A1, D1, F1) in the second year.

Owing to the lack of the mastoid process (which does not develop until the second year), the stylomastoid foramen (B19) and the emerging facial nerve are relatively near the surface and unprotected.

G Resin cast of head and neck arteries *full-term fetus, from the left*

In this cast of fetal arteries, note in the front of the neck the dense arterial pattern indicating the thyroid gland (G), and above and in front of it the fine vessels outlining the tongue (T).

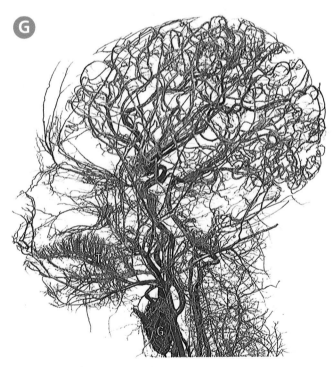

Hydrocephalus, scalp wounds, see pages 80–82.

Skull ⓐ *coloured left half of the skull in sagittal section*

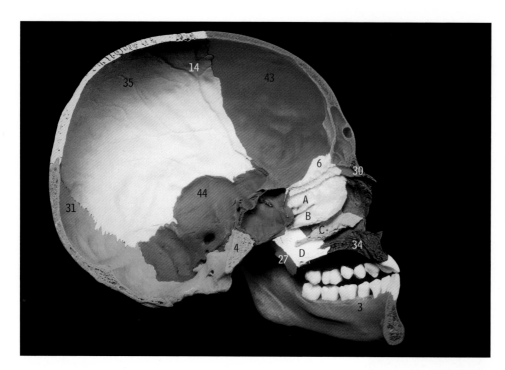

A Superior nasal concha
B Middle nasal concha
C Inferior nasal concha
D Palatine bone
See page 17 for additional label numbers.

NB: The perpendicular plate of the ethmoid has been removed to expose the conchae.

ⓑ *cleared specimen from the front, illuminated from behind*

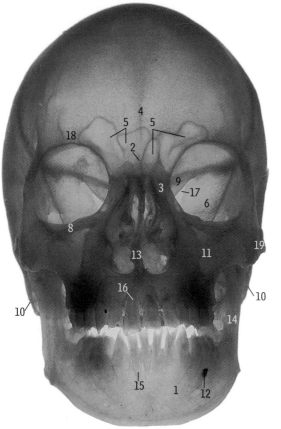

ⓒ *radiograph of facial bones, occipitofrontal view*

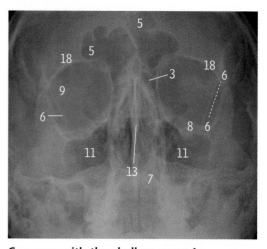

Compare with the skull on page 1.

1	Body of mandible	**10**	Mastoid process
2	Crista galli	**11**	Maxillary sinus
3	Ethmoidal air cells	**12**	Mental foramen
4	Frontal crest	**13**	Nasal septum
5	Frontal sinus	**14**	Ramus of mandible
6	Greater wing of sphenoid bone	**15**	Root of lower lateral incisor
7	Inferior nasal concha	**16**	Root of upper central incisor
8	Infra-orbital margin	**17**	Superior orbital fissure
9	Lesser wing of sphenoid bone	**18**	Supra-orbital margin
		19	Zygomatic arch

Blow-out fractures of the orbit, mastoiditis, see pages 80–82.

Skull *left half of the skull in sagittal section*

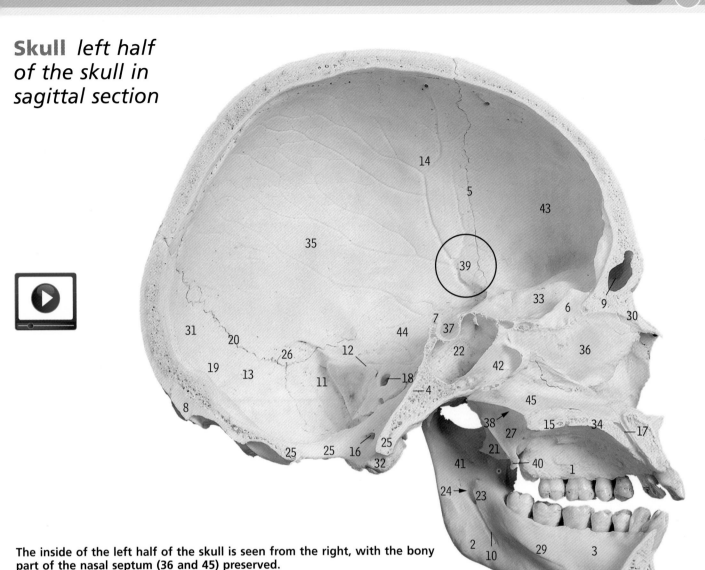

The inside of the left half of the skull is seen from the right, with the bony part of the nasal septum (36 and 45) preserved.

1 Alveolar process of maxilla
2 Angle of mandible
3 Body of mandible
4 Clivus
5 Coronal suture
6 Crista galli of ethmoid bone
7 Dorsum sellae
8 External occipital protuberance
9 Frontal sinus
10 Groove for mylohyoid nerve
11 Groove for sigmoid sinus
12 Groove for superior petrosal sinus
13 Groove for transverse sinus
14 Grooves for middle meningeal vessels (anterior division)
15 Horizontal plate of palatine bone
16 Hypoglossal canal
17 Incisive canal
18 Internal acoustic meatus in petrous part of temporal bone
19 Internal occipital protuberance
20 Lambdoid suture
21 Lateral pterygoid plate
22 Left sphenoidal sinus
23 Lingula

24 Mandibular foramen
25 Margin of foramen magnum
26 Mastoid (posterior inferior) angle of parietal bone
27 Medial pterygoid plate
28 Mental protuberance
29 Mylohyoid line
30 Nasal bone
31 Occipital bone
32 Occipital condyle
33 Orbital part of frontal bone
34 Palatine process of maxilla
35 Parietal bone
36 Perpendicular plate of ethmoid bone
37 Pituitary fossa (sella turcica)
38 Posterior nasal aperture (choana)
39 Pterion (encircled)
40 Pterygoid hamulus of medial pterygoid plate
41 Ramus of mandible
42 Right sphenoidal sinus
43 Squamous part of frontal bone
44 Squamous part of temporal bone
45 Vomer

The bony part of the nasal septum consists of the vomer (45) and the perpendicular plate of the ethmoid bone (36). The anterior part of the septum consists of the septal cartilage (pages 58 and 59).

In this skull, the sphenoidal sinuses (42 and 22) are large, and the right one (42) has extended to the left of the midline. The pituitary fossa (37) projects down into the left sinus (22).

The grooves for the middle meningeal vessels (14) pass upwards and backwards. The circle (39) marks the region of the pterion, and corresponds to the position shown on the outside of the skull on page 4.

Extradural haemorrhage, pituitary tumour, see pages 80–82.

Mandible

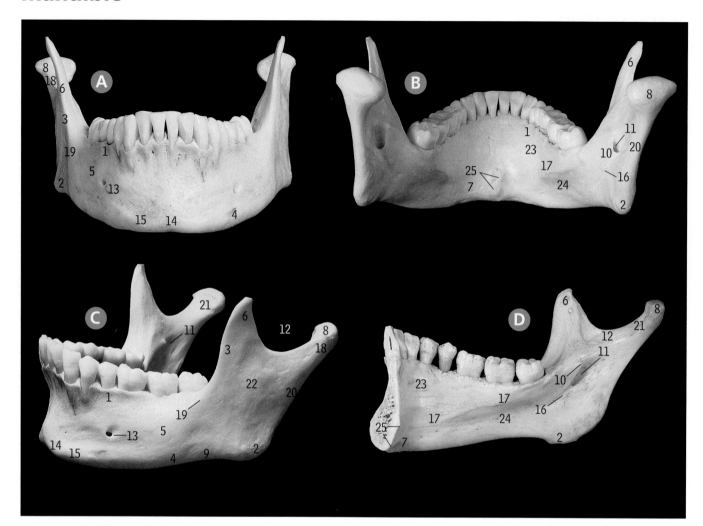

A from the front

B from behind

C from the left and front

D internal view from the left

1	Alveolar part	**14**	Mental protuberance
2	Angle	**15**	Mental tubercle
3	Anterior border of ramus	**16**	Mylohyoid groove
4	Base	**17**	Mylohyoid line
5	Body	**18**	Neck
6	Coronoid process	**19**	Oblique line
7	Digastric fossa	**20**	Posterior border of ramus
8	Head	**21**	Pterygoid fovea
9	Inferior border of ramus	**22**	Ramus
10	Lingula	**23**	Sublingual fossa
11	Mandibular foramen	**24**	Submandibular fossa
12	Mandibular notch	**25**	Superior and inferior mental
13	Mental foramen		spines (genial tubercles)

The head (8) and the neck (18, including the pterygoid fovea, 21) constitute the condyle.

The alveolar part (1) contains the sockets for the roots of the teeth.

The base (4) is the inferior border of the body (5), and becomes continuous with the inferior border (9) of the ramus (22).

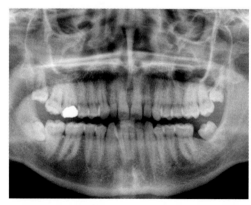

Orthopantomogram

Impacted wisdom tooth, mastoiditis, see pages 80–82.

Mandible *muscle attachments*

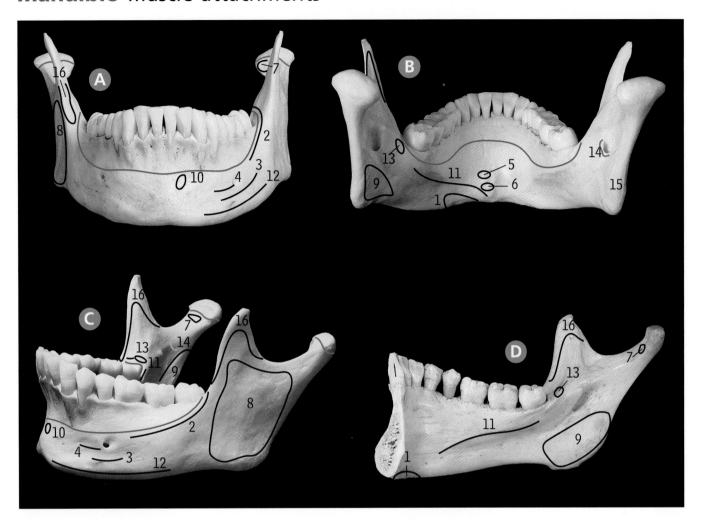

A from the front

B from behind

C from the left and front

D internal view from the left

Green line = capsular attachment of temporomandibular joint; blue line = limit of attachment of the oral mucous membrane; pale green line = ligament attachment

1 Anterior belly of digastric	**10** Mentalis
2 Buccinator	**11** Mylohyoid
3 Depressor anguli oris	**12** Platysma
4 Depressor labii inferioris	**13** Pterygomandibular raphe and
5 Genioglossus	superior constrictor
6 Geniohyoid	**14** Sphenomandibular ligament
7 Lateral pterygoid	**15** Stylomandibular ligament
8 Masseter	**16** Temporalis
9 Medial pterygoid	

The lateral pterygoid (A7) is attached to the pterygoid fovea on the neck of the mandible (and also to the capsule of the temporomandibular joint and the articular disc – see page 42, A27, A28).

The medial pterygoid (B9, C9) is attached to the medial surface of the angle of the mandible, below the groove for the mylohyoid nerve.

Masseter (C8) is attached to the lateral surface of the ramus.

Temporalis (C16) is attached over the coronoid process, extending back as far as the deepest part of the mandibular notch and downwards over the front of the ramus almost as far as the last molar tooth.

Buccinator (C2) is attached opposite the three molar teeth, at the back reaching the pterygomandibular raphe (C13).

Genioglossus (B5) is attached to the upper mental spine and geniohyoid (B6) to the lower.

Mylohyoid (11) is attached to the mylohyoid line.

The attachment of the lateral temporomandibular ligament to the lateral aspect of the neck of the condyle is not shown.

Fractured mandible, see pages 80–82.

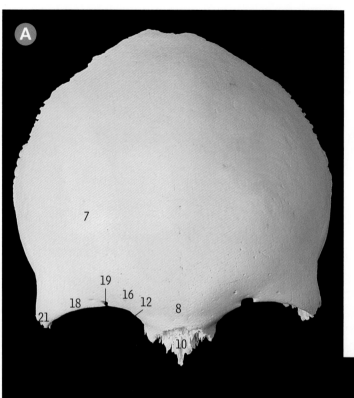

Frontal bone

A external surface from the front

B external surface from the left

C from below

D internal surface from above and behind (right half removed; ethmoidal notch is inferior)

1	Anterior ethmoidal canal (position of groove)	**13**	Posterior ethmoidal canal (position of groove)
2	Ethmoidal notch	**14**	Roof of ethmoidal air cells
3	Foramen caecum	**15**	Sagittal crest
4	Fossa for lacrimal gland	**16**	Superciliary arch
5	Frontal crest	**17**	Superior temporal line
6	Frontal sinus	**18**	Supra-orbital margin
7	Frontal tuberosity	**19**	Supra-orbital notch or foramen
8	Glabella	**20**	Trochlear fovea (or tubercle)
9	Inferior temporal line	**21**	Zygomatic process
10	Nasal spine		
11	Orbital part		
12	Position of frontal notch or foramen		

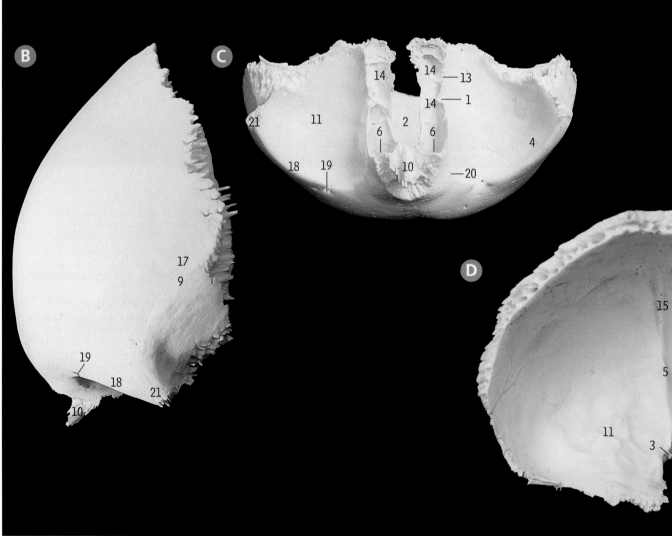

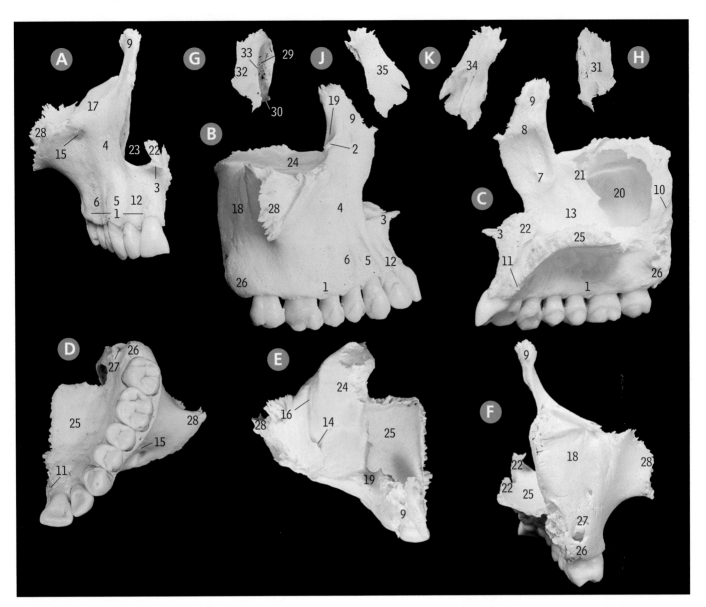

Right maxilla

A from the front

B from the lateral side

C from the medial side

D from below

E from above

F from behind

1	Alveolar process	**15**	Infra-orbital foramen
2	Anterior lacrimal crest	**16**	Infra-orbital groove
3	Anterior nasal spine	**17**	Infra-orbital margin
4	Anterior surface	**18**	Infratemporal surface
5	Canine eminence	**19**	Lacrimal groove
6	Canine fossa	**20**	Maxillary hiatus and sinus
7	Conchal crest	**21**	Middle meatus
8	Ethmoidal crest	**22**	Nasal crest
9	Frontal process	**23**	Nasal notch
10	Greater palatine canal (position of groove)	**24**	Orbital surface
		25	Palatine process
11	Incisive canal	**26**	Tuberosity
12	Incisive fossa	**27**	Unerupted third molar tooth
13	Inferior meatus		
14	Infra-orbital canal	**28**	Zygomatic process

Right lacrimal bone

G from the lateral (orbital) side

H from the medial (nasal) side

29 Lacrimal groove
30 Lacrimal hamulus
31 Nasal surface
32 Orbital surface
33 Posterior lacrimal crest

Right nasal bone

J from the lateral side

K from the medial side

34 Internal surface and groove for anterior ethmoidal nerve
35 Lateral surface

Right palatine bone

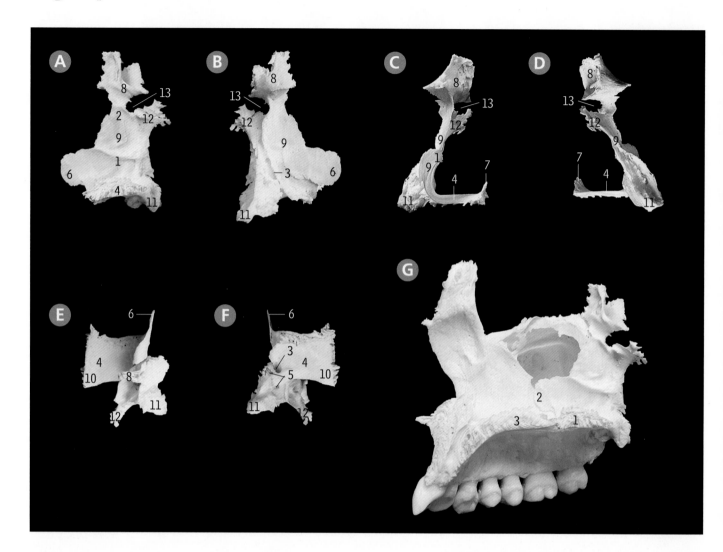

A from the medial side

B from the lateral side

C from the front

D from behind

E from above

F from below

G Articulation of the right maxilla and the palatine bone, from the medial side

1 Horizontal plate of palatine
2 Maxillary process of palatine
3 Palatine process of maxilla

1 Conchal crest
2 Ethmoidal crest
3 Greater palatine groove
4 Horizontal plate
5 Lesser palatine canals
6 Maxillary process
7 Nasal crest
8 Orbital process
9 Perpendicular plate
10 Posterior nasal spine
11 Pyramidal process
12 Sphenoidal process
13 Sphenopalatine notch

Right temporal bone

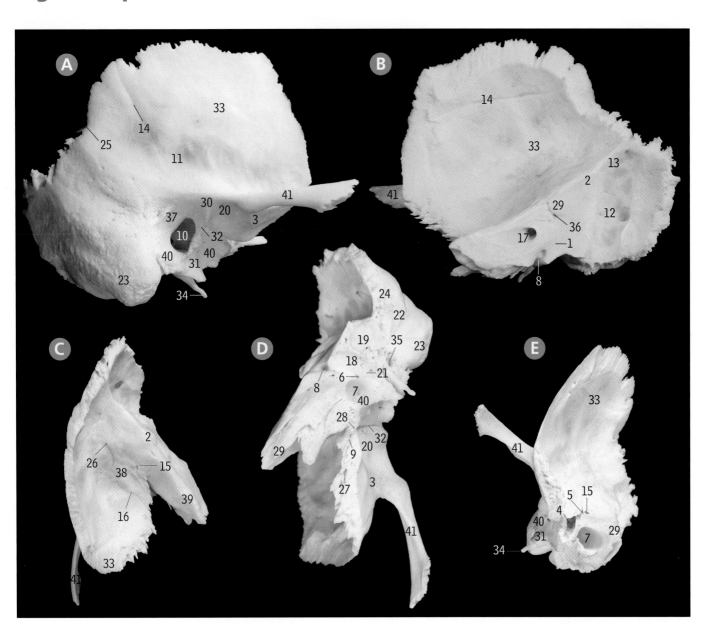

A external aspect

B internal aspect

C from above

D from below

E from the front

1 Aqueduct of vestibule
2 Arcuate eminence
3 Articular tubercle
4 Auditory (eustachian) tube
5 Canal for tensor tympani
6 Canaliculus for tympanic branch of glossopharyngeal nerve
7 Carotid canal
8 Cochlear canaliculus
9 Edge of tegmen tympani
10 External acoustic meatus
11 Groove for middle temporal artery
12 Groove for sigmoid sinus
13 Groove for superior petrosal sinus
14 Grooves for branches of middle meningeal vessels

15 Hiatus and groove for greater petrosal nerve
16 Hiatus and groove for lesser petrosal nerve
17 Internal acoustic meatus
18 Jugular fossa
19 Jugular surface
20 Mandibular fossa
21 Mastoid canaliculus for auricular branch of vagus nerve
22 Mastoid notch
23 Mastoid process
24 Occipital groove
25 Parietal notch
26 Petrosquamous fissure (from above)
27 Petrosquamous fissure (from below)

28 Petrotympanic fissure
29 Petrous part
30 Postglenoid tubercle
31 Sheath of styloid process
32 Squamotympanic fissure
33 Squamous part
34 Styloid process
35 Stylomastoid foramen
36 Subarcuate fossa
37 Suprameatal triangle
38 Tegmen tympani
39 Trigeminal impression on apex of petrous part
40 Tympanic part
41 Zygomatic process

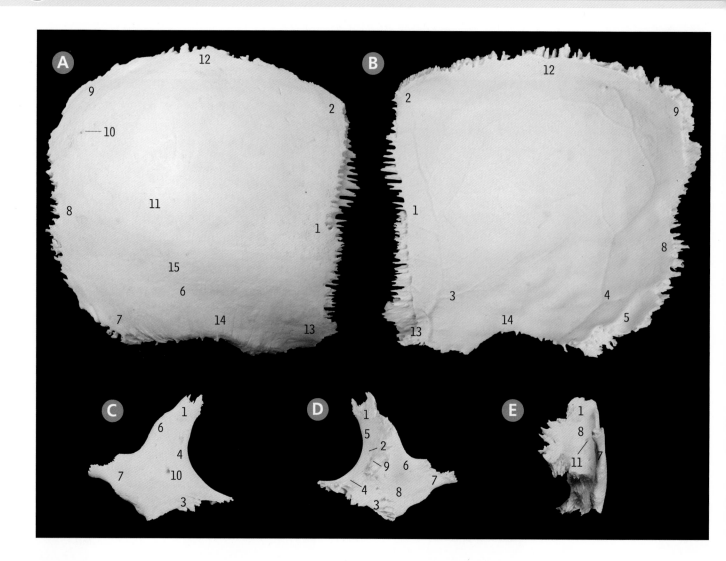

Right parietal bone

A external surface

B internal surface

1 Frontal (anterior) border
2 Frontal (antero-superior) angle
3 Furrows for frontal branch of middle meningeal vessels (anterior division)
4 Furrows for parietal branch of middle meningeal vessels (posterior division)
5 Groove for sigmoid sinus at mastoid angle
6 Inferior temporal line
7 Mastoid (postero-inferior) angle
8 Occipital (posterior) border
9 Occipital (postero-superior) angle
10 Parietal foramen
11 Parietal tuberosity
12 Sagittal (superior) border
13 Sphenoidal (antero-inferior) angle
14 Squamosal (inferior) border
15 Superior temporal line

Right zygomatic bone

C lateral surface

D from the medial side

E from behind

1 Frontal process
2 Marginal tubercle
3 Maxillary border
4 Orbital border
5 Orbital surface
6 Temporal border
7 Temporal process
8 Temporal surface
9 Zygomatico-orbital foramen
10 Zygomaticofacial foramen
11 Zygomaticotemporal foramen

The zygomatic process of the temporal bone (page 4, 37) and the temporal process of the zygomatic bone (C7, D7) form the zygomatic arch (page 4, 35).

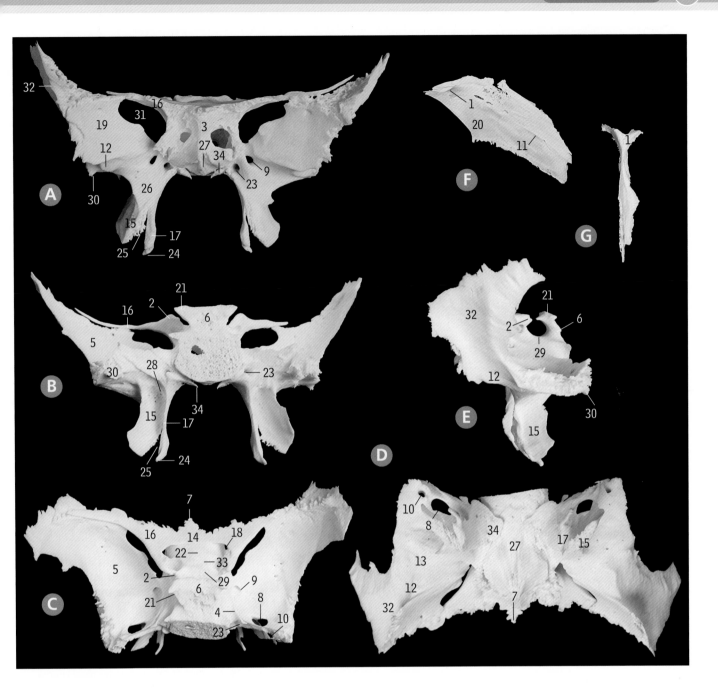

Sphenoid bone

A from the front

B from behind

C from above and behind

D from below

E from the left

Vomer

F from the right

G from behind

1 Ala of vomer
2 Anterior clinoid process
3 Body with openings of sphenoidal sinuses
4 Carotid groove
5 Cerebral surface of greater wing
6 Dorsum sellae
7 Ethmoidal spine
8 Foramen ovale
9 Foramen rotundum
10 Foramen spinosum
11 Groove for nasopalatine nerve and vessels
12 Infratemporal crest of greater wing
13 Infratemporal surface of greater wing
14 Jugum
15 Lateral pterygoid plate
16 Lesser wing
17 Medial pterygoid plate
18 Optic canal
19 Orbital surface of greater wing
20 Posterior border of vomer
21 Posterior clinoid process
22 Prechiasmatic groove
23 Pterygoid canal
24 Pterygoid hamulus
25 Pterygoid notch
26 Pterygoid process
27 Rostrum
28 Scaphoid fossa
29 Sella turcica (pituitary fossa)
30 Spine
31 Superior orbital fissure
32 Temporal surface of greater wing
33 Tuberculum sellae
34 Vaginal process

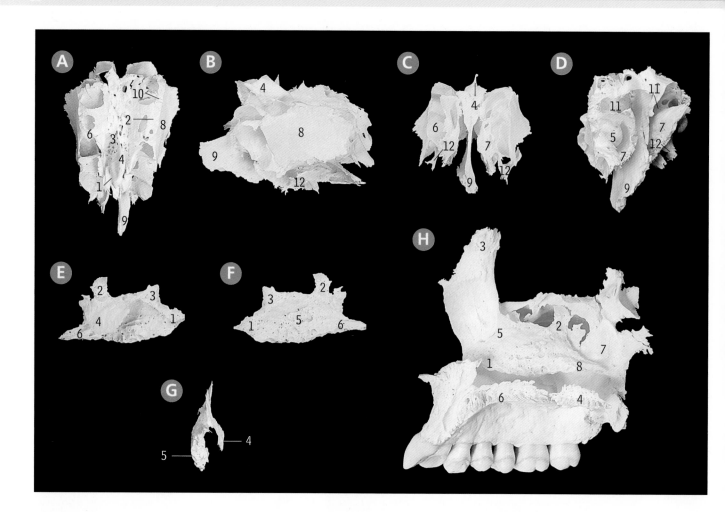

Ethmoid bone

A from above

B from the left

C from the front

D from the left, below and behind

1 Ala of crista galli
2 Anterior ethmoidal groove
3 Cribriform plate
4 Crista galli
5 Ethmoidal bulla
6 Ethmoidal labyrinth (containing ethmoidal air cells)
7 Middle nasal concha
8 Orbital plate
9 Perpendicular plate
10 Posterior ethmoidal groove
11 Superior nasal concha (meatus)
12 Uncinate process

Right inferior nasal concha

E from the lateral side

F from the medial side

G from behind

1 Anterior end
2 Ethmoidal process
3 Lacrimal process
4 Maxillary process
5 Medial surface
6 Posterior end

Maxilla

H Articulation of right maxilla, palatine bone and inferior nasal concha, from the medial side

1 Anterior end of inferior nasal concha
2 Ethmoidal process of inferior nasal concha
3 Frontal process of maxilla
4 Horizontal plate of palatine
5 Lacrimal process of inferior nasal concha
6 Palatine process of maxilla
7 Perpendicular plate of palatine
8 Posterior end of inferior nasal concha

Occipital bone

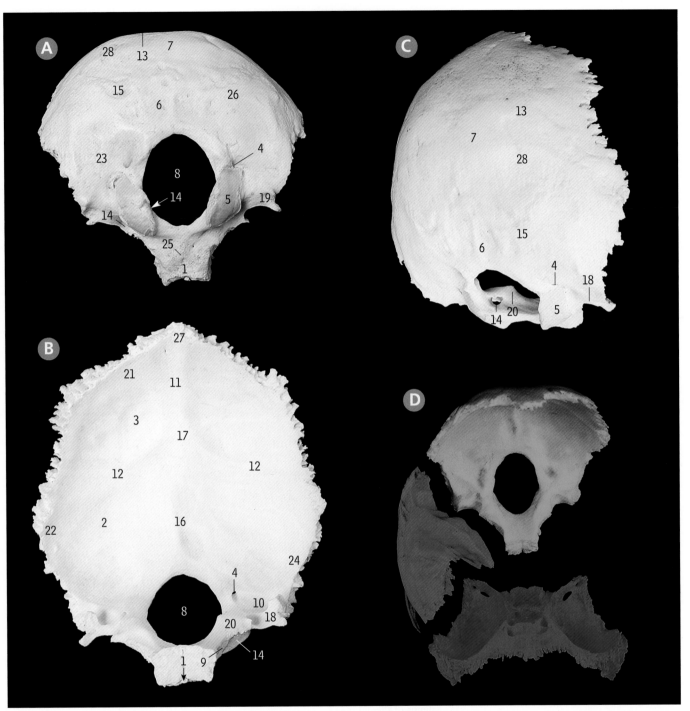

A external surface from below

B internal surface

C external surface from the right and below

D bones of the base of the skull

orange, occipital; red, temporal; blue, sphenoid

1 Basilar part	
2 Cerebellar fossa	
3 Cerebral fossa	
4 Condylar fossa (and condylar canal in B and C)	
5 Condyle	
6 External occipital crest	
7 External occipital protuberance	
8 Foramen magnum	
9 Groove for inferior petrosal sinus	
10 Groove for sigmoid sinus	
11 Groove for superior sagittal sinus	
12 Groove for transverse sinus	
13 Highest nuchal line	
14 Hypoglossal canal	
15 Inferior nuchal line	
16 Internal occipital crest	
17 Internal occipital protuberance	
18 Jugular notch	
19 Jugular process	
20 Jugular tubercle	
21 Lambdoid margin	
22 Lateral angle	
23 Lateral part	
24 Mastoid margin	
25 Pharyngeal tubercle	
26 Squamous part	
27 Superior angle	
28 Superior nuchal line	

Neck *surface markings of the front and right side*

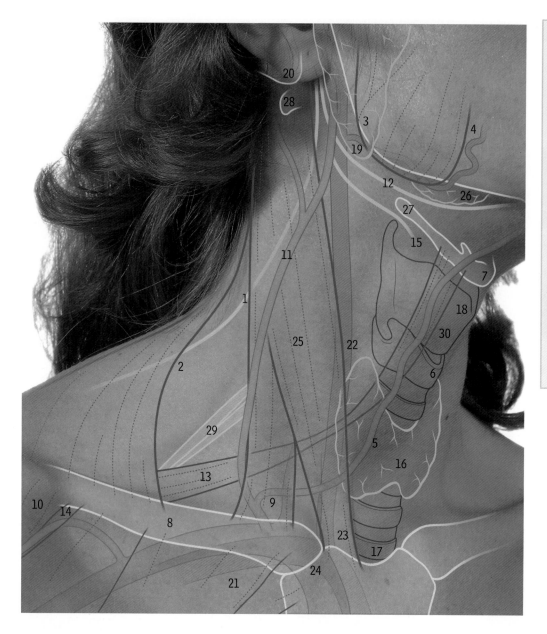

The pulsation of the common carotid artery (22, opposite page, 8) can be felt by backward pressure in the angle between the lower anterior border of sternocleidomastoid and the side of the larynx and trachea.

The cricoid cartilage (6) is about 5 cm (2 in) above the jugular notch of the manubrium of the sternum (17).

The lower end of the internal jugular vein lies behind the interval between the sternal (23) and clavicular (9) heads of sternocleidomastoid (when viewed from the front), just above the point where it joins the subclavian vein to form the brachiocephalic vein (24).

The trunks of the brachial plexus (29) can be felt as a cord-like structure in the lower part of the posterior triangle.

1 Accessory nerve emerging from sternocleidomastoid	**10** Deltoid	**22** Site for palpation of common carotid artery
2 Accessory nerve passing under anterior border of trapezius	**11** External jugular vein	**23** Sternal head of sternocleidomastoid
3 Angle of mandible	**12** Hypoglossal nerve	**24** Sternoclavicular joint and union of internal jugular and subclavian veins to form brachiocephalic vein
4 Anterior border of masseter and facial artery	**13** Inferior belly of omohyoid	
5 Anterior jugular vein	**14** Infraclavicular fossa and cephalic vein	**25** Sternocleidomastoid
6 Arch of cricoid cartilage	**15** Internal laryngeal nerve	**26** Submandibular gland
7 Body of hyoid bone	**16** Isthmus of thyroid gland	**27** Tip of greater horn of hyoid bone
8 Clavicle	**17** Jugular notch and trachea	**28** Tip of transverse process of atlas
9 Clavicular head of sternocleidomastoid	**18** Laryngeal prominence (Adam's apple)	**29** Upper trunk of brachial plexus
	19 Lowest part of parotid gland	**30** Vocal cord position
	20 Mastoid process	
	21 Pectoralis major	

Torticollis, varicella-zoster virus infection, see pages 80–82.

Side of the neck *right side, deep dissection*

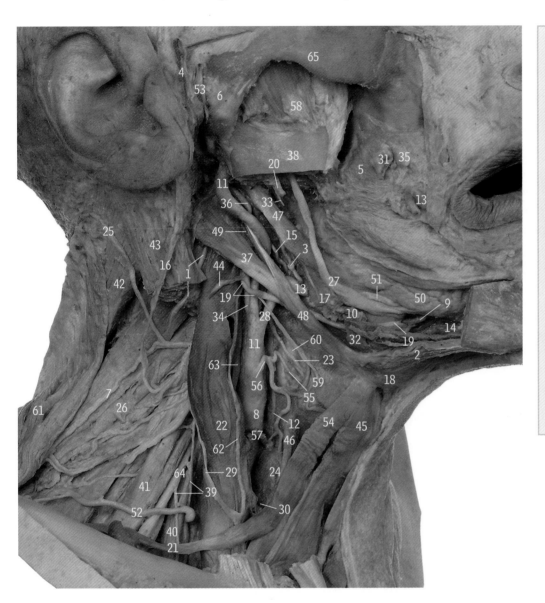

The lingual nerve (27) lies superficial to hyoglossus (17) and at this level is a flattened band rather than a typical round nerve, with the deep part of the submandibular gland (10) below it. The nerve crosses underneath the submandibular duct (51), lying first lateral to the duct and then medial to it.

The thyrohyoid membrane (60) is pierced by the internal laryngeal nerve (23) and the superior laryngeal artery (55).

Apart from supplying muscles of the tongue, the hypoglossal nerve (19) gives branches to geniohyoid (14) and thyrohyoid (59) and forms the upper root of the ansa cervicalis (62). These three branches consist of the fibres from the first cervical nerve that have joined the hypoglossal nerve higher in the neck; they are not derived from the hypoglossal nucleus. The C1 fibres in the upper root of the ansa contribute to the supply of sternohyoid (45) and omohyoid (21, 54).

1 Accessory nerve	**34** Occipital artery
2 Anterior belly of digastric and nerve	**35** Parotid duct
3 Ascending palatine artery	**36** Posterior auricular artery
4 Auriculotemporal nerve	**37** Posterior belly of digastric
5 Buccinator	**38** Ramus of mandible
6 Capsule of temporomandibular joint	**39** Roots of phrenic nerve
7 Cervical nerves to trapezius	**40** Scalenus anterior
8 Common carotid artery	**41** Scalenus medius
9 Deep lingual artery	**42** Splenius capitis
10 Deep part of submandibular gland	**43** Sternocleidomastoid (cut)
11 External carotid artery	**44** Sternocleidomastoid branch of occipital artery
12 External laryngeal nerve	**45** Sternohyoid
13 Facial artery	**46** Sternothyroid
14 Geniohyoid	**47** Styloglossus
15 Glossopharyngeal nerve	**48** Stylohyoid

16 Great auricular nerve	**51** Submandibular duct
17 Hyoglossus	**52** Superficial (transverse) cervical artery
18 Hyoid bone	**53** Superficial temporal artery
19 Hypoglossal nerve	**54** Superior belly of omohyoid
20 Inferior alveolar nerve	**55** Superior laryngeal artery
21 Inferior belly of omohyoid	**56** Superior thyroid artery
22 Internal jugular vein	**57** Superior thyroid vein
23 Internal laryngeal nerve	**58** Temporalis
24 Lateral lobe of thyroid gland	**59** Thyrohyoid and nerve
25 Lesser occipital nerve	**60** Thyrohyoid membrane
26 Levator scapulae	**61** Trapezius
27 Lingual nerve	**62** Upper root of ansa cervicalis
28 Linguofacial trunk	**63** Vagus nerve
29 Lower root of ansa cervicalis	**64** Ventral ramus of fifth cervical nerve
30 Middle thyroid vein	**65** Zygomatic arch
31 Molar salivary glands	
32 Mylohyoid and nerve	
33 Nerve to mylohyoid	

Front of the neck *deeper dissection*

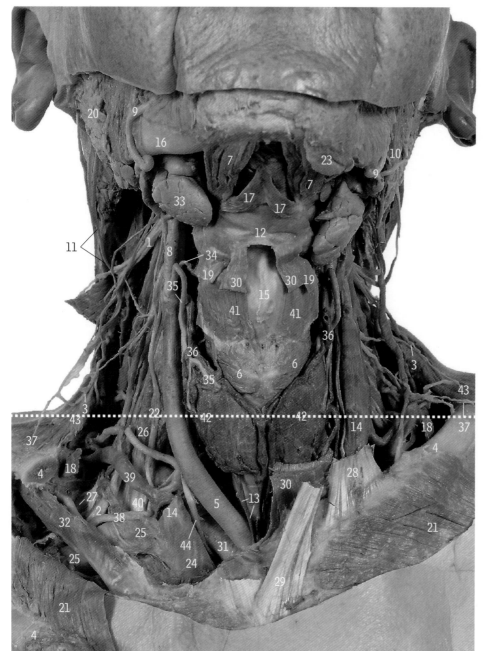

1 Accessory nerve
2 Brachial plexus (roots)
3 Cervical nerves to trapezius
4 Clavicle
5 Common carotid artery
6 Cricothyroid
7 Digastric, anterior belly
8 External carotid artery
9 Facial artery
10 Facial vein
11 Great auricular nerve
12 Hyoid bone, body
13 Inferior thyroid vein
14 Internal jugular vein
15 Laryngeal prominence
16 Mandible
17 Mylohyoid, anomalous fibres
18 Omohyoid, inferior belly
19 Omohyoid, superior belly
20 Parotid gland
21 Pectoralis major
22 Phrenic nerve
23 Platysma
24 Right brachiocephalic vein
25 Right subclavian vein
26 Scalenus anterior
27 Scalenus medius
28 Sternocleidomastoid, clavicular head
29 Sternocleidomastoid, sternal head
30 Sternohyoid
31 Subclavian artery
32 Subclavius
33 Submandibular gland
34 Superior laryngeal artery
35 Superior thyroid artery
36 Superior thyroid vein
37 Supraclavicular nerve
38 Suprascapular artery
39 Suprascapular vein
40 Tendon of scalenus anterior
41 Thyrohyoid
42 Thyroid gland, lateral lobe
43 Trapezius
44 Vagus nerve

On the right hand side, the clavicle (4) has been cut and removed to reveal the underlying subclavius (32). Dotted line is the level of axial CT (shown on the right).

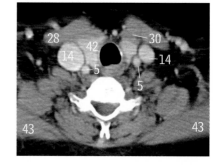

Accessory nerve palsy, goitre, sialectasis, submandibular tumour, see pages 80–82.

Right side of the neck

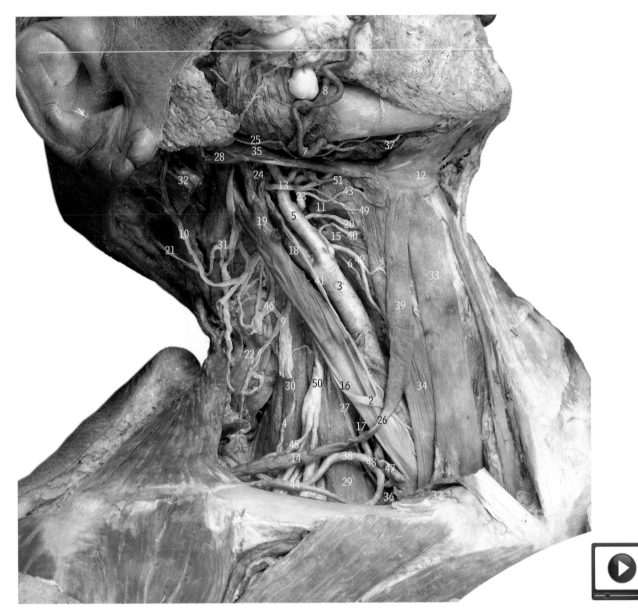

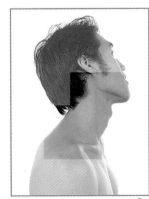

1 Accessory nerve
2 Ansa cervicalis
3 Common carotid artery
4 Dorsal scapular nerve
5 External carotid artery
6 External laryngeal nerve
7 Facial artery
8 Facial vein
9 Fourth cervical nerve ventral rami
10 Great auricular nerve
11 Greater horn of hyoid bone
12 Hyoid bone
13 Hypoglossal nerve
14 Inferior belly of omohyoid
15 Inferior constrictor of pharynx
16 Inferior root of ansa cervicalis
17 Inferior thyroid artery
18 Internal carotid artery
19 Internal jugular vein (double at upper end)
20 Internal laryngeal nerve penetrating thyrohyoid membrane
21 Lesser occipital nerve
22 Levator scapulae
23 Lingual artery
24 Lingual vein
25 Marginal mandibular branch of facial nerve
26 Omohyoid tendon
27 Phrenic nerve
28 Posterior belly of digastric
29 Scalenus anterior
30 Scalenus medius
31 Second cervical nerve ventral rami
32 Sternocleidomastoid (cut)
33 Sternohyoid
34 Sternothyroid
35 Stylohyoid
36 Subclavian vein
37 Submental artery
38 Transverse cervical artery (superficial)
39 Superior belly of omohyoid
40 Superior laryngeal artery
41 Superior root of ansa cervicalis
42 Superior thyroid artery
43 Suprahyoid artery on hyoglossus
44 Suprascapular artery
45 Suprascapular nerve
46 Third cervical nerve ventral rami
47 The right lymphatic duct termination
48 Thyrocervical trunk
49 Thyrohyoid muscle and nerve to thyrohyoid
50 Upper trunk of brachial plexus
51 Vena comitans of hypoglossal nerve

Branchial cysts, carotid artery stenosis, see pages 80–82.

Left side of the neck *from the left and front*

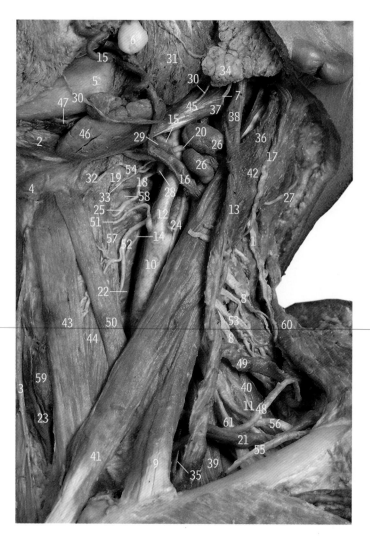

Platysma and the deep cervical fascia have been removed.

In 20% of faces, as in this specimen, the marginal mandibular branch of the facial nerve (30) arches downwards off the face for part of its course and overlies the submandibular gland (46).

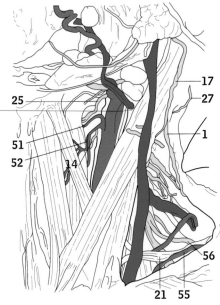

1	Accessory nerve	**20**	Hypoglossal nerve	**38**	Posterior branch of
2	Anterior belly of digastric	**21**	Inferior belly of omohyoid		retromandibular vein
3	Anterior jugular vein	**22**	Inferior constrictor of pharynx	**39**	Scalenus anterior

1 Accessory nerve
2 Anterior belly of digastric
3 Anterior jugular vein
4 Body of hyoid bone
5 Body of mandible
6 Buccal fat pad
7 Cervical branch of facial nerve
8 Cervical nerves to trapezius
9 Clavicular head of sternocleidomastoid
10 Common carotid artery
11 Dorsal scapular nerve
12 External carotid artery
13 External jugular vein
14 External laryngeal nerve
15 Facial artery
16 Facial vein
17 Great auricular nerve
18 Greater horn of hyoid bone (underlying 25)
19 Hyoglossus

20 Hypoglossal nerve
21 Inferior belly of omohyoid
22 Inferior constrictor of pharynx
23 Inferior thyroid vein
24 Internal carotid artery and superior root of ansa cervicalis
25 Internal laryngeal nerve
26 Jugulodigastric lymph nodes
27 Lesser occipital nerve
28 Lingual artery
29 Lingual vein
30 Marginal mandibular branch of facial nerve
31 Masseter
32 Mylohyoid
33 Nerve to thyrohyoid
34 Parotid gland
35 Phrenic nerve (on scalenus anterior)
36 Posterior auricular vein
37 Posterior belly of digastric

38 Posterior branch of retromandibular vein
39 Scalenus anterior
40 Scalenus medius
41 Sternal head of sternocleidomastoid
42 Sternocleidomastoid
43 Sternohyoid
44 Sternothyroid
45 Stylohyoid
46 Submandibular gland
47 Submental artery and vein
48 Superficial (transverse) cervical artery
49 Superficial (transverse) cervical vein
50 Superior belly of omohyoid
51 Superior laryngeal artery
52 Superior thyroid artery
53 Supraclavicular nerve (cut upper edge)
54 Suprahyoid artery

55 Suprascapular artery
56 Suprascapular nerve
57 Thyrohyoid
58 Thyrohyoid membrane
59 Thyroid gland (left lobe)
60 Trapezius
61 Upper trunk of brachial plexus

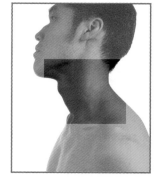

Carotid artery bruits, carotid artery variants, cervical lymph node enlargement, see pages 80–82.

Right lower face and upper neck B *submandibular region*
A *parotid and upper cervical regions*

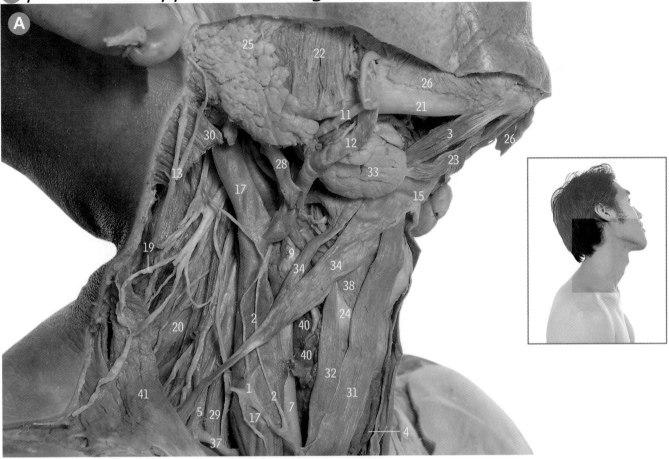

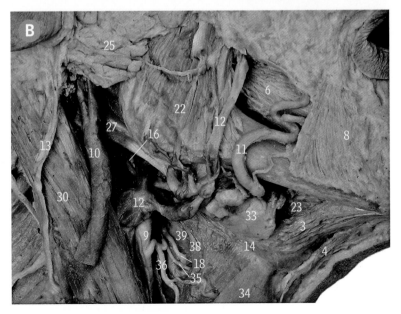

1	Ansa cervicalis, inferior branch	**23**	Mylohyoid
2	Ansa cervicalis, superior branch	**24**	Oblique line of the thyroid cartilage
3	Anterior belly of digastric	**25**	Parotid gland and facial nerve branches at anterior border
4	Anterior jugular vein		
5	Brachial plexus (roots)	**26**	Platysma
6	Buccinator	**27**	Posterior belly of digastric
7	Common carotid artery	**28**	Retromandibular vein
8	Depressor anguli oris	**29**	Scalenus anterior
9	External carotid artery	**30**	Sternocleidomastoid
10	External jugular vein	**31**	Sternohyoid
11	Facial artery	**32**	Sternothyroid
12	Facial vein	**33**	Submandibular gland
13	Great auricular nerve	**34**	Superior belly of omohyoid (bifid-variation)
14	Greater horn of hyoid bone		
15	Hyoid bone	**35**	Superior laryngeal artery
16	Hypoglossal nerve	**36**	Superior thyroid artery
17	Internal jugular vein	**37**	Suprascapular artery
18	Internal laryngeal nerve	**38**	Thyrohyoid
19	Lesser occipital nerve	**39**	Thyrohyoid membrane
20	Levator scapulae	**40**	Thyroid gland (right lobe)
21	Mandible		
22	Masseter	**41**	Trapezius

Mumps, parotidectomy (removal of parotid gland), parotid tumours, see pages 80–82.

Left lower face and upper neck

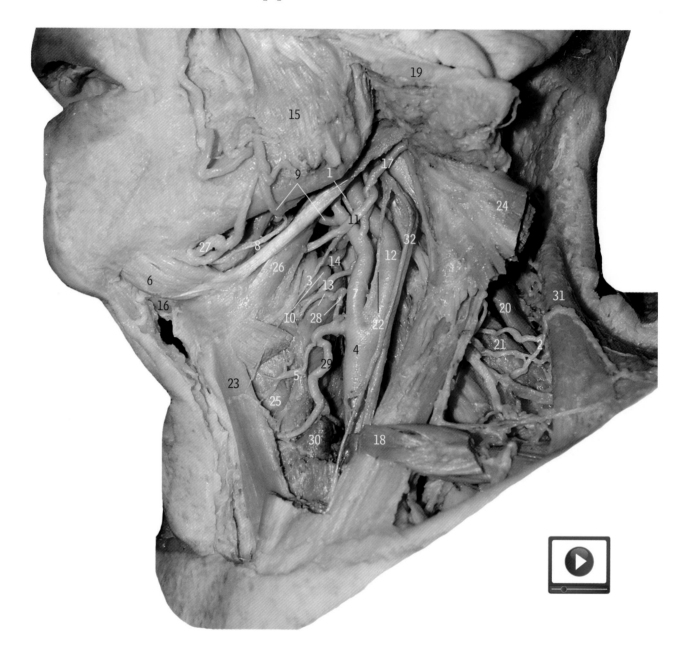

1 Ascending pharyngeal artery	**12** Internal carotid artery	**23** Sternohyoid muscle
2 Branches of cervical plexus	**13** Internal laryngeal nerve	**24** Sternocleidomastoid muscle (reflected)
3 C1 (descendens hypoglossi)	**14** Lingual artery	**25** Sternothyroid muscle (cut)
4 Common carotid artery	**15** Masseter muscle	**26** Stylohyoid muscle
5 Cricothyroid artery	**16** Mylohyoid muscle	**27** Submental artery
6 Digastric muscle (anterior belly)	**17** Occipital artery	**28** Superior laryngeal artery
7 External carotid artery	**18** Omohyoid muscle (reflected)	**29** Superior thyroid artery
8 Facial nerve, marginal branch	**19** Parotid gland (reflected)	**30** Thyroid gland (lateral lobe)
9 Facial artery	**20** Scalenus posterior muscle	**31** Trapezius muscle
10 Greater horn of the hyoid bone	**21** Scalenus medius muscle	**32** Vagus nerve
11 Hypoglossal nerve	**22** Sinus nerve to carotid sinus and body	

Carotid endarterectomy, see pages 80–82.

Right side of the neck *deep dissection*

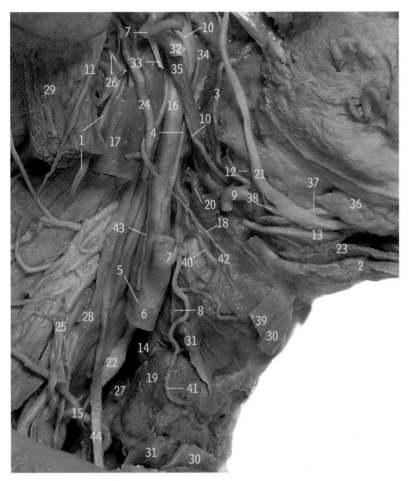

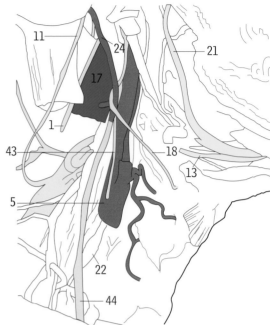

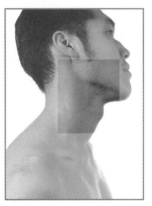

1 Accessory nerve (cut)	**23** Mylohyoid
2 Anterior belly of digastric	**24** Occipital artery
3 Ascending palatine artery	**25** Phrenic nerve
4 Ascending pharyngeal artery	**26** Posterior belly of digastric (cut)
5 Carotid sinus	**27** Recurrent laryngeal nerve
6 Common carotid artery	**28** Scalenus anterior
7 External carotid artery	**29** Sternocleidomastoid
8 External laryngeal nerve	**30** Sternohyoid
9 Facial artery	**31** Sternothyroid
10 Glossopharyngeal nerve	**32** Styloglossus
11 Great auricular nerve	**33** Stylohyoid (cut end displaced
12 Hyoglossus	medially)
13 Hypoglossal nerve (cut)	**34** Stylohyoid ligament
14 Inferior constrictor	**35** Stylopharyngeus
15 Inferior thyroid artery	**36** Sublingual gland
16 Internal carotid artery	**37** Submandibular duct
17 Internal jugular vein	**38** Submandibular ganglion
18 Internal laryngeal nerve	**39** Superior belly of omohyoid
19 Lateral lobe of thyroid gland	**40** Superior laryngeal artery
20 Lingual artery	**41** Superior thyroid artery
21 Lingual nerve	**42** Thyrohyoid and nerve
22 Middle cervical sympathetic	**43** Upper root of ansa cervicalis
ganglion	**44** Vagus nerve

The hypoglossal nerve (13) passes downwards, curling around the occipital artery (24) and lying superficial to the external carotid (7) and lingual (20) arteries.

The glossopharyngeal nerve (10) passes downwards and forwards, curling round the lateral side of stylopharyngeus (35).

The removal of parts of the sternohyoid (30), omohyoid (39) and sternothyroid (31) displays the lateral lobe of the thyroid gland (19). Note the inferior thyroid artery (15) behind the lower part of the lobe, with the recurrent laryngeal nerve (27) passing deep to this looping vessel to enter the pharynx beneath the inferior constrictor (14).

Prevertebral region

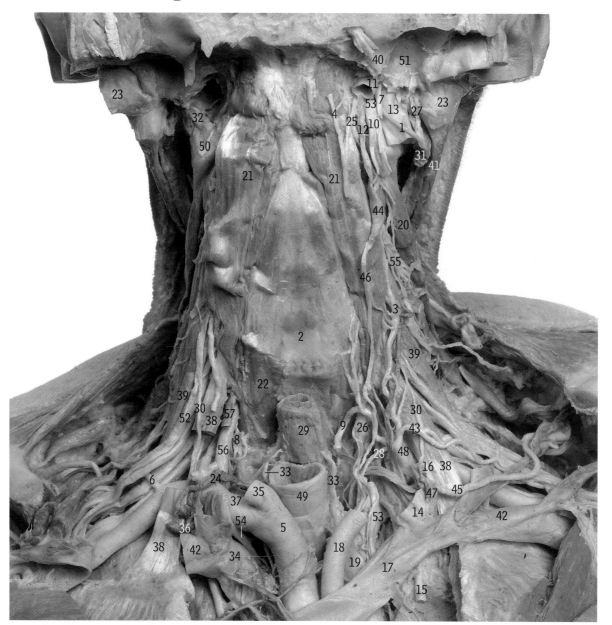

1 Accessory nerve (spinal root)	**21** Longus capitis	**39** Scalenus medius
2 Anterior longitudinal ligament	**22** Longus colli	**40** Spine of sphenoid bone
3 Ascending cervical artery and vein	**23** Mastoid process	**41** Sternocleidomastoid
4 Ascending pharyngeal artery	**24** Mediastinal lymphatic trunk	**42** Subclavian vein
5 Brachiocephalic artery	**25** Meningeal branch of ascending	**43** Superficial cervical artery
6 Dorsal scapular artery	pharyngeal artery	**44** Superior cervical ganglion
7 Glossopharyngeal nerve	**26** Middle cervical ganglion	**45** Suprascapular artery
8 Inferior cervical ganglion	**27** Occipital artery	**46** Sympathetic trunk
9 Inferior thyroid artery	**28** Oesophageal branch of inferior thyroid	**47** Thoracic duct
10 Inferior vagal ganglion	artery	**48** Thyrocervical trunk
11 Internal carotid artery	**29** Oesophagus	**49** Trachea
12 Internal carotid nerve	**30** Phrenic nerve	**50** Transverse process of atlas
13 Internal jugular vein, upper end	**31** Posterior belly of digastric	**51** Tympanic part of temporal bone
14 Internal jugular vein, lower end	**32** Rectus capitis lateralis	**52** Upper trunk of brachial plexus
15 Internal thoracic artery	**33** Recurrent laryngeal nerve	**53** Vagus nerve, on left
16 Jugular lymphatic trunk	**34** Right brachiocephalic vein	**54** Vagus nerve, on right
17 Left brachiocephalic vein	**35** Right common carotid artery	**55** Ventral ramus of third cervical nerve
18 Left common carotid artery	**36** Right lymphatic duct	**56** Vertebral artery
19 Left subclavian artery	**37** Right subclavian artery	**57** Vertebral vein
20 Levator scapulae	**38** Scalenus anterior	

Horner's syndrome, see pages 80–82.

Root of the neck

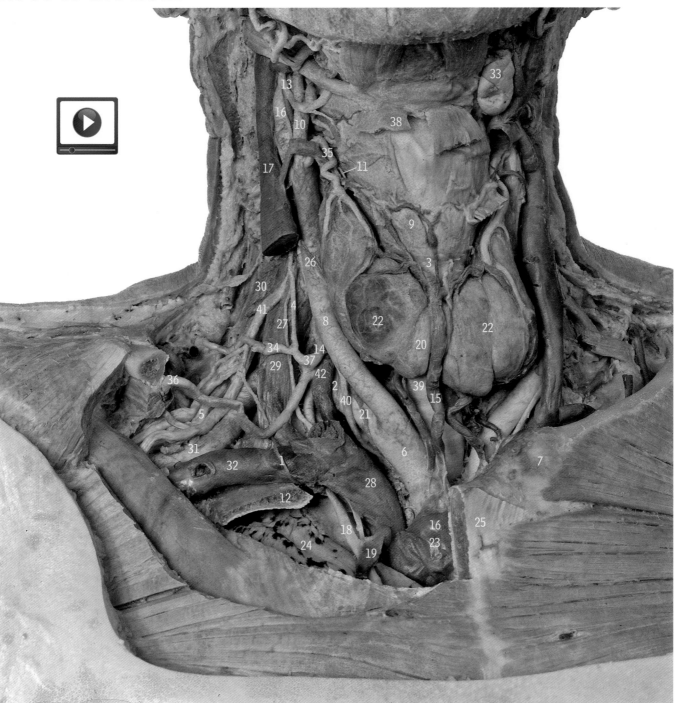

1	Accessory phrenic nerve	**15**	Inferior thyroid veins
2	Ansa subclavia	**16**	Internal carotid artery
3	Arch of cricoid cartilage	**17**	Internal jugular vein
4	Ascending cervical artery	**18**	Internal thoracic artery
5	Brachial plexus	**19**	Internal thoracic vein
6	Brachiocephalic artery	**20**	Isthmus of thyroid gland
7	Capsule of sternoclavicular joint	**21**	Jugular lymphatic trunk
8	Common carotid artery	**22**	Lateral lobe of thyroid gland
9	Cricothyroid muscle	**23**	Left brachiocephalic vein
10	External carotid artery	**24**	Lung apex
11	External laryngeal nerve	**25**	Manubrium of sternum
12	First rib (sectioned)	**26**	Middle thyroid vein
13	Hypoglossal nerve	**27**	Phrenic nerve
14	Inferior thyroid artery	**28**	Right brachiocephalic vein

29	Scalenus anterior
30	Scalenus medius
31	Subclavian artery
32	Subclavian vein
33	Submandibular gland
34	Superficial (transverse) cervical artery
35	Superior thyroid artery and vein
36	Suprascapular artery
37	Thyrocervical trunk
38	Sternohyoid
39	Trachea
40	Vagus nerve
41	Ventral ramus of fifth cervical nerve
42	Vertebral vein

Internal jugular vein catheterisation, subclavian vein catheterisation, see pages 80–82.

Face *surface markings on the front and right side*

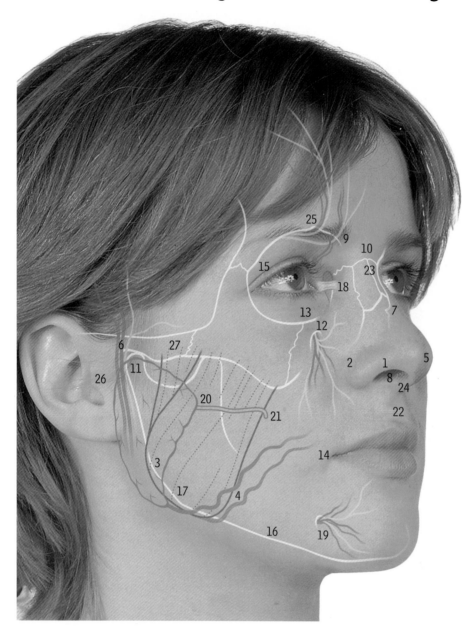

1 Ala
2 Alar groove (nasolabial groove)
3 Angle of mandible
4 Anterior border of masseter and facial vessels
5 Apex of external nose
6 Auriculotemporal nerve and superficial temporal vessels
7 Dorsum of nose
8 External aperture (anterior naris)
9 Frontal notch and supratrochlear nerve and vessels
10 Glabella of nose
11 Head of mandible
12 Infra-orbital foramen, nerve and vessels
13 Infra-orbital margin
14 Lateral angle of mouth
15 Lateral part of supra-orbital margin
16 Lower border of body of mandible
17 Lower border of ramus of mandible
18 Medial palpebral ligament anterior to lacrimal sac
19 Mental foramen, nerve and vessels
20 Parotid duct emerging from gland
21 Parotid duct turning medially at anterior border of masseter
22 Philtrum
23 Root of nose
24 Septum of nose (nasal columella)
25 Supra-orbital notch (or foramen), nerve and vessels
26 Tragus
27 Zygomatic arch

The pulsation of the superficial temporal artery (6) is palpable in front of the tragus of the ear (26).

The parotid duct (20 and 21) lies under the middle-third of a line drawn from the tragus of the ear (26) to the midpoint of the philtrum (22).

The pulsation of the facial artery (4) is palpable where the vessel crosses the lower border of the mandible at the anterior margin of the masseter muscle, about 2.5 cm (1 in) in front of the angle of the mandible (3).

Ophthalmic herpes zoster, see pages 80–82.

Face *superficial dissection from the front and the right*

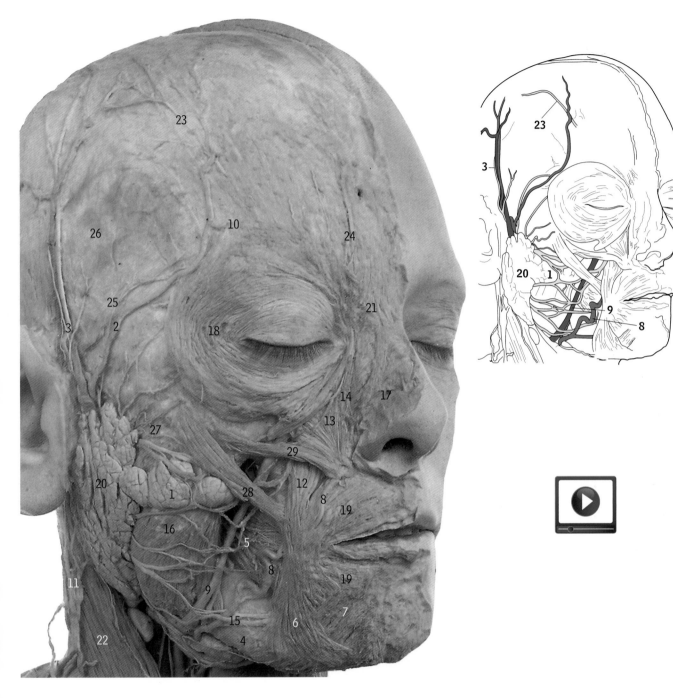

1. Accessory parotid gland overlying parotid duct
2. Anterior branch of superficial temporal artery
3. Auriculotemporal nerve and superficial temporal vessels
4. Body of mandible
5. Buccinator and buccal branches of facial nerve
6. Depressor anguli oris
7. Depressor labii inferioris
8. Facial artery
9. Facial vein
10. Frontalis part of occipitofrontalis
11. Great auricular nerve
12. Levator anguli oris
13. Levator labii superioris
14. Levator labii superioris alaeque nasi
15. Marginal mandibular branch of facial nerve
16. Masseter
17. Nasalis
18. Orbicularis oculi
19. Orbicularis oris
20. Parotid gland
21. Procerus
22. Sternocleidomastoid
23. Supra-orbital nerve
24. Supratrochlear nerve
25. Temporal branch of facial nerve
26. Temporalis underlying temporal fascia
27. Zygomatic branch of facial nerve
28. Zygomaticus major
29. Zygomaticus minor

Facial nerve palsy, intracranial spread of infection, surgical flaps of the scalp, see pages 80–82.

Face *superficial dissection from the right*

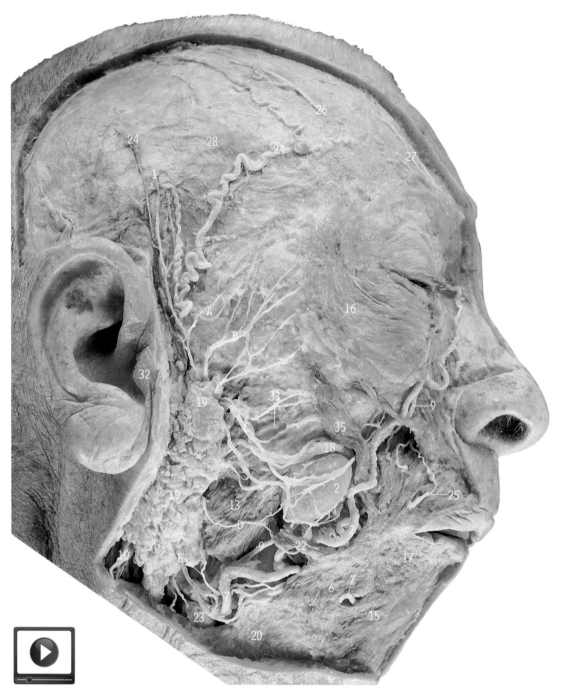

After removal of skin and some fat (A, B, C, D, E = temporal, zygomatic, buccal, mandibular and cervical branches of facial nerve, respectively).

1 Auriculotemporal nerve	**9** Facial vein	**19** Parotid gland	**28** Temporal fascia
2 Buccal fat pad	**10** Great auricular nerve	**20** Platysma	**29** Temporal line, inferior
3 Buccal nerve (V3)	**11** Infra-orbital nerve	**21** Retromandibular vein	**30** Temporal line, superior
4 Buccinator	**12** Mandible, body	**22** Risorius, overlying facial	**31** Temporalis
5 Capsule of	**13** Masseter	artery and vein	**32** Tragus
temporomandibular joint	**14** Mental nerve	**23** Submandibular gland	**33** Transverse facial artery
6 Depressor anguli oris	**15** Mentalis	**24** Superficial temporal vessels	**34** Zygomatic arch
7 Facial artery	**16** Orbicularis oculi	**25** Superior labial artery	**35** Zygomaticus major
8 Facial nerve (A, B, C, D, E	**17** Orbicularis oris	**26** Supraorbital nerve	
branches)	**18** Parotid duct	**27** Supratrochlear nerve	

Right temporal fossa

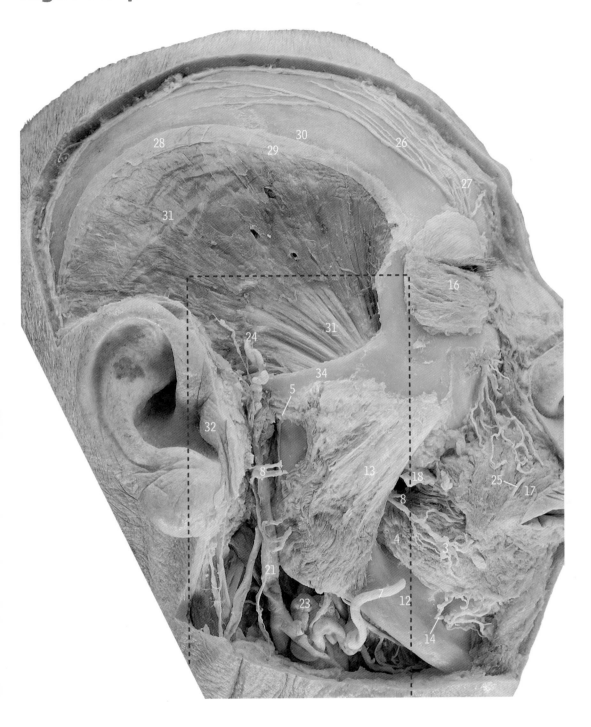

After removal of temporal fascia, parotid gland and most branches of the facial nerve. Dotted line indicates field of deeper dissections shown on next page.

Infratemporal fossa *progressively deeper dissections*

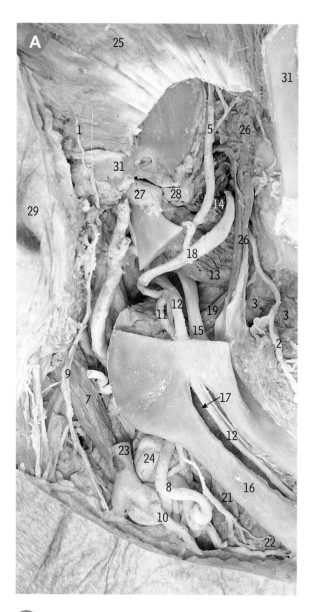

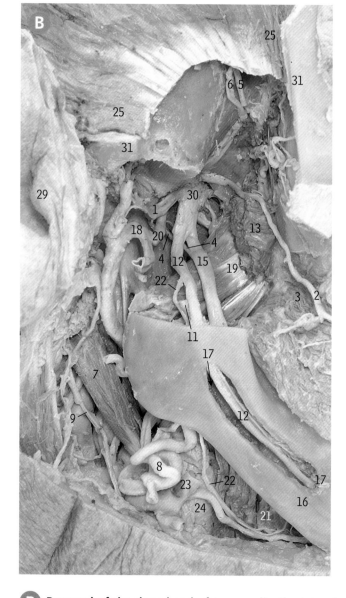

A Removal of the masseter, part of the zygomatic arch, most of the superficial and inferior parts of temporalis, the superior half of the mandibular ramus (except the neck and condyle) and the pterygoid venous plexus reveals the superficial contents of the infratemporal fossa.

B Removal of the deep head of temporalis, the lateral pterygoid and the neck and condyle of the mandible exposes the deepest structures.

1	Auriculotemporal nerve	**13**	Lateral pterygoid, inferior head
2	Buccal nerve (V3)	**14**	Lateral pterygoid, superior head
3	Buccinator	**15**	Lingual nerve
4	Chorda tympani	**16**	Mandible, body
5	Deep temporal artery	**17**	Mandibular canal (opened)
6	Deep temporal nerve	**18**	Maxillary artery
7	Digastric, posterior belly	**19**	Medial pterygoid
8	Facial artery	**20**	Middle meningeal artery
9	Facial nerve, cervical branch	**21**	Mylohyoid
10	Facial vein	**22**	Nerve to mylohyoid
11	Inferior alveolar artery		
12	Inferior alveolar nerve		

23	Retromandibular vein
24	Submandibular gland
25	Temporalis
26	Temporalis, deep head (sphenomandibularis)
27	Temporomandibular joint, capsule
28	Temporomandibular joint, disc
29	Tragus
30	Trigeminal nerve, mandibular division (V3)
31	Zygomatic arch

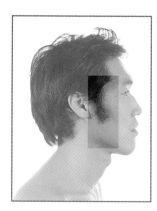

A Coronal section of cadaveric face *temporalis heads*

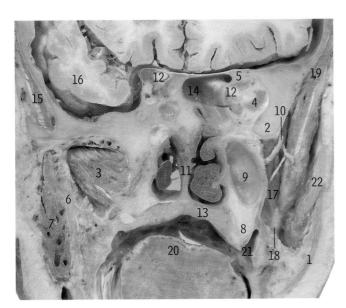

1 Buccinator
2 Greater wing of sphenoid
3 Lateral pterygoid
4 Lateral rectus
5 Lesser wing of sphenoid
6 Mandible
7 Masseter
8 Maxilla
9 Maxillary air (paranasal) sinus
10 Maxillary artery, muscular branches
11 Nasal septum
12 Optic nerve
13 Palate
14 Sphenoidal sinus
15 Temporal bone
16 Temporal lobe, brain
17 Temporalis, deep head (sphenomandibularis – Zenker 1955)
18 Temporalis, insertion
19 Temporalis, superficial head
20 Tongue
21 Vestibule of oral cavity
22 Zygoma

C Endoscopic view of nasal septum (choanae)

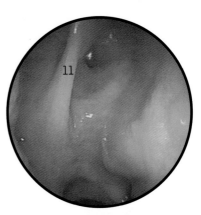

B Coronal MR image of face *muscles of mastication*

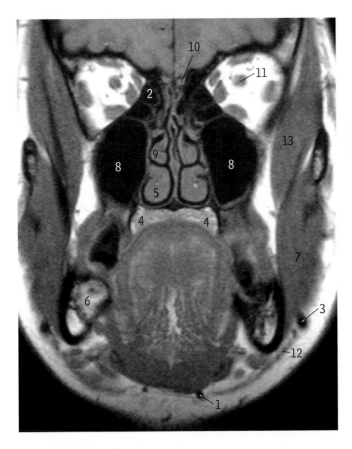

1 Anterior jugular vein
2 Ethmoid air cells
3 Facial artery
4 Hard palate
5 Inferior concha
6 Mandible
7 Masseter
8 Maxillary sinus
9 Middle concha
10 Olfactory tract
11 Optic nerve
12 Platysma
13 Temporalis

Inferior alveolar nerve block, see pages 80–82.

Right trigeminal, facial and petrosal nerves *with associated ganglia*

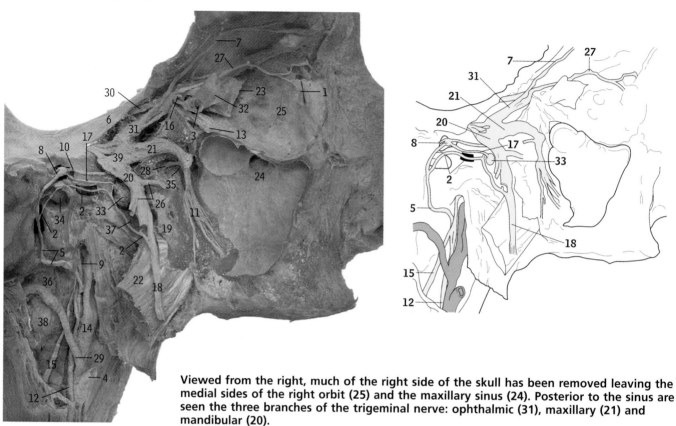

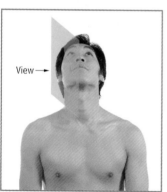

View →

Viewed from the right, much of the right side of the skull has been removed leaving the medial sides of the right orbit (25) and the maxillary sinus (24). Posterior to the sinus are seen the three branches of the trigeminal nerve: ophthalmic (31), maxillary (21) and mandibular (20).

1 Bristle in lacrimal canaliculus
2 Chorda tympani
3 Ciliary ganglion
4 External carotid artery
5 Facial nerve
6 Free margin of tentorium cerebelli
7 Frontal nerve
8 Geniculate ganglion of facial nerve
9 Glossopharyngeal nerve
10 Greater petrosal nerve
11 Greater and lesser palatine nerves
12 Hypoglossal nerve
13 Inferior rectus

14 Internal carotid artery
15 Internal jugular vein and accessory nerve
16 Lacrimal nerve
17 Lesser petrosal nerve
18 Lingual nerve
19 Lower head of lateral pterygoid and lateral pterygoid plate
20 Mandibular nerve
21 Maxillary nerve
22 Medial pterygoid
23 Medial rectus
24 Medial wall of maxillary sinus and ostium
25 Medial wall of orbit

26 Muscular branches of mandibular nerve
27 Nasociliary nerve
28 Nerve of pterygoid canal
29 Occipital artery
30 Oculomotor nerve
31 Ophthalmic nerve
32 Optic nerve
33 Otic ganglion
34 Position of tympanic membrane
35 Pterygopalatine ganglion
36 Rectus capitis lateralis
37 Tensor veli palatini
38 Transverse process of atlas
39 Trigeminal ganglion

The greater petrosal nerve (10) is a branch of the geniculate ganglion of the facial nerve (8) and can be remembered as the nerve of tear secretion (though it also supplies nasal glands). It carries preganglionic fibres from the superior salivary nucleus in the pons, and runs in the groove on the floor of the middle cranial fossa (page 11, 25) to enter the foramen lacerum and become the nerve of the pterygoid canal (28) which joins the pterygopalatine ganglion (35). Postganglionic fibres leave the ganglion to join the maxillary nerve and enter the orbit by the zygomatic branch which communicates with the lacrimal nerve, supplying the gland.

The lesser petrosal nerve (17), although having a communication with the facial nerve, is a branch of the glossopharyngeal nerve, being derived from the tympanic branch which supplies the mucous membrane of the middle ear by the tympanic plexus (page 60, C19). Its fibres are derived from the inferior salivary nucleus in the pons, and after leaving the middle ear and running in its groove on the floor of the middle cranial fossa (17, and page 11, 26), the nerve reaches the otic ganglion (33) via the foramen ovale. From the ganglion secretomotor fibres join the mandibular nerve (20) to be distributed to the parotid gland by filaments from the auriculotemporal nerve.

The chorda tympani (2) arises from the facial nerve before the latter leaves the stylomastoid foramen (5, upper leader line). It crosses the upper part of the tympanic membrane (34) underneath its mucosal covering and runs through the temporal bone, emerging from the petrotympanic fissure (page 9, 35) to join the lingual nerve (18). It carries preganglionic fibres to the submandibular ganglion (page 59, C35) for the submandibular and sublingual salivary glands, and also taste fibres for the anterior two-thirds of the tongue.

The otic ganglion (33), which normally adheres to the deep surface of the mandibular nerve (20), has been teased off from the nerve and a black marker has been placed behind it.

Pharynx *posterior surface, from behind*

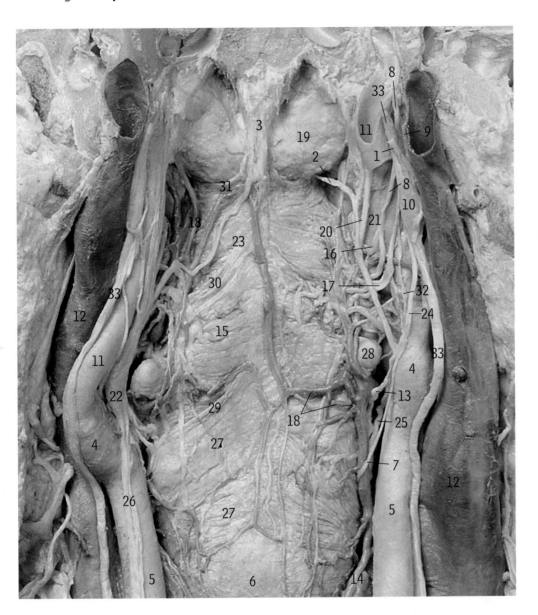

1 Accessory nerve
2 Ascending pharyngeal artery
3 Attachment of pharyngeal raphe to pharyngeal tubercle of base of skull
4 Carotid sinus
5 Common carotid artery
6 Cricopharyngeal part of inferior constrictor
7 External laryngeal nerve
8 Glossopharyngeal nerve
9 Hypoglossal nerve
10 Inferior ganglion of vagus nerve
11 Internal carotid artery
12 Internal jugular vein
13 Internal laryngeal nerve
14 Lateral lobe of thyroid gland
15 Middle constrictor
16 Pharyngeal branch of glossopharyngeal nerve
17 Pharyngeal branch of vagus nerve

18 Pharyngeal veins
19 Pharyngobasilar fascia
20 Posterior meningeal artery
21 Stylopharyngeus
22 Superior cervical sympathetic ganglion
23 Superior constrictor
24 Superior laryngeal branch of vagus nerve
25 Superior thyroid artery
26 Sympathetic trunk
27 Thyropharyngeal part of inferior constrictor
28 Tip of greater horn of hyoid bone
29 Upper border of inferior constrictor
30 Upper border of middle constrictor
31 Upper border of superior constrictor
32 Vagal branch to carotid body
33 Vagus nerve

The vertebral column has been removed to reveal the carotid sheath and constrictor muscles of the pharynx.

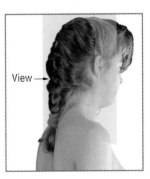

View →

Gag reflex, see pages 80–82.

Posterior pharyngeal wall *from behind*

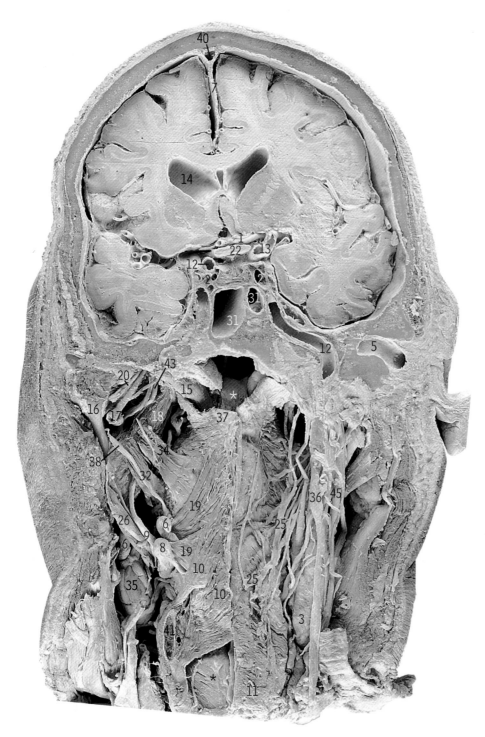

Slightly oblique coronal section of the head and neck in the plane of the posterior pharyngeal wall, with the right side slightly posterior to the left.

Sections of the posterior pharyngeal wall have been removed (asterisks – superiorly the pharyngobasilar fascia and inferiorly the lower border of the inferior constrictor) to reveal parts of the nasopharynx and the laryngopharynx, respectively.

Refer to the key on page 47 for the numbers on this figure.

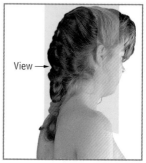

View →

Pharyngeal pouch, tonsillectomy, see pages 80–82.

Ⓐ 'Opened' pharynx *from behind*

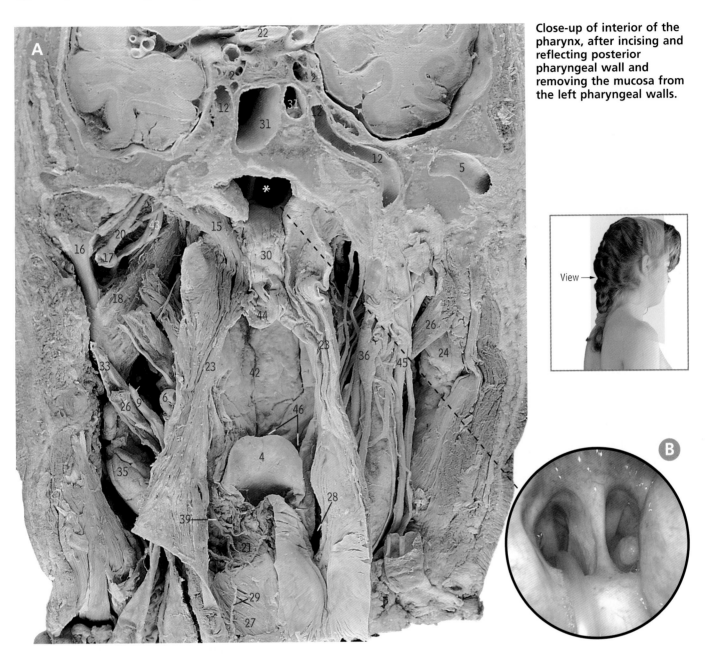

Close-up of interior of the pharynx, after incising and reflecting posterior pharyngeal wall and removing the mucosa from the left pharyngeal walls.

View →

Ⓑ

1	Anterior cerebral artery
2	Cavernous sinus
3	Common carotid
4	Epiglottis
5	External auditory canal
6	Facial artery
7	Falx cerebri
8	Hyoid-tip of greater horn
9	Hypoglossal nerve
10	Inferior constrictor
11	Inferior constrictor-cricopharyngeus part
12	Internal carotid
13	Internal carotid giving off middle cerebral
14	Lateral ventricle
15	Levator veli palatini
16	Mandible, neck

17	Maxillary artery
18	Medial pterygoid
19	Middle constrictor
20	Middle meningeal artery
21	Oblique arytenoid
22	Optic chiasm
23	Palatopharyngeus
24	Parotid gland
25	Pharyngeal plexus of veins
26	Posterior belly of digastric
27	Posterior crico-arytenoid
28	Piriform fossa (recess)
29	Recurrent laryngeal nerve
30	Soft palate, nasal surface
31	Sphenoidal sinus
32	Styloglossus muscle
33	Stylohyoid muscle

34	Stylopharyngeus, with glossopharyngeal nerve
35	Submandibular gland
36	Superior cervical ganglion
37	Superior constrictor
38	Superior pharyngeal branch of vagus
39	Superior laryngeal nerve, internal branch
40	Superior sagittal sinus
41	Thyroid cartilage lamina, cut
42	Tongue, dorsum, posterior third
43	Trigeminal nerve, mandibular division
44	Uvula
45	Vagus
46	Vallecula

Ⓑ Endoscopic view of choanae and posterior nasal septum

NB: Nasogastric tube in situ

Pharyngitis, see pages 80–82.

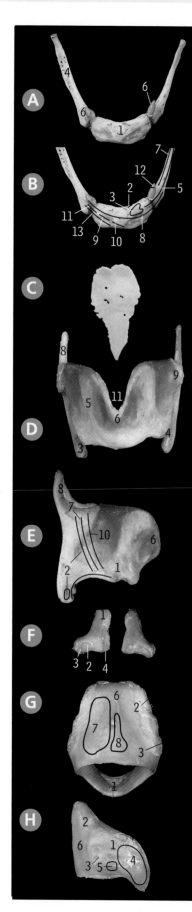

Hyoid bone

A from above and in front

B with muscle attachments

1 Body
2 Genioglossus
3 Geniohyoid
4 Greater horn
5 Hyoglossus
6 Lesser horn
7 Middle constrictor
8 Mylohyoid
9 Omohyoid
10 Sternohyoid
11 Stylohyoid
12 Stylohyoid ligament
13 Thyrohyoid

Epiglottis

C cartilage, from the front

Thyroid

D cartilage, from the front

E from the right, with attachments

1 Cricothyroid
2 Inferior constrictor
3 Inferior horn
4 Inferior tubercle
5 Lamina
6 Laryngeal prominence (Adam's apple)
7 Sternothyroid
8 Superior horn
9 Superior tubercle
10 Thyrohyoid
11 Thyroid notch

Arytenoid cartilages

F from behind

1 Apex
2 Articular surface for cricoid cartilage
3 Muscular process
4 Vocal process

Cricoid cartilage and muscle attachments

G from behind and below

H from the right

1 Arch
2 Articular surface for arytenoid cartilage
3 Articular surface for inferior horn of thyroid cartilage
4 Cricothyroid
5 Inferior constrictor
6 Lamina
7 Posterior crico-arytenoid
8 Tendon of oesophagus

Laryngeal *surface anatomy*

I lateral view

J anterior view

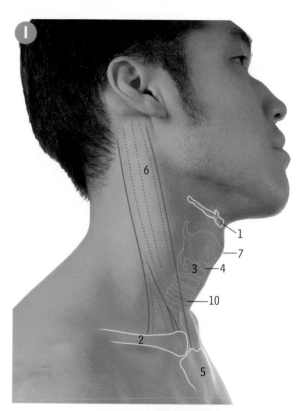

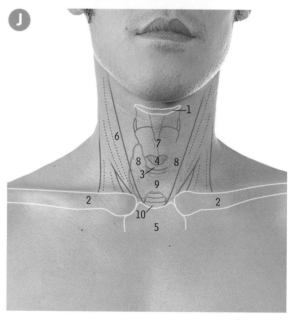

1 Body of hyoid bone
2 Clavicle
3 Cricoid cartilage
4 Cricothyroid ligament/ membrane
5 Manubrium
6 Sternocleidomastoid muscle
7 Thyroid cartilage, laryngeal prominence
8 Thyroid gland, lateral lobe
9 Thyroid gland, isthmus
10 Tracheal ring

Tracheostomy, see pages 80–82.

A Tongue and the inlet of the larynx *from above*

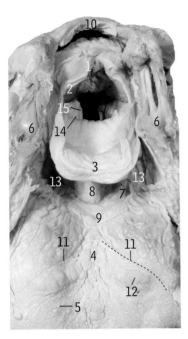

1 Corniculate cartilage in aryepiglottic fold
2 Cuneiform cartilage in aryepiglottic fold
3 Epiglottis
4 Foramen caecum
5 Fungiform papilla
6 Hyoid, greater horn
7 Lateral glossoepiglottic fold
8 Median glossoepiglottic fold
9 Pharyngeal part of dorsum of tongue
10 Posterior wall of pharynx
11 Sulcus terminalis, unilaterally indicated by dashed line
12 Vallate papilla
13 Vallecula
14 Vestibular fold (false vocal cord)
15 Vocal fold (true vocal cord)

B Larynx *from behind*

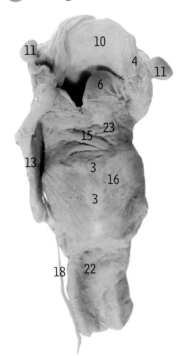

See label list below right for B.

Intrinsic muscles of the larynx

C *from the left*

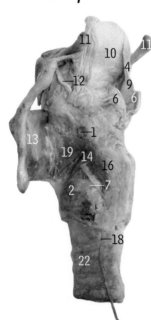

D *from the posterior oblique view*

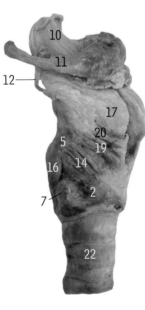

E *from the right*

1 Anastomosis of internal and recurrent laryngeal nerves (galen's anastomosis)
2 Arch of cricoid cartilage
3 Area on lamina of cricoid cartilage for attachment of oesophagus
4 Aryepiglottic fold
5 Aryepiglottic muscle
6 Corniculate cartilage
7 Cricothyroid joint
8 Cricothyroid muscle (origin from thyroid cartilage)
9 Cuneiform cartilage
10 Epiglottis
11 Greater horn of hyoid bone
12 Internal laryngeal nerve
13 Lamina of thyroid cartilage
14 Lateral crico-arytenoid muscle
15 Oblique arytenoid cartilage
16 Posterior crico-arytenoid muscle
17 Quadrangular ligament
18 Recurrent laryngeal nerve
19 Thyro-arytenoid muscle
20 Thyro-epiglottic muscle
21 Thyrohyoid membrane
22 Trachea
23 Transverse arytenoid muscle

In D, the thyroid cartilage has been reflected forward, and in E the right lamina of the thyroid cartilage has been removed.

Endotracheal intubation, recurrent laryngeal nerve palsy, see pages 80–82.

A Larynx *in sagittal section, from the right*

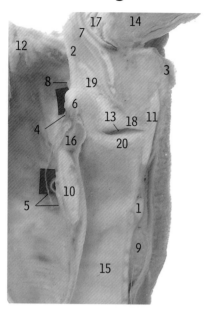

The vocal fold (vocal cord, 20) lies below the vestibular fold (false vocal cord, 18).

1	Arch of cricoid cartilage	**9**	Isthmus of thyroid gland
2	Aryepiglottic fold and inlet of larynx	**10**	Lamina of cricoid cartilage
3	Body of hyoid bone	**11**	Lamina of thyroid cartilage
4	Branches of internal laryngeal nerve anastomosing with recurrent laryngeal nerve	**12**	Pharyngeal wall
		13	Sinus of larynx (laryngeal ventricle)
5	Branches of recurrent laryngeal nerve	**14**	Tongue
		15	Trachea
6	Corniculate cartilage and apex of arytenoid cartilage	**16**	Transverse arytenoid muscle
		17	Vallecula
7	Epiglottis	**18**	Vestibular fold
8	Internal laryngeal nerve entering piriform recess	**19**	Vestibule of larynx
		20	Vocal fold

The space between the vestibular and vocal folds is the sinus of the larynx (A13), and this is continuous with the saccule, a small pouch that extends upwards for a few millimetres between the vestibular fold and the inner surface of the thyroarytenoid muscle.

The fissure between the two vestibular folds (A18) is the rima of the vestibule. The fissure between the vocal folds is the rima of the glottis.

The vestibular folds are often called the false vocal cords.

The intrinsic muscles of the larynx are supplied by the recurrent laryngeal nerve, except the cricothyroid (page 49, C8) which is supplied by the external laryngeal nerve (page 29, 12).

B Larynx *internal views*

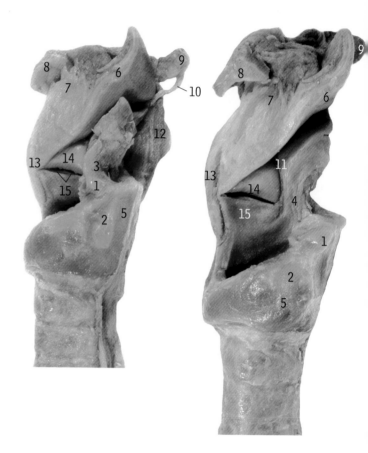

1	Articular facet on cricoid for left arytenoid cartilage	**8**	Hyoid arch, cross-section
2	Articular site of thyroid and cricoid cartilages	**9**	Hyoid, greater horn
		10	Internal laryngeal nerve
3	Arytenoid cartilage, left, lateral surface	**11**	Quadrangular membrane
		12	Thyrohyoid membrane
4	Arytenoid cartilage, right, medial surface	**13**	Thyroid cartilage, lamina, cross-section
5	Cricoid cartilage, lamina	**14**	Vestibular fold (false vocal cord)
6	Epiglottis	**15**	Vocal fold (true vocal cord)
7	Hyoepiglottic ligament		

Endoscopic view of cricoid and tracheal rings

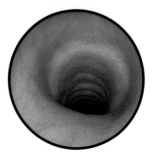

Cranial fossae Ⓐ *with dura mater intact* Ⓑ *with some dura removed*

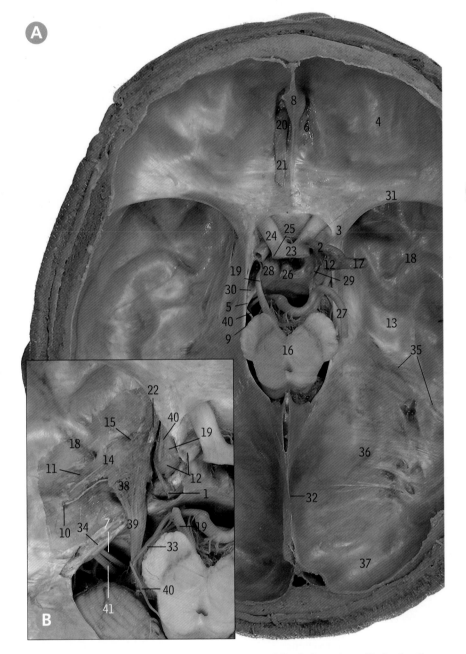

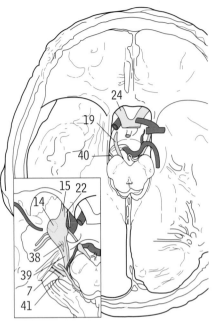

1 Abducent nerve	**16** Midbrain (superior colliculus level)	**31** Sphenoparietal sinus (at posterior border of lesser wing of sphenoid bone)
2 Anterior cerebral artery	**17** Middle cerebral artery	
3 Anterior clinoid process	**18** Middle meningeal vessels	**32** Straight sinus (at junction of falx cerebri and tentorium cerebelli)
4 Anterior cranial fossa	**19** Oculomotor nerve (cut)	
5 Attached margin of tentorium cerebelli	**20** Olfactory bulb	**33** Superior cerebellar artery
6 Cribriform plate of ethmoid bone	**21** Olfactory tract	**34** Superior petrosal sinus
7 Facial nerve	**22** Ophthalmic nerve	**35** Superior petrosal sinus (at attached margin of tentorium cerebelli)
8 Falx cerebri attached to crista galli	**23** Optic chiasma	
9 Free margin of tentorium cerebelli	**24** Optic nerve	**36** Tentorium cerebelli
10 Hiatus for greater petrosal nerve	**25** Optic tract	**37** Transverse sinus (at attached margin of tentorium cerebelli)
11 Hiatus for lesser petrosal nerve	**26** Pituitary stalk	
12 Internal carotid artery	**27** Posterior cerebral artery	**38** Trigeminal ganglion
13 Lateral part of middle cranial fossa	**28** Posterior clinoid process	**39** Trigeminal nerve
14 Mandibular nerve	**29** Posterior communicating artery	**40** Trochlear nerve
15 Maxillary nerve	**30** Roof of cavernous sinus	**41** Vestibulocochlear nerve

Cavernous sinus thrombosis, see pages 80–82.

Sagittal section of the head

A *right half, from the left*

B *endoscopic view of nasopharynx*

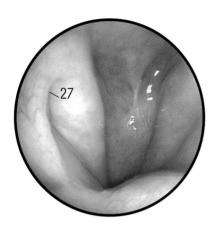

The falx cerebri (10) separates the two cerebral hemispheres. The tentorium cerebelli (39) separates the posterior parts of the cerebral hemispheres from the cerebellum (5).

C *MRI (magnetic resonance image)*

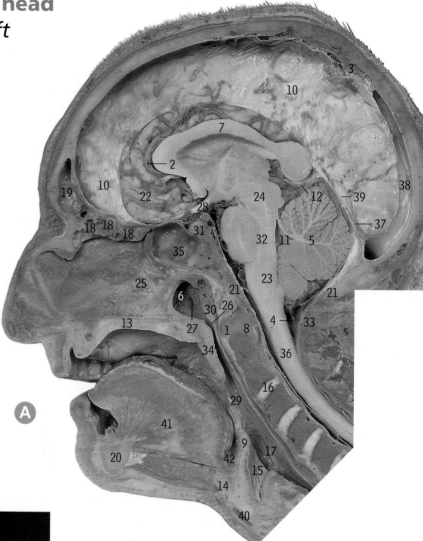

A

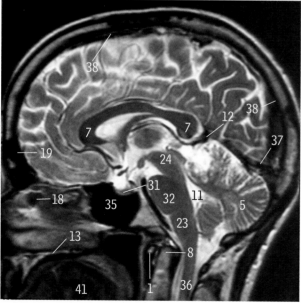

1	Anterior arch of atlas	**22**	Medial surface of right cerebral hemisphere
2	Anterior cerebral artery	**23**	Medulla oblongata
3	Arachnoid granulations	**24**	Midbrain
4	Cerebellomedullary cistern (cisterna magna)	**25**	Nasal septum (bony part)
5	Cerebellum	**26**	Nasopharynx
6	Choana (posterior nasal aperture)	**27**	Opening of auditory tube
7	Corpus callosum	**28**	Optic chiasma
8	Dens of axis	**29**	Oral part of pharynx (oropharynx)
9	Epiglottis	**30**	Pharyngeal (nasopharyngeal) tonsil (adenoids)
10	Falx cerebri	**31**	Pituitary gland
11	Fourth ventricle	**32**	Pons
12	Great cerebral vein (of Galen)	**33**	Posterior arch of atlas
13	Hard palate	**34**	Soft palate
14	Hyoid bone	**35**	Sphenoidal sinus
15	Inlet of larynx	**36**	Spinal cord
16	Intervertebral disc between axis and third cervical vertebra	**37**	Straight sinus
		38	Superior sagittal sinus
17	Laryngeal part of pharynx	**39**	Tentorium cerebelli
18	Left ethmoidal air cells	**40**	Thyroid cartilage
19	Left frontal sinus	**41**	Tongue
20	Mandible	**42**	Vallecula
21	Margin of foramen magnum		

Adenoid (pharyngeal tonsil) enlargement, pituitary apoplexy, see pages 80–82.

A Cerebral dura mater and cranial nerves

1 Abducent nerve
2 Arachnoid granulations
3 Attached margin of tentorium cerebelli
4 Choana (posterior nasal aperture)
5 Clivus
6 Dens of axis
7 Falx cerebri
8 Free margin of tentorium cerebelli
9 Glossopharyngeal, vagus and accessory nerves
10 Inferior sagittal sinus
11 Internal carotid artery
12 Margin of foramen magnum
13 Medulla oblongata
14 Motor root of facial nerve
15 Nasal septum
16 Oculomotor nerve
17 Olfactory tract
18 Optic nerve
19 Pituitary gland
20 Posterior arch of atlas
21 Rootlets of hypoglossal nerve
22 Sensory root (nervus intermedius) of facial nerve
23 Sphenoidal sinus
24 Sphenoparietal sinus
25 Spinal cord
26 Spinal part of accessory nerve
27 Straight sinus
28 Superior sagittal sinus
29 Tentorium cerebelli
30 Transverse sinus
31 Trigeminal nerve
32 Trochlear nerve
33 Vertebral artery
34 Vestibulocochlear nerve

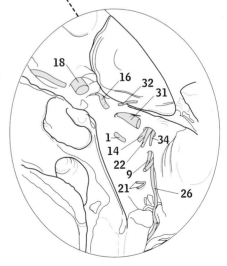

In this oblique view from the left and behind, the brain has been removed and a window has been cut in the posterior part of the falx cerebri (7) to show the upper surface of the tentorium cerebelli (29).

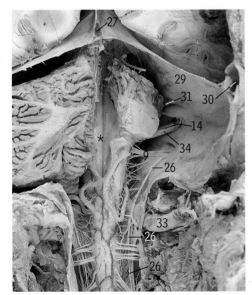

B Right posterior cranial fossa *viewed from behind*

After removal of posterior skull, dura, upper cervical vertebral laminae, all of right cerebellar hemisphere and much of left to expose the floor of the fourth ventricle (asterisk).

Craniotomy, subdural haemorrhage, see pages 80–82.

Left eye

A surface features

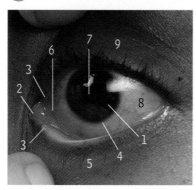

With the eyelids in the normal open position, the lower margin of the upper lid (9) overlaps approximately the upper half of the iris (1); the margin of the lower lid (5) is level with the lower margin of the iris (1).

1 Iris behind cornea
2 Lacrimal caruncle
3 Lacrimal papilla
4 Limbus (corneoscleral junction)
5 Lower lid
6 Plica semilunaris
7 Pupil behind cornea
8 Sclera
9 Upper lid

The cornea is the transparent anterior part of the outer coat of the eyeball and is continuous with the sclera (8) at the limbus (4).

The pupil (7) is the central aperture of the iris (1), the circular pigmented diaphragm that lies in front of the lens.

Each lacrimal papilla (3) contains the lacrimal punctum, the minute opening of the lacrimal canaliculus (B8) which runs medially to open into the lacrimal sac, lying deep to the medial palpebral ligament (B10) and continuing downwards as the nasolacrimal duct (B12) within the nasolacrimal canal.

B Nasolacrimal duct

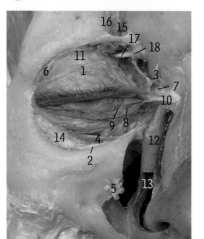

1 Aponeurosis of levator palpebrae superioris
2 Cut edge of orbital septum and periosteum
3 Dorsal nasal artery
4 Inferior oblique
5 Infra-orbital nerve
6 Lacrimal gland
7 Lacrimal sac (upper extremity)
8 Lower lacrimal canaliculus
9 Lower lacrimal papilla and punctum
10 Medial palpebral ligament
11 Muscle fibres of levator palpebrae superioris
12 Nasolacrimal duct
13 Opening of nasolacrimal duct (anterior wall removed) in inferior meatus of nose
14 Orbital fat pad
15 Supra-orbital artery
16 Supra-orbital nerve
17 Tendon of superior oblique
18 Trochlea

In B, the facial muscles and part of the skull have been dissected away to display the nasolacrimal duct (12) opening into the inferior meatus of the nose (13).

C Macrodacryocystogram

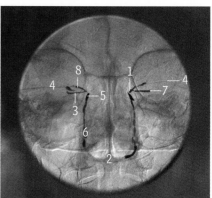

1 Common canaliculus
2 Hard palate
3 Inferior canaliculus
4 Lacrimal catheters
5 Lacrimal sac
6 Nasolacrimal duct
7 Site of lacrimal punctum
8 Superior canaliculus

1 Anterior cerebral artery
2 Anterior communicating artery
3 Anterior ethmoidal artery and nerve
4 Cribriform plate of ethmoid bone
5 Eyeball
6 Frontal nerve
7 Infratrochlear nerve and ophthalmic artery
8 Internal carotid artery
9 Lacrimal artery
10 Lacrimal gland
11 Lacrimal nerve
12 Lateral rectus
13 Levator palpebrae superioris (cut)
14 Medial rectus
15 Middle cerebral artery
16 Nasociliary nerve
17 Ophthalmic artery
18 Optic chiasma
19 Optic nerve (with overlying short ciliary nerves in left orbit)
20 Posterior ciliary artery
21 Superior oblique
22 Superior rectus (cut)
23 Supra-orbital artery
24 Supra-orbital nerve
25 Supratrochlear nerve
26 Trochlear nerve

D Orbits from above

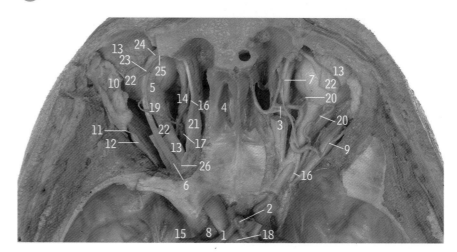

Central retinal artery occlusion, corneal arcus, corneal reflex, meibomian cyst, ophthalmoscopy, pupillary reflex, see pages 80–82.

Internal view left orbit

A medial wall view

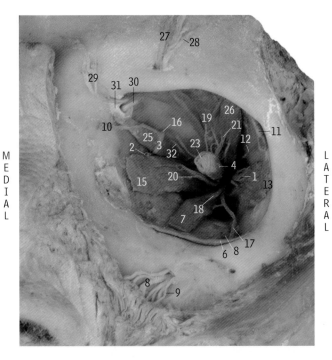

B lateral wall view

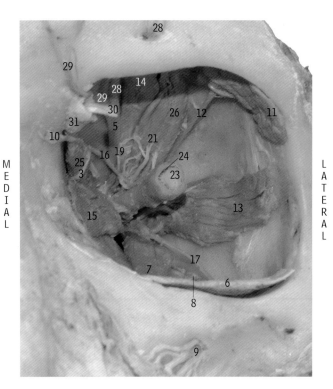

C frontal view

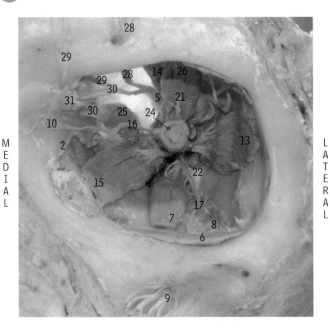

1 Abducent nerve	18 Nerve to inferior rectus
2 Anterior ethmoidal artery	19 Nerve to levator palpebrae
3 Anterior ethmoidal nerve	superioris
4 Dural sheath of optic nerve	20 Nerve to medial rectus
5 Frontal nerve	21 Nerve to superior rectus
6 Inferior oblique	22 Oculomotor nerve
7 Inferior rectus	23 Optic nerve surrounding
8 Infra-orbital artery	central artery of retina
9 Infra-orbital nerve	24 Subarachnoid space
10 Infratrochlear nerve	25 Superior oblique
11 Lacrimal gland	26 Superior rectus
12 Lacrimal nerve	27 Supra-orbital artery
13 Lateral rectus	28 Supra-orbital nerve
14 Levator palpebrae superioris	29 Supratrochlear nerve
15 Medial rectus	30 Tendon of superior oblique
16 Nasociliary nerve	31 Trochlea
17 Nerve to inferior oblique	32 Trochlear nerve

Meibomian cyst, periorbital and subconjunctival haemorrhage, glaucoma, see pages 80–82.

Superior view of right orbit

A *superficial*

B *deep, with muscle reflection*

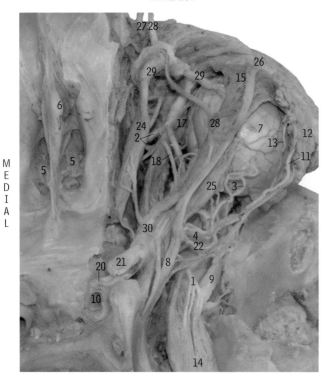

ANTERIOR

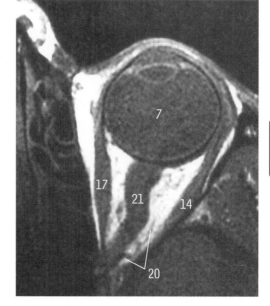

ANTERIOR

1 Abducent nerve
2 Anterior ethmoidal artery and nerve
3 Ciliary arteries
4 Ciliary ganglion
5 Cribriform plate of ethmoid bone
6 Crista galli
7 Eyeball
8 Frontal nerve
9 Infra-orbital nerve
10 Internal carotid artery
11 Lacrimal artery
12 Lacrimal gland
13 Lacrimal nerve
14 Lateral rectus (reflected)
15 Levator palpebrae superioris
16 Long ciliary nerve
17 Medial rectus
18 Nasociliary nerve
19 Nerve to superior rectus
20 Ophthalmic artery
21 Optic nerve
22 Posterior ciliary artery
23 Short ciliary nerves
24 Superior oblique
25 Superior rectus
26 Supra-orbital nerve
27 Supratrochlear artery
28 Supratrochlear nerve
29 Tendon of superior oblique
30 Trochlear nerve

Abducent nerve palsy, oculomotor nerve palsy, orbital cellulitis, trochlear nerve palsy, see pages 80–82.

Lateral view of right orbit
A *superficial* **B** *deep*

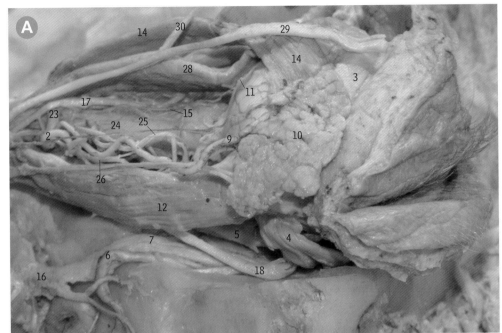

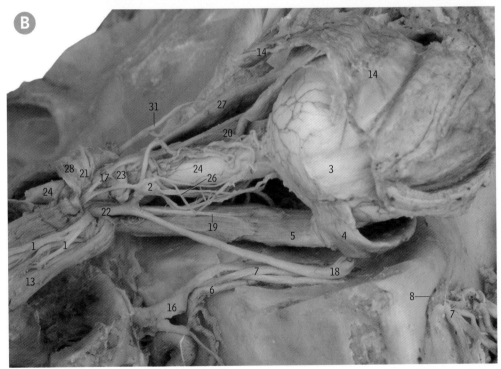

1 Abducent nerve
2 Ciliary ganglion
3 Eyeball
4 Inferior oblique
5 Inferior rectus
6 Infra-orbital artery
7 Infra-orbital nerve
8 Infra-orbital foramen
9 Lacrimal artery
10 Lacrimal gland
11 Lacrimal nerve
12 Lateral rectus
13 Lateral rectus (reflected backwards)
14 Levator palpebrae superioris
15 Long ciliary nerve
16 Maxillary branch of trigeminal nerve
17 Nasociliary nerve
18 Nerve to inferior oblique
19 Nerve to inferior rectus
20 Nerve to medial rectus
21 Nerve to superior rectus
22 Oculomotor nerve, inferior division
23 Ophthalmic artery
24 Optic nerve
25 Short ciliary artery
26 Short ciliary nerves
27 Superior oblique
28 Superior rectus
29 Supra-orbital nerve
30 Supratrochlear nerve
31 Trochlear nerve

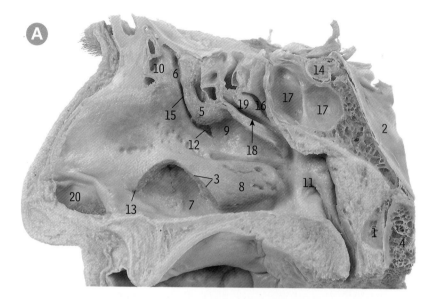

A Lateral wall of the right nasal cavity

1 Anterior arch of atlas
2 Clivus
3 Cut edge of inferior nasal concha
4 Dens of axis
5 Ethmoidal bulla
6 Ethmoidal infundibulum
7 Inferior meatus
8 Inferior nasal concha
9 Middle meatus
10 Opening of anterior ethmoidal air cells
11 Opening of auditory tube
12 Opening of maxillary sinus
13 Opening of nasolacrimal duct
14 Pituitary gland
15 Semilunar hiatus
16 Sphenoethmoidal recess
17 Sphenoidal sinus
18 Superior meatus
19 Superior nasal concha
20 Vestibule

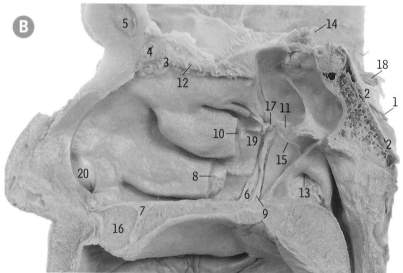

B Right nasal cavity and pterygopalatine ganglion
from the left

1 Abducent nerve
2 Clivus
3 Cribriform plate of ethmoid
4 Ethmoidal air cell (anterior)
5 Frontal sinus
6 Greater palatine nerve
7 Incisive foramen
8 Inferior nasal concha, cut edge of mucoperiosteum
9 Lesser palatine nerves
10 Middle nasal concha, cut
11 Nerve of pterygoid canal
12 Olfactory nerve fibres
13 Opening of auditory tube
14 Optic nerve
15 Pharyngeal branch to ganglion
16 Premaxilla
17 Pterygopalatine ganglion
18 Trigeminal nerve
19 Vertical plate of palatine bone
20 Vestibule

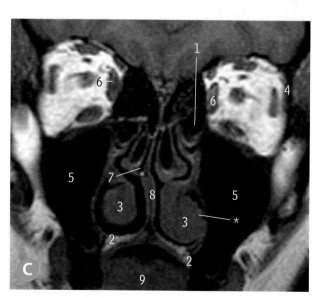

C Face
coronal MR image

1 Ethmoid air cells
2 Hard palate
3 Inferior concha
4 Lacrimal gland
5 Maxillary sinus
6 Medial rectus muscle
7 Middle meatus
8 Nasal septum
9 Tongue

*NB: This is a variant concha bullosa

Middle ear pressure equalisation, nasal polyps, nasogastric intubation, see pages 80–82.

Right trigeminal nerve branches *from the midline*

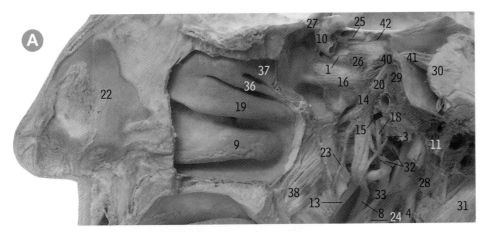

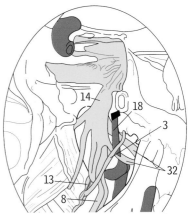

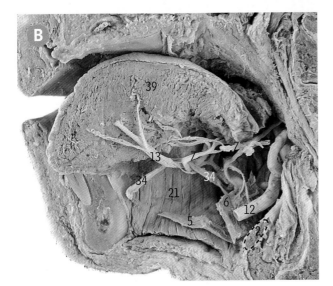

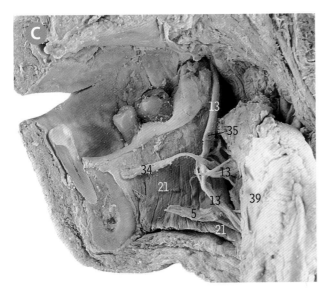

A sagittal section just left of midline

B **C** sagittal sections just right of the midline after removal of geniohyoid muscle, sublingual gland and oral mucosa. Tongue reflected medially in C.

1 Abducent nerve
2 Body of hyoid bone
3 Chorda tympani
4 External carotid artery
5 Geniohyoid
6 Hyoglossus
7 Hypoglossal nerve
8 Inferior alveolar nerve
9 Inferior nasal concha
10 Internal carotid artery
11 Jugular bulb
12 Lingual artery
13 Lingual nerve
14 Mandibular branch of trigeminal nerve
15 Marker in auditory tube
16 Maxillary branch of trigeminal nerve
17 Medial pterygoid
18 Middle meningeal artery
19 Middle nasal concha
20 Motor root of trigeminal nerve
21 Mylohyoid
22 Nasal septum (cartilaginous part)
23 Nerve to medial pterygoid
24 Nerve to mylohyoid
25 Oculomotor nerve
26 Ophthalmic branch of trigeminal nerve
27 Optic nerve
28 Parotid gland
29 Petrous part of temporal bone
30 Pons
31 Posterior belly of digastric
32 Roots of auriculotemporal nerve
33 Sphenomandibular ligament and maxillary artery
34 Submandibular duct
35 Submandibular ganglion
36 Superior nasal concha
37 Supreme nasal concha
38 Tensor veli palatini
39 Tongue
40 Trigeminal ganglion
41 Trigeminal nerve
42 Trochlear nerve

Hypoglossal nerve palsy, oral pathology, tongue carcinoma, see pages 80–82.

A Right external ear

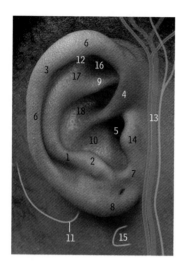

1 Antihelix
2 Antitragus
3 Auricular tubercle
4 Crus of helix
5 External acoustic meatus
6 Helix
7 Intertragic notch
8 Lobule
9 Lower crus of antihelix
10 Lower part of concha
11 Mastoid process
12 Scaphoid fossa
13 Superficial temporal vessels and auriculotemporal nerve
14 Tragus
15 Transverse process of atlas
16 Triangular fossa
17 Upper crus of antihelix
18 Upper part of concha

B Right tympanic membrane
as seen using auriscope

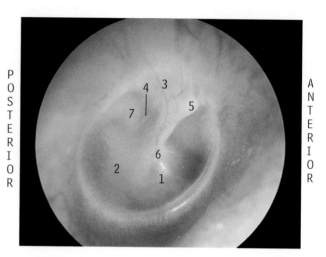

1 Cone of light (light reflex)
2 Pars tensa
3 Pars flaccida
4 Chorda tympani
5 Malleus, lateral process
6 Umbo
7 Incus, long process

C Right temporal bone and ear

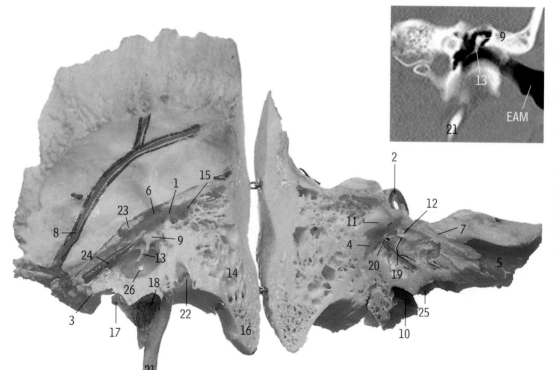

The bone has been bisected and opened out like a book, with some removal of the upper part of the petrous part. The section has opened up the tympanic (middle ear) cavity. On the left side of the figure the lateral wall of the middle ear, which includes the tympanic membrane (26), is seen from the medial side, while on the right the main features of the medial wall are in view.

1 Aditus to mastoid antrum
2 Anterior (superior) semicircular canal
3 Bony part of auditory tube
4 Canal for facial nerve (yellow)
5 Carotid canal (red)
6 Epitympanic recess
7 Groove for greater petrosal nerve (yellow)
8 Groove for middle meningeal vessels
9 Incus
10 Jugular bulb (blue)
11 Lateral semicircular canal
12 Lesser petrosal nerve
13 Malleus
14 Mastoid air cells
15 Mastoid antrum
16 Mastoid process
17 Part of carotid canal (red)
18 Part of jugular bulb (blue)
19 Promontory with overlying tympanic plexus
20 Stapes in oval window and stapedius muscle
21 Styloid process
22 Stylomastoid foramen
23 Tegmen tympani
24 Tensor tympani muscle in its canal
25 Tympanic branch of glossopharyngeal nerve entering its canaliculus
26 Tympanic membrane

Hyperacusis, perforated drum, otalgia (referred pain), see pages 80–82.

Ear *right temporal bone*

A middle ear and the facial nerve and branches

B enlarged view of A

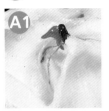
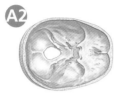

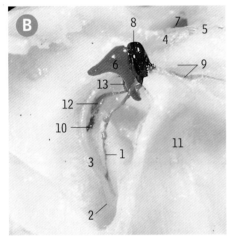

This dissection is seen from the right and above, looking forwards and medially. Bone has been removed to show the upper parts of the malleus (8) and incus (6), which normally project up into the epitympanic recess. The upper part of the facial canal (2) has been opened to show the facial nerve (3) giving off the chorda tympani (1) and the nerve to stapedius (10). The geniculate ganglion of the facial nerve (4) is seen giving off the greater petrosal nerve (5).

1 Chorda tympani
2 Facial canal leading to stylomastoid foramen
3 Facial nerve
4 Geniculate ganglion of facial nerve
5 Greater petrosal nerve
6 Incus
7 Internal acoustic meatus
8 Malleus
9 Margin of auditory tube
10 Nerve to stapedius
11 Paraffin wax (for support) overlying tympanic membrane
12 Stapedius
13 Stapes

The stapedius (12) tendon emerges from a small conical projection on the posterior wall of the tympanic cavity, the pyramid (here dissected away).

Ear

C right temporal bone; middle ear and inner ear, enlarged

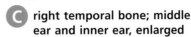
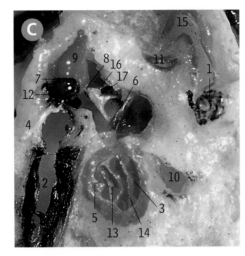

This dissection is viewed from above, looking slightly backwards and laterally. Within the cavity of the middle ear are the three auditory ossicles – malleus (12), incus (9) and stapes (17). The tympanic membrane and external acoustic meatus are not seen but lie below the label 7. The cochlea has been opened up to show its internal bony structure (3, 5, 13 and 14).

1 Anterior (superior) semicircular canal
2 Auditory tube
3 Bony canal of cochlea
4 Chorda tympani
5 Cupola of cochlea
6 Footplate of stapes in oval window of vestibule
7 Incudomalleolar joint
8 Incudostapedial joint
9 Incus
10 Internal acoustic meatus
11 Lateral semicircular canal
12 Malleus
13 Modiolus of cochlea
14 Osseous spiral lamina of cochlea
15 Posterior semicircular canal
16 Stapedius tendon
17 Stapes

Right ear

D from above, diagram of parts

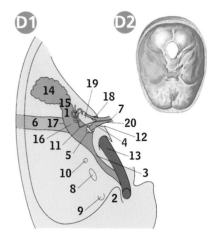

1 Aditus to mastoid antrum
2 Anterior clinoid process
3 Auditory tube
4 Cochlear nerve
5 Cochlear part of inner ear
6 External acoustic meatus
7 Facial nerve
8 Foramen ovale
9 Foramen rotundum
10 Foramen spinosum
11 Geniculate ganglion of facial nerve
12 Internal acoustic meatus
13 Internal carotid artery emerging from foramen lacerum
14 Mastoid air cells
15 Mastoid antrum
16 Middle ear
17 Tympanic membrane
18 Vestibular nerve
19 Vestibular part of inner ear
20 Vestibulocochlear nerve

E Inner ear CT (3D reconstruction)

1 Anterior (superior) semicircular canals (SSC)
2 Common crus
3 Labyrinthine segment of facial nerve
4 Superior vestibular nerve
5 Cochlear nerve
6 Vestibulocochlear nerve
7 Abducent nerve CN VI
8 Cochlea
9 Vestibule
10 Oval window
11 Lateral SCC
12 Lateral SCC, ampulla
13 Posterior SCC

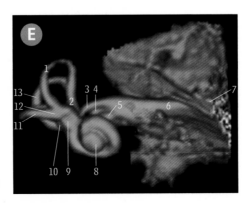
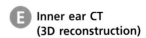

Labyrinthitis, see pages 80–82.

A Cranial vault and falx *from below*

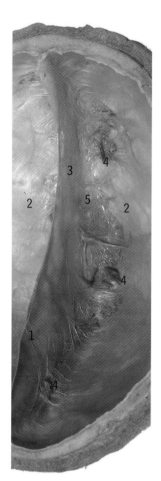

B Brain *from above*

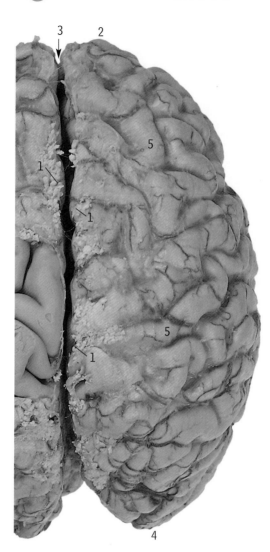

C Brain *right cerebral hemisphere, from above*

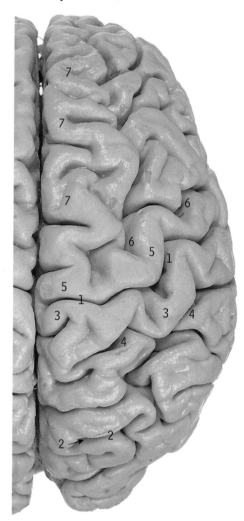

Looking up into the cranial vault from below, the falx cerebri (3) is seen to be continuous with the dura over the vault (2), and has been cut off at the back (1) from the tentorium cerebelli.

1 Cut edge of falx cerebri
2 Dura mater over cranial vault
3 Falx cerebri
4 Superior cerebral veins
5 Superior sagittal sinus

The right cerebral hemisphere is seen with the overlying arachnoid mater and arachnoid granulations (1) adjacent to the longitudinal fissure (3). Over the small part of the left hemisphere shown, a window has been cut in the arachnoid revealing the subarachnoid space.

1 Arachnoid granulations
2 Frontal pole
3 Longitudinal fissure
4 Occipital pole
5 Superolateral surface

Removal of the arachnoid and the underlying vessels displays the gyri and sulci. Only a small number are named here; the most important are the central sulcus (1) and the precentral and postcentral gyri (5 and 3).

1 Central sulcus
2 Parieto-occipital sulcus
3 Postcentral gyrus
4 Postcentral sulcus
5 Precentral gyrus
6 Precentral sulcus
7 Superior frontal gyrus

Subarachnoid haemorrhage, see pages 80–82.

Brain **A** *from the right* **B** *right cerebral hemisphere, from the right*

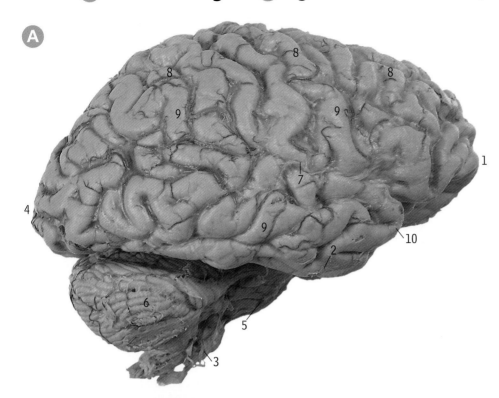

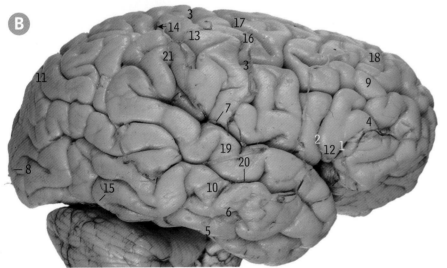

As in B (page 62), the arachnoid mater has been left intact and vessels are seen beneath it; the larger ones are veins (as at 7).

1 Frontal pole
2 Inferior cerebral veins
3 Medulla oblongata and vertebral artery
4 Occipital pole
5 Pons and basilar artery
6 Right cerebellar hemisphere
7 Superficial middle cerebral vein overlying lateral sulcus
8 Superior cerebral veins
9 Superolateral surface of right cerebral hemisphere
10 Temporal pole

The arachnoid mater has been removed, leaving some of the larger branches of the middle cerebral artery (unlabelled) after they have emerged from the lateral sulcus (7). Only the main gyri and sulci are named here: the most important are the precentral and postcentral gyri (16 and 13) and the central and lateral sulci (3 and 7).

1 Anterior ramus of lateral sulcus
2 Ascending ramus of lateral sulcus
3 Central sulcus
4 Inferior frontal gyrus
5 Inferior temporal gyrus
6 Inferior temporal sulcus
7 Lateral sulcus (posterior ramus)
8 Lunate sulcus
9 Middle frontal gyrus
10 Middle temporal gyrus
11 Parieto-occipital sulcus
12 Pars triangularis
13 Postcentral gyrus
14 Postcentral sulcus
15 Pre-occipital notch
16 Precentral gyrus
17 Precentral sulcus
18 Superior frontal gyrus
19 Superior temporal gyrus
20 Superior temporal sulcus
21 Supramarginal gyrus

The central sulcus (C1 (page 62) and B3, above) marks the boundary between the frontal and parietal lobes.

An arbitrary line from the pre-occipital notch (B15) to the parieto-occipital sulcus (B11) marks the boundary between the parietal and occipital lobes, and the part of the hemisphere in front of this line and below the lateral sulcus (strictly, the posterior ramus of the lateral sulcus, B7) forms the temporal lobe.

The precentral and postcentral gyri (B16 and 13) contain the classically described primary 'motor' and 'sensory' areas of the cortex.

The motor speech (Broca) areas (usually in the left cerebral hemisphere) are in the region of the ascending and anterior rami of the lateral sulcus and the pars triangularis (B2, 1 and 12).

The auditory areas of the cortex probably comprise parts of the superior temporal gyrus (B19), especially the upper surface of it within the lateral sulcus (B7).

Ⓐ Brain *from below*

This is the view of the under-surface of the brain as typically seen when first removed from the skull, without any dissection. Arachnoid mater, torn in places and with blood vessels beneath it, remains on the outer surface.

1   Abducent nerve
2   Anterior perforated substance
3   Arachnoid mater overlying mamillary bodies
4   Basilar artery
5   Cerebellar hemisphere
6   Crus of cerebral peduncle (midbrain)
7   Facial nerve
8   Frontal pole
9   Gyrus rectus
10   Inferior surface of frontal lobe
11   Inferior surface of temporal lobe
12   Internal carotid artery
13   Longitudinal fissure
14   Medulla oblongata
15   Oculomotor nerve
16   Olfactory bulb
17   Olfactory tract
18   Optic chiasma
19   Optic nerve
20   Pituitary stalk (infundibulum)
21   Pons
22   Posterior communicating artery
23   Spinal part of accessory nerve
24   Temporal pole
25   Trigeminal nerve
26   Uncus
27   Vertebral artery
28   Vestibulocochlear nerve

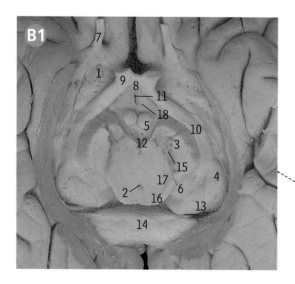

Ⓑ Optic tract and geniculate bodies *from below*

The brainstem has been mostly removed, leaving only the upper part of the midbrain. The most medial parts of each cerebral hemisphere have also been dissected away. To find the geniculate bodies (4 and 6), which are on the under-surface of the posterior part (pulvinar, 13) of the thalamus, identify the optic chiasma (8) and then follow the optic tract (10) backwards round the side of the midbrain (3).

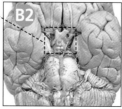

1   Anterior perforated substance
2   Aqueduct of midbrain
3   Crus of midbrain
4   Lateral geniculate body
5   Mamillary body
6   Medial geniculate body
7   Olfactory tract
8   Optic chiasma
9   Optic nerve
10   Optic tract

11   Pituitary stalk (infundibulum)
12   Posterior perforated substance
13   Pulvinar of thalamus
14   Splenium of corpus callosum
15   Substantia nigra of midbrain
16   Tectum of midbrain
17   Tegmentum of midbrain
18   Tuber cinereum

A Brain *from below*

A1

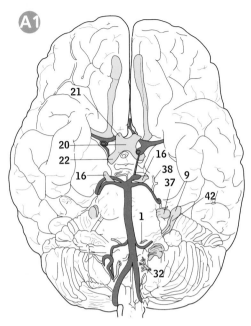

A2

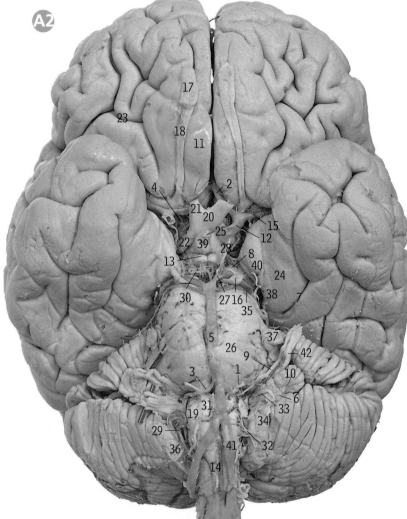

1 Abducent nerve
2 Anterior cerebral artery
3 Anterior inferior cerebellar artery
4 Anterior perforated substance
5 Basilar artery
6 Choroid plexus from lateral recess of fourth ventricle
7 Collateral sulcus
8 Crus of cerebral peduncle
9 Facial nerve
10 Flocculus of cerebellum
11 Gyrus rectus
12 Internal carotid artery
13 Mamillary body
14 Medulla oblongata
15 Middle cerebral artery
16 Oculomotor nerve
17 Olfactory bulb
18 Olfactory tract
19 Olive of medulla oblongata
20 Optic chiasma
21 Optic nerve
22 Optic tract
23 Orbital sulcus
24 Parahippocampal gyrus
25 Pituitary stalk (infundibulum)
26 Pons
27 Posterior cerebral artery
28 Posterior communicating artery
29 Posterior inferior cerebellar artery
30 Posterior perforated substance
31 Pyramid of medulla oblongata
32 Rootlets of hypoglossal nerve (superficial to marker)
33 Roots of glossopharyngeal, vagus and accessory nerves
34 Spinal part of accessory nerve
35 Superior cerebellar artery
36 Tonsil of cerebellum
37 Trigeminal nerve
38 Trochlear nerve
39 Tuber cinereum and median eminence
40 Uncus
41 Vertebral artery
42 Vestibulocochlear nerve

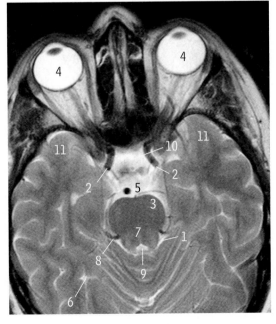

B Brain

axial MR image showing cisterns

1 Ambient cistern
2 Carotid artery, internal
3 Cerebral peduncle
4 Globe (eyeball)
5 Interpeduncular cistern
6 Lateral ventricle, posterior horn
7 Midbrain
8 Posterior cerebral artery
9 Quadrigeminal cistern
10 Suprachiasmatic cistern
11 Temporal lobe

A Right half of the brain *in a midline sagittal section, from the left*

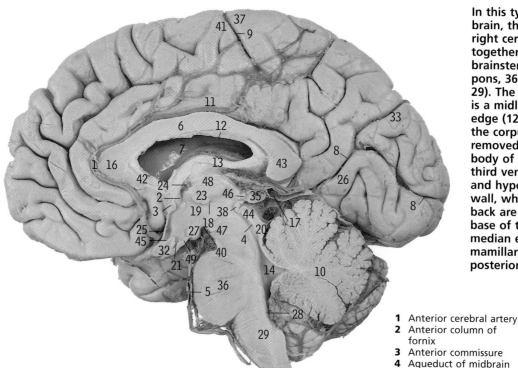

In this typical half-section of the brain, the medial surface of the right cerebral hemisphere is seen, together with the sectioned brainstem (midbrain, 4, 20, 44, 47; pons, 36; and medulla oblongata, 29). The septum pellucidum, which is a midline structure and whose cut edge (12) is seen below the body of the corpus callosum (6), has been removed to show the interior of the body of the lateral ventricle (7). The third ventricle has the thalamus (48) and hypothalamus (19) in its lateral wall, while in its floor from front to back are the optic chiasma (32), the base of the pituitary stalk (21), the median eminence (49), the mamillary bodies (27), and the posterior perforated substance (40).

B Carotid arteriogram
digitally subtracted arterial phase of carotid arteriogram, lateral projection

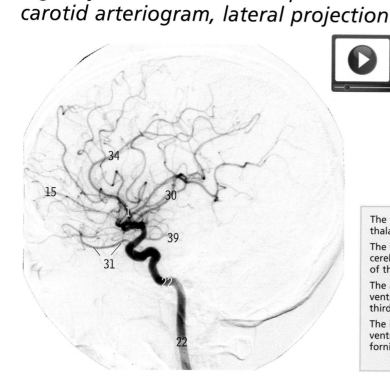

1 Anterior cerebral artery	**27** Mamillary body
2 Anterior column of fornix	**28** Median aperture of fourth ventricle
3 Anterior commissure	**29** Medulla oblongata
4 Aqueduct of midbrain	**30** Middle cerebral artery
5 Basilar artery	**31** Ophthalmic artery
6 Body of corpus callosum	**32** Optic chiasma
7 Body of lateral ventricle	**33** Parieto-occipital sulcus
8 Calcarine sulcus	**34** Pericallosal artery
9 Central sulcus	**35** Pineal body
10 Cerebellum	**36** Pons
11 Cingulate gyrus	**37** Postcentral gyrus
12 Cut edge of septum pellucidum	**38** Posterior commissure
13 Fornix	**39** Posterior communicating artery
14 Fourth ventricle	**40** Posterior perforated substance
15 Frontopolar artery	**41** Precentral gyrus
16 Genu of corpus callosum	**42** Rostrum of corpus callosum
17 Great cerebral vein	**43** Splenium of corpus callosum
18 Hypothalamic sulcus	**44** Superior colliculus of midbrain
19 Hypothalamus	**45** Supra-optic recess
20 Inferior colliculus of midbrain	**46** Suprapineal recess
21 Infundibular recess (base of pituitary stalk)	**47** Tegmentum of midbrain
22 Internal carotid artery	**48** Thalamus
23 Interthalamic connexion	**49** Tuber cinereum and median eminence
24 Interventricular foramen and choroid plexus	
25 Lamina terminalis	
26 Lingual gyrus	

The third ventricle is the cavity which has in its lateral wall the thalamus (A48) and hypothalamus (A19).

The fourth ventricle (A14) is largely between the pons (A36) and cerebellum (A10), although its lower end is behind the upper part of the medulla oblongata (A29) (see page 53, B).

The aqueduct of the midbrain (A4) connects the third and fourth ventricles; cerebrospinal fluid normally flows through it from the third to the fourth ventricle.

The interventricular foramen (A24) connects the third to the lateral ventricle, and is bounded in front by the anterior column of the fornix (A2) and behind by the thalamus (A48).

C Brain *median sagittal MR image*

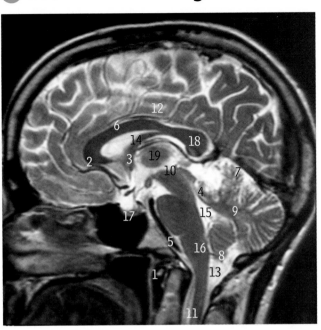

1 Anterior arch of atlas
2 Anterior cerebral artery
3 Anterior commissure
4 Aqueduct of Sylvius
5 Basilar artery
6 Body of corpus callosum
7 Cerebellar folia
8 Cerebellar tonsil
9 Cerebellum
10 Cerebral peduncle of midbrain
11 Cervical spinal cord
12 Cingulate gyrus
13 Cisterna magna
14 Fornix
15 Fourth ventricle
16 Medulla oblongata
17 Pituitary gland
18 Splenium of corpus callosum
19 Thalamus in lateral wall third ventricle

D *Cranial nerves*

E *Endoscopy – base of brain*

In this ventral view of the central part of the brain, the right vertebral artery (on the left of the picture) has been removed almost at the junction with its fellow (22). The filaments of the first nerve (olfactory) are not seen entering the olfactory bulb (10) as they are torn off when removing the brain. The roots forming the glossopharyngeal, vagus and accessory nerves (6, 21 and 2) cannot be clearly identified from one another, but the spinal part of the accessory nerve (2) is seen running up beside the medulla to join the cranial part.

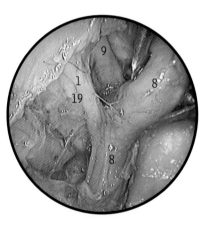

1 Abducent nerve
2 Accessory nerve, spinal root
3 Basilar artery
4 Crus of cerebral peduncle
5 Facial nerve
6 Glossopharyngeal nerve
7 Hypoglossal nerve
8 Internal carotid artery
9 Oculomotor nerve
10 Olfactory bulb
11 Olive of medulla oblongata
12 Optic nerve
13 Pituitary stalk
14 Pons
15 Posterior cerebral artery
16 Posterior communicating artery
17 Pyramid of medulla oblongata
18 Superior cerebellar artery
19 Trigeminal nerve
20 Trochlear nerve
21 Vagus nerve
22 Vertebral artery
23 Vestibulocochlear nerve

The oculomotor nerve (D9) emerges on the medial side of the crus of the cerebral peduncle (D4), and the trochlear nerve (D20) winds round the lateral side of the peduncle. Both nerves pass between the posterior cerebral and superior cerebellar arteries (D15 and 18).

The trochlear nerve (D20) is the only cranial nerve to emerge from the dorsal surface of the brainstem and to decussate after emergence.

The trigeminal nerve (D19) emerges from the lateral side of the pons (D14).

The abducent nerve (D1) emerges between the pons and the pyramid (D14 and 17).

The facial and vestibulocochlear nerves (D5 and 23) emerge from the lateral pontomedullary angle.

The glossopharyngeal and vagus nerves (D6, 21) and the cranial root of the accessory nerve emerge from the medulla oblongata lateral to the olive (D11).

The hypoglossal nerve (D7) emerges as two series of rootlets from the medulla oblongata between the pyramid (D17) and the olive (D11).

The spinal part of the accessory nerve emerges from the lateral surface of the upper five or six cervical segments of the spinal cord, dorsal to the denticulate ligament (page 69, G27).

Arteries of the base of the brain Ⓐ *injected arteries*
Ⓑ *arterial circle (Willis) and basilar artery*

Ⓒ *MR angiogram of arterial circle (Willis)*

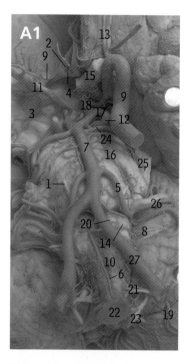

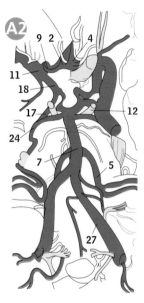

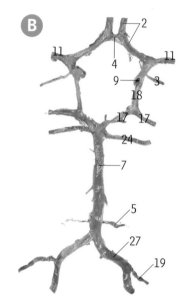

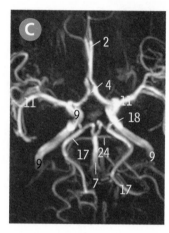

Part of the right cerebral hemisphere (on the left of the picture) has been removed to show the right middle cerebral artery (11).

The anastomosing vessels have been removed from the base of the brain and spread out in their relative positions.

Ⓓ *Intracranial endoscopy at the base of the brain*

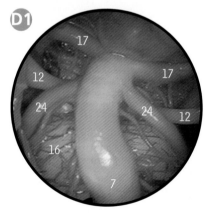

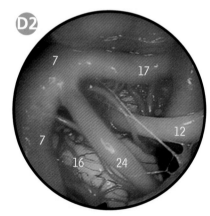

1 Abducent nerve	**8** Filaments of glossopharyngeal, vagus and accessory nerves	**16** Pons
2 Anterior cerebral artery	**9** Internal carotid artery	**17** Posterior cerebral artery
3 Anterior choroidal artery	**10** Medulla oblongata	**18** Posterior communicating artery
4 Anterior communicating artery	**11** Middle cerebral artery	**19** Posterior inferior cerebellar artery
5 Anterior inferior cerebellar artery	**12** Oculomotor nerve	**20** Pyramid
6 Anterior spinal artery	**13** Olfactory tract	**21** Rootlets of first cervical nerve
7 Basilar artery with pontine branches	**14** Olive	**22** Spinal cord
	15 Optic nerve	

23 Spinal part of accessory nerve	
24 Superior cerebellar artery	
25 Trigeminal nerve	
26 Unusually large branch of 5 overlying facial and vestibulocochlear nerves	
27 Vertebral artery	

Berry aneurysm, see pages 80–82.

F Brainstem and floor of the fourth ventricle

In this view of the dorsal surface of the brainstem, it has been cut off from the rest of the brain at the top of the midbrain, just above the superior colliculi (15). The cerebellum has been removed by transecting the superior (14), middle (12) and inferior (6) cerebellar peduncles.

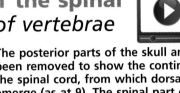

1 Cuneate tubercle	7 Inferior colliculus	14 Superior cerebellar peduncle
2 Cut edge of superior medullary velum	8 Lateral recess	15 Superior colliculus
3 Facial colliculus	9 Medial eminence	16 Trochlear nerve
4 Gracile tubercle	10 Median sulcus	17 Vagal triangle
5 Hypoglossal triangle	11 Medullary striae	18 Vestibular area
6 Inferior cerebellar peduncle	12 Middle cerebellar peduncle	
	13 Obex	

G Brainstem and upper part of the spinal cord *from behind after removal of vertebrae*

The posterior parts of the skull and upper vertebrae have been removed to show the continuity of the brainstem with the spinal cord, from which dorsal nerve rootlets are seen to emerge (as at 9). The spinal part of the accessory nerve (27) runs up through the foramen magnum (20) to join the cranial part in the jugular foramen (24). Ventral nerve rootlets (as at 33), ventral to the denticulate ligament (5), unite to form a ventral nerve root which joins with a dorsal nerve root (8, whose formative rootlets dorsal to the ligament have been cut off from the cord in order to make the ventral roots visible) to form a spinal nerve immediately beyond the dorsal root ganglion (7). The nerve immediately divides into ventral and dorsal rami (as at 32 and 6).

1 Arachnoid mater	18 Lateral mass of atlas
2 Atlanto-occipital joint	19 Longus capitis
3 Capsule of lateral atlanto-axial joint	20 Margin of foramen magnum
4 Choroid plexus emerging from lateral recess of fourth ventricle	21 Posterior inferior cerebellar artery
5 Denticulate ligament	22 Posterior spinal arteries
6 Dorsal ramus of third cervical nerve	23 Rectus capitis lateralis
7 Dorsal root ganglion of fourth cervical nerve	24 Roots of glossopharyngeal, vagus and cranial part of accessory nerves and jugular foramen
8 Dorsal root of fourth cervical nerve	25 Scalenus anterior
9 Dorsal rootlets of second cervical nerve	26 Sigmoid sinus
10 Dura mater	27 Spinal part of accessory nerve
11 External carotid artery	28 Spinous process of seventh cervical vertebra
12 First cervical nerve and posterior arch of atlas	29 Transverse process of atlas
13 Floor of the fourth ventricle	30 Vagus nerve
14 Internal acoustic meatus with facial and vestibulocochlear nerves and labyrinthine artery	31 Vein from vertebral venous plexuses
15 Internal carotid artery	32 Ventral ramus of third cervical nerve
16 Internal jugular vein	33 Ventral rootlets of fourth cervical nerve
17 Lamina of sixth cervical vertebra	34 Vertebral artery

The lower part of the diamond-shaped floor of the fourth ventricle containing the hypoglossal and vagal triangles (F5 and 17) is part of the medulla oblongata; the rest of the floor is part of the pons.

The gracile and cuneate tubercles (F4 and 1) are caused by the underlying gracile and cuneate nuclei, where the fibres of the gracile and cuneate tracts (posterior white columns) end by synapsing with the cells of the nuclei. The fibres from these cells form the medial lemniscus which runs through the brainstem to the thalamus.

The facial colliculus (F3), at the lower end of the medial eminence (F9) in the floor of the fourth ventricle, is caused by fibres of the facial nerve overlying the abducent nerve nucleus; it is not produced by the facial nerve nucleus, which lies at a deeper level in the pons.

After emerging from the foramen in the transverse process of the atlas the vertebral artery (G34) winds backwards round the lateral mass of the atlas (G18) on its posterior arch before turning upwards to enter the skull, via the foramen magnum.

Cerebral hemispheres Ⓐ *sectioned horizontally* Ⓑ *axial MR image*

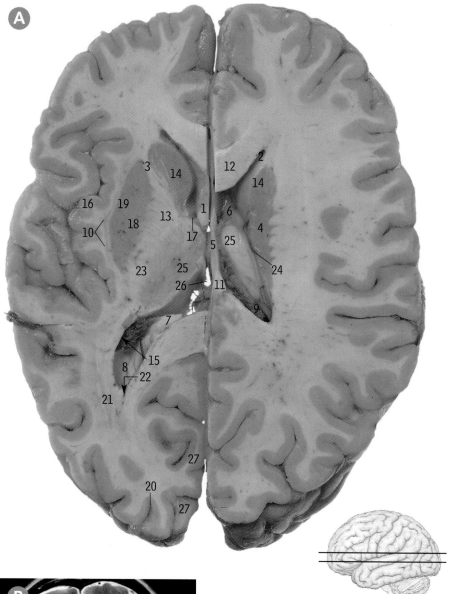

Viewed from above, the left cerebral hemisphere has been sectioned on a level with the interventricular foramen (17), and that on the right about 1.5 cm higher. The most important feature seen in the left hemisphere is the internal capsule (3, 13 and 23), situated between the caudate (14) and lentiform (18 and 19) nuclei and the thalamus (25). On the right side, a large part of the corpus callosum (11) has been removed, so opening up the lateral ventricle (6) from above and showing the caudate nucleus (14 and 4) arching backwards over the thalamus (25), with the thalamostriate vein (24) and choroid plexus (9) in the shallow groove between them.

1 Anterior column of fornix
2 Anterior horn of lateral ventricle
3 Anterior limb of internal capsule
4 Body of caudate nucleus
5 Body of fornix
6 Body of lateral ventricle
7 Bulb
8 Calcar avis
9 Choroid plexus
10 Claustrum
11 Corpus callosum
12 Forceps minor (corpus callosum)
13 Genu of internal capsule
14 Head of caudate nucleus
15 Inferior horn of lateral ventricle
16 Insula
17 Interventricular foramen
18 Lentiform nucleus: globus pallidus
19 Lentiform nucleus: putamen
20 Lunate sulcus
21 Optic radiation
22 Posterior horn of lateral ventricle
23 Posterior limb of internal capsule
24 Thalamostriate vein
25 Thalamus
26 Third ventricle
27 Visual area of cortex

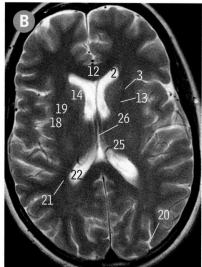

The anterior limb of the internal capsule (3) is bounded medially by the head of the caudate nucleus (14) and laterally by the lentiform nucleus (putamen and globus pallidus, 18 and 19).

The genu of the internal capsule (13) lies at the most medial edge of the globus pallidus (18).

The posterior limb of the internal capsule (23) is bounded medially by the thalamus (25) and laterally by the lentiform nucleus (18 and 19).

Corticonuclear fibres (motor fibres from the cerebral cortex to the motor nuclei of cranial nerves) pass through the genu of the internal capsule (13).

Corticospinal fibres (motor fibres from the cerebral cortex to anterior horn cells of the spinal cord) pass through the anterior two-thirds of the posterior limb of the internal capsule (23).

The genu and the posterior limb of the internal capsule, supplied by the striate branches of the anterior and middle cerebral arteries and by the anterior choroidal artery, are of the greatest clinical importance as they are the common sites for cerebral haemorrhage or thrombosis ('stroke').

Brain Ⓐ coronal section, from the front Ⓑ coronal MR image

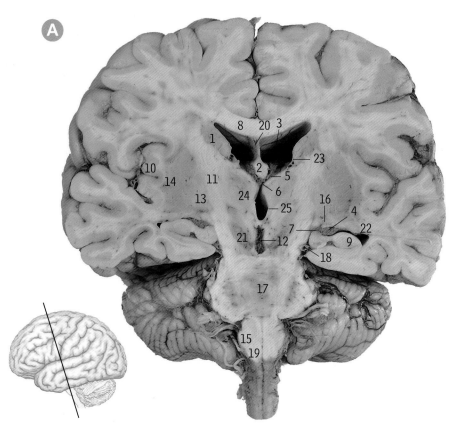

This coronal section is not quite vertical but passes slightly backwards, through the third ventricle (25) and bodies of the lateral ventricles (3) from a level about 0.5 cm behind the interventricular foramina, and down through the pons (17) and the pyramid of the medulla (19). It has been cut in this way to show the path of the important corticospinal (motor) fibres passing down through the internal capsule (11) and pons (17) to form the pyramid of the medulla (19). Compare with features in the MR image.

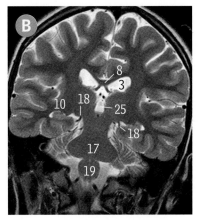

1 Body of caudate nucleus	**6** Choroid plexus of third ventricle	**13** Lentiform nucleus: globus pallidus	**19** Pyramid of medulla oblongata
2 Body of fornix	**7** Choroidal fissure	**14** Lentiform nucleus: putamen	**20** Septum pellucidum
3 Body of lateral ventricle	**8** Corpus callosum	**15** Olive of medulla oblongata	**21** Substantia nigra
4 Choroid plexus of inferior horn of lateral ventricle	**9** Hippocampus	**16** Optic tract	**22** Tail of caudate nucleus
5 Choroid plexus of lateral ventricle	**10** Insula	**17** Pons	**23** Thalamostriate vein
	11 Internal capsule	**18** Posterior cerebral artery	**24** Thalamus
	12 Interpeduncular cistern		**25** Third ventricle

Ⓒ Sectioned cerebral hemispheres and the brainstem

from above and behind

The cerebral hemispheres have been sectioned horizontally just above the level of the interventricular foramina, and the posterior parts of the hemispheres have been removed, together with the whole of the cerebellum, to show the tela choroidea (12) of the posterior part of the roof of the third ventricle and the underlying internal cerebral veins (10).

1 Anterior horn of lateral ventricle	**4** Floor of fourth ventricle	**10** Internal cerebral vein
2 Anterior limb of internal capsule	**5** Forceps minor	**11** Posterior limb of internal capsule
3 Choroid plexus and junction of inferior and posterior horn of lateral ventricle	**6** Genu of internal capsule	**12** Tela choroidea of roof of third ventricle
	7 Head of caudate nucleus	**13** Thalamus
	8 Inferior colliculus	**14** Third ventricle
	9 Insula	**15** Trochlear nerve

Arteriovenous fistulae, see pages 80–82.

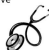

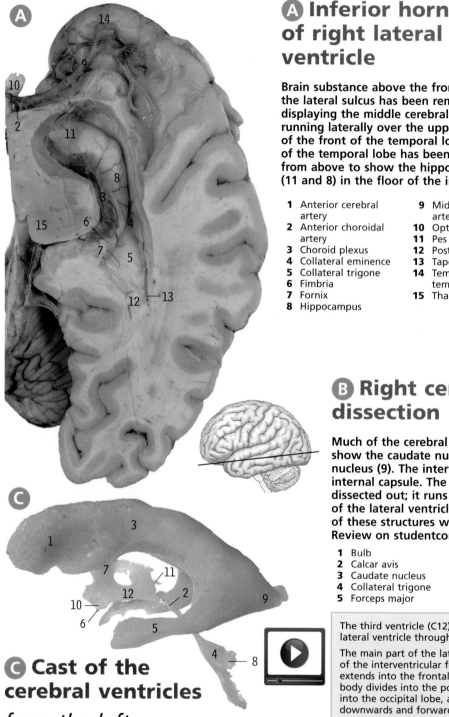

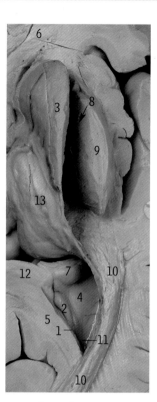

Ⓐ Inferior horn of right lateral ventricle

Brain substance above the front part of the lateral sulcus has been removed, displaying the middle cerebral artery (9) running laterally over the upper surface of the front of the temporal lobe (14). Part of the temporal lobe has been opened up from above to show the hippocampus (11 and 8) in the floor of the inferior horn.

1 Anterior cerebral artery	9 Middle cerebral artery
2 Anterior choroidal artery	10 Optic nerve
3 Choroid plexus	11 Pes hippocampi
4 Collateral eminence	12 Posterior horn
5 Collateral trigone	13 Tapetum
6 Fimbria	14 Temporal pole of temporal lobe
7 Fornix	15 Thalamus
8 Hippocampus	

Ⓑ Right cerebral hemisphere dissection *from above*

Much of the cerebral substance has been dissected away to show the caudate nucleus (3), thalamus (13) and lentiform nucleus (9). The intervening gap (8) is occupied by the internal capsule. The optic radiation (10) has also been dissected out; it runs backwards lateral to the posterior horn of the lateral ventricle. Compare this three-dimensional view of these structures with the brain section in the Systemic Review on studentconsult.com.

1 Bulb	6 Forceps minor	11 Posterior horn of lateral ventricle
2 Calcar avis	7 Fornix	
3 Caudate nucleus	8 Internal capsule	12 Splenium of corpus callosum
4 Collateral trigone	9 Lentiform nucleus	
5 Forceps major	10 Optic radiation	13 Thalamus

Ⓒ Cast of the cerebral ventricles

from the left

In this side view, the left lateral ventricle largely overlaps the right one.

1 Anterior horn of lateral ventricle	8 Lateral recess
2 Aqueduct of midbrain	9 Posterior horn of lateral ventricle
3 Body of lateral ventricle	10 Supra-optic recess of third ventricle
4 Fourth ventricle	
5 Inferior horn of lateral ventricle	11 Suprapineal recess of third ventricle
6 Infundibular recess of third ventricle	12 Third ventricle (with gap for interthalamic connexion)
7 Interventricular foramen	

The third ventricle (C12) communicates at its upper front end with each lateral ventricle through the interventricular foramen (C7).

The main part of the lateral ventricle is the body (C3). The part in front of the interventricular foramen (C7) is the anterior horn (C1), which extends into the frontal lobe of the brain. At its posterior end, the body divides into the posterior horn (C9), which extends backwards into the occipital lobe, and the inferior horn (C5), which passes downwards and forwards into the temporal lobe.

The lower posterior part of the third ventricle (C12) communicates with the fourth ventricle (C4) through the aqueduct of the midbrain (C2).

The floor of the inferior horn consists of the hippocampus (A11 and 8) medially and the collateral eminence (A4) laterally. At its junction with the posterior horn (A12 and B11) the eminence broadens into the collateral trigone (A5, B4).

The collateral eminence (A4) is produced by the inward projection of the collateral sulcus.

In the medial wall of the posterior horn, the bulb (B1) is produced by fibres of the corpus callosum, and the calcar avis (B2) by the inward projection of the calcarine sulcus.

A Cranial nerve *I – olfactory*

A1

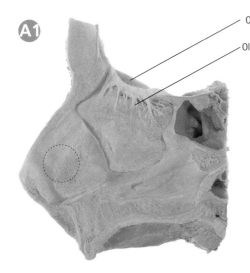

Olfactory bulbs

Olfactory nerves

A2

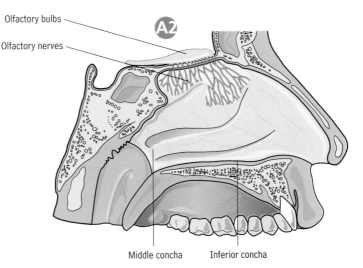

Middle concha   Inferior concha

See pages 58, 64 and 65.

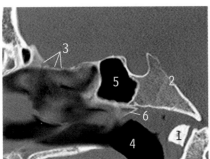

1 Anterior arch of C1
2 Clivus
3 Cribriform plate
4 Nasopharynx
5 Sphenoidal air sinus
6 Vomer

Endoscopy of olfactory mucosa

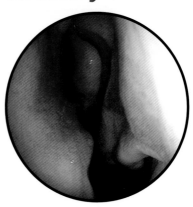

B Cranial nerve *II – optic (seen from above)*

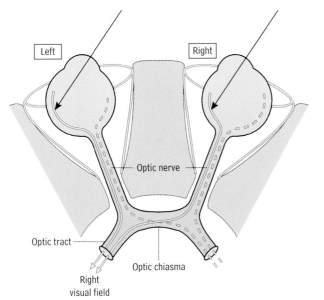

Left

Right

Optic nerve

Optic tract

Optic chiasma

Right visual field

See pages 53, 57, 58 and 65.

C Fundus of eye

ophthalmoscopic photograph of a retina

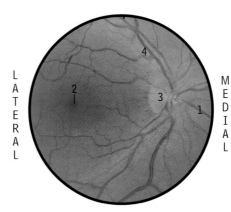

L A T E R A L

M E D I A L

1 Inferior nasal branches of central vein and artery
2 Macula with central fovea
3 Optic disc
4 Superior temporal branches of central vein and artery

Anosmia, epistaxis, ophthalmoscopy, retinoscopy, tonsillitis, see pages 80–82.

Cranial nerves *III – oculomotor, IV – trochlear, VI – abducent*

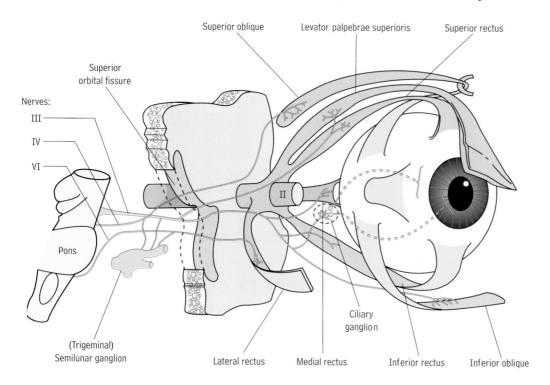

Superior oblique
Levator palpebrae superioris
Superior rectus
Superior orbital fissure
Nerves:
III
IV
VI
Pons
(Trigeminal) Semilunar ganglion
Lateral rectus
Medial rectus
Ciliary ganglion
Inferior rectus
Inferior oblique
II

See pages 53, 54–57 and 65 for III.
See pages 54–57 and 65 for IV.
See pages 53, 54–57 and 65 for VI.

Ciliary ganglion

1 Abducent nerve
2 Ciliary ganglion
3 Eyeball
4 Frontal nerve
5 Inferior oblique
6 Inferior rectus
7 Infra-orbital artery
8 Infra-orbital nerve
9 Lacrimal artery
10 Lateral rectus, reflected
11 Levator palpebrae superioris
12 Maxillary artery
13 Maxillary branch of trigeminal nerve
14 Nasociliary nerve
15 Nerve to inferior rectus
16 Oculomotor nerve
17 Ophthalmic artery
18 Optic nerve in anterior cranial fossa
19 Optic nerve in orbit
20 Sensory root to ciliary ganglion
21 Short ciliary arteries
22 Short ciliary nerves
23 Sphenopalatine nerve
24 Superior rectus
25 Supra-orbital nerve
26 Supratrochlear nerve

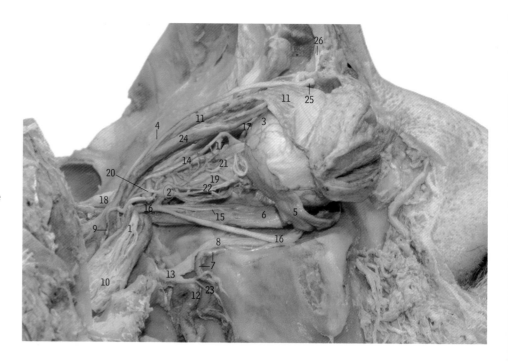

Abducent nerve palsy, accommodation reflex, oculomotor nerve palsy, trochlear nerve palsy, see pages 80–82.

Cranial nerve
A V – trigeminal (overview)

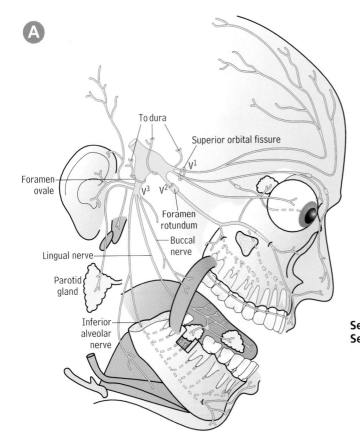

To dura
Superior orbital fissure
V¹
Foramen ovale
V³   V²
Foramen rotundum
Buccal nerve
Lingual nerve
Parotid gland
Inferior alveolar nerve

B V¹ ophthalmic division of trigeminal

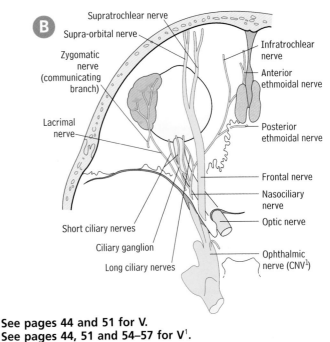

Supratrochlear nerve
Supra-orbital nerve
Infratrochlear nerve
Zygomatic nerve (communicating branch)
Anterior ethmoidal nerve
Lacrimal nerve
Posterior ethmoidal nerve
Frontal nerve
Nasociliary nerve
Short ciliary nerves
Optic nerve
Ciliary ganglion
Long ciliary nerves
Ophthalmic nerve (CNV¹)

See pages 44 and 51 for V.
See pages 44, 51 and 54–57 for V¹.

C V² maxillary division of trigeminal

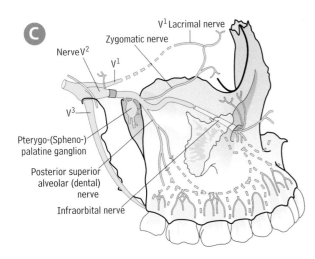

V¹ Lacrimal nerve
Zygomatic nerve
Nerve V²
V¹
V³
Pterygo-(Spheno-)palatine ganglion
Posterior superior alveolar (dental) nerve
Infraorbital nerve

See pages 44 and 51 for V².
See pages 42, 44, 59 and 76 for V³.

D V³ mandibular division of trigeminal

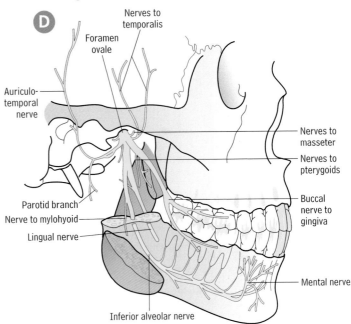

Nerves to temporalis
Foramen ovale
Auriculo-temporal nerve
Nerves to masseter
Nerves to pterygoids
Buccal nerve to gingiva
Parotid branch
Nerve to mylohyoid
Lingual nerve
Mental nerve
Inferior alveolar nerve

Trigeminal nerve *branches and associated parasympathetic ganglia*

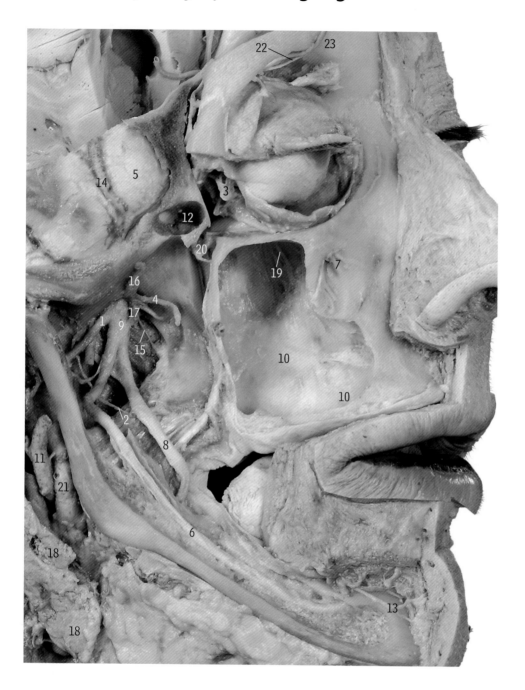

1 Auriculotemporal nerve
2 Chorda tympani
3 Ciliary ganglion
4 Deep temporal nerve
5 Dura mater
6 Inferior alveolar nerve within canal
7 Infra-orbital nerve
8 Lingual nerve
9 Mandibular nerve
10 Maxillary air sinus (opened)
11 Maxillary artery
12 Maxillary nerve

13 Mental nerve
14 Middle meningeal artery
15 Nerve to lateral pterygoid
16 Nerve to masseter
17 Otic ganglion
18 Parotid gland
19 Posterior superior alveolar nerves
20 Pterygopalatine ganglion
21 Retromandibular vein
22 Supra-orbital nerve
23 Supratrochlear nerve

A Cranial nerve *VII – facial*

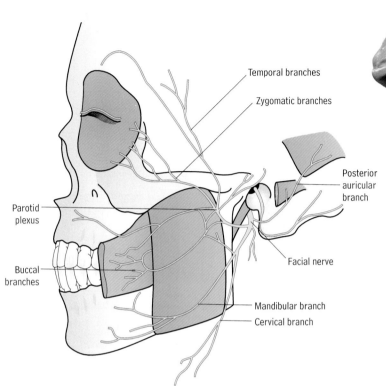

Temporal branches

Zygomatic branches

Posterior auricular branch

Parotid plexus

Facial nerve

Buccal branches

Mandibular branch

Cervical branch

B Nasal cartilage

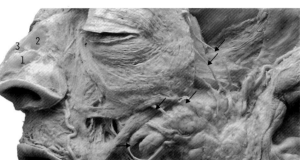

1 Lateral crus of alar cartilage
2 Lateral nasal cartilage
3 Septal angle

NB: Facial nerve branches exit the parotid gland (arrows).

See pages 39–41, 53, 61 and 67.

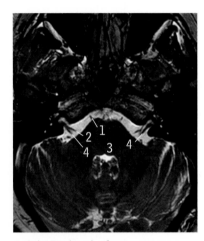

Axial MR, level of pontomedullary junction

1 Abducent nerve (CN VI)
2 Facial nerve (CN VII)
3 Pons
4 Vestibulocochlear nerve (CN VIII)

C Cranial nerve *VIII – vestibulocochlear*

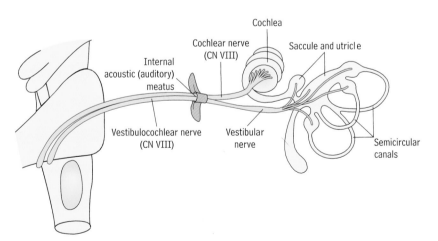

Cochlea

Cochlear nerve (CN VIII)

Saccule and utricle

Internal acoustic (auditory) meatus

Vestibulocochlear nerve (CN VIII)

Vestibular nerve

Semicircular canals

See pages 51, 53, 61 and 67.

Acoustic neuroma, facial nerve palsy, hyperacusis, otalgia, see pages 80–82.

Cranial nerve **Ⓐ** *IX – glossopharyngeal* **Ⓑ** *X – vagus*

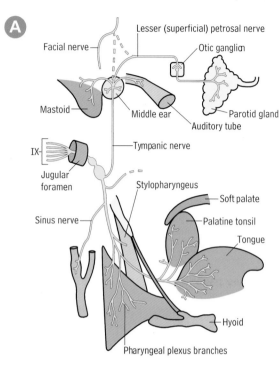

Ⓐ

Facial nerve
Lesser (superficial) petrosal nerve
Otic ganglion
Mastoid
Middle ear
Parotid gland
Auditory tube
IX
Tympanic nerve
Jugular foramen
Stylopharyngeus
Soft palate
Palatine tonsil
Sinus nerve
Tongue
Hyoid
Pharyngeal plexus branches

See pages 44–47, 53 and 67.

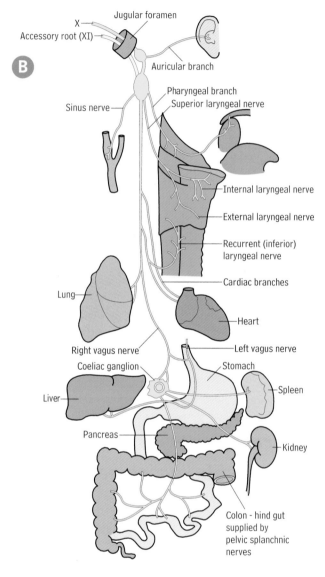

Ⓑ

X
Accessory root (XI)
Jugular foramen
Auricular branch
Pharyngeal branch
Superior laryngeal nerve
Sinus nerve
Internal laryngeal nerve
External laryngeal nerve
Recurrent (inferior) laryngeal nerve
Cardiac branches
Lung
Heart
Right vagus nerve
Left vagus nerve
Coeliac ganglion
Stomach
Liver
Spleen
Pancreas
Kidney
Colon - hind gut supplied by pelvic splanchnic nerves

See pages 44–47, 53, 67 and 69.

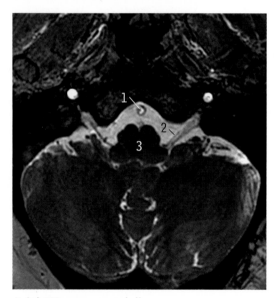

Axial MR, upper medulla

1 Basilar artery
2 Hypoglossal nerve rootlets
3 Medulla

Parotid tumours, recurrent laryngeal nerve palsy, see pages 80–82.

Cranial nerve   Ⓐ *XI – accessory*   Ⓑ *XII – hypoglossal*

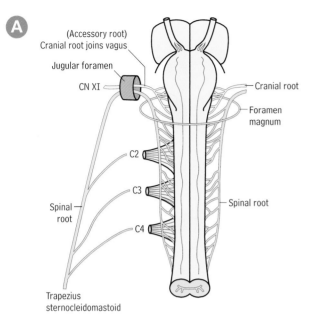

Ⓐ

(Accessory root)
Cranial root joins vagus

Jugular foramen

CN XI

Cranial root

Foramen magnum

C2

C3

C4

Spinal root

Spinal root

Trapezius
sternocleidomastoid

See pages 53 and 67.

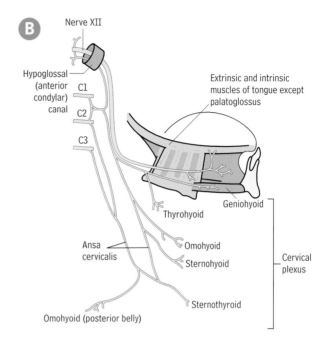

Ⓑ

Nerve XII

Hypoglossal (anterior condylar) canal

C1

C2

C3

Extrinsic and intrinsic muscles of tongue except palatoglossus

Thyrohyoid

Geniohyoid

Ansa cervicalis

Omohyoid

Sternohyoid

Cervical plexus

Sternothyroid

Omohyoid (posterior belly)

See pages 47, 59 and 67.

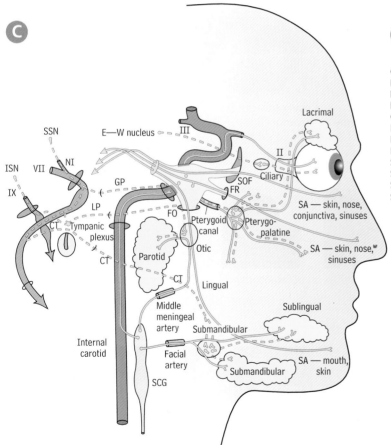

Ⓒ

Lacrimal

SSN

E—W nucleus

III

E—W nucleus

II

ISN   VII   NI

GP

SOF

FR

Ciliary

ISN

IX

LP

SA — skin, nose, conjunctiva, sinuses

CT   Tympanic plexus

FO

Pterygoid canal

Pterygo-palatine

Otic

SA — skin, nose, sinuses

CT

Parotid

CT

Lingual

Middle meningeal artery

Sublingual

Internal carotid

Submandibular

Facial artery

SCG

Submandibular

SA — mouth, skin

Ⓒ Cranial autonomics

CT	chorda tympani
E–W	Edinger–Westphal
FO	foramen ovale
FR	foramen rotundum
GP	greater petrosal
ISN	inferior salivatory nucleus
LP	lesser petrosal
NI	nervus intermedius
SA	somatic afferent
SCG	superior cervical ganglion
SOF	superior orbital fissure
SSN	superior salivatory nucleus

Accessory nerve palsy, gag reflex, hypoglossal nerve palsy, see pages 80–82.

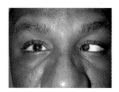

Head, neck and brain

Clinical thumbnails, see website for details and further clinical images to download into your own notes.

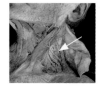

Abducent nerve palsy

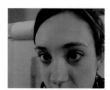

Accessory nerve palsy

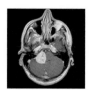

Accommodation reflex

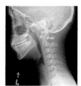

Acoustic neuroma

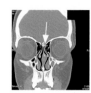

Adenoid enlargement

Anosmia

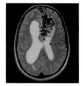

Arteriovenous fistulae

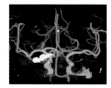

Berry aneurysm

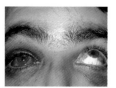

Blow-out fractures of the orbit

Branchial cysts

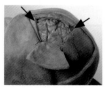

Burr holes

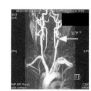

Carotid artery bruits

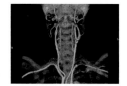

Carotid artery stenosis

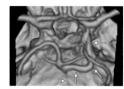

Carotid artery variants

Carotid endarterectomy

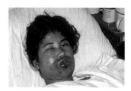

Cavernous sinus thrombosis

Central retinal artery occlusion

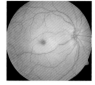

Cervical lymph node enlargement

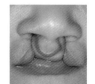

Cleft lip and palate

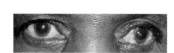

Corneal arcus

Corneal reflex

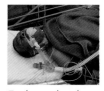

Craniotomy

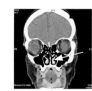

Endotracheal intubation

Epistaxis

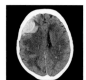

Extradural haemorrhage

Facial nerve (Bell's) palsy

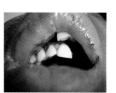

Fractured mandible

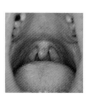

Gag reflex

Glaucoma

Goitre

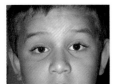
Horner's syndrome

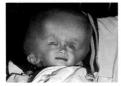
Hydrocephalus

Hyperacusis

Hypoglossal nerve palsy

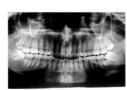
Impacted wisdom tooth

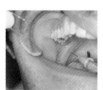
Inferior alveolar nerve block

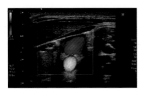
Internal jugular vein catheterisation

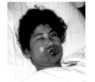
Intracranial spread of infection – face

Intracranial spread of infection – scalp

Labyrinthitis

Mastoiditis

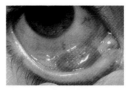
Meibomian cyst (chalazion)

Middle ear pressure equalisation

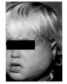
Mumps

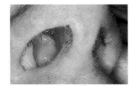
Nasal polyps

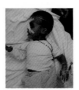
Nasogastric intubation

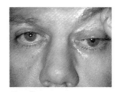
Oculomotor nerve palsy

Ophthalmic herpes zoster

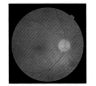
Ophthalmoscopy

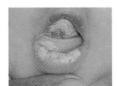
Oral pathology

Orbital cellulitis

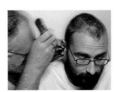
Otalgia (referred pain)

Parotid tumours

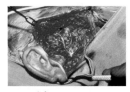
Parotidectomy

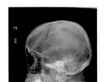
Pepperpot skull

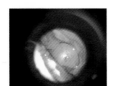
Perforated drum

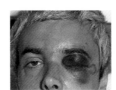
Periorbital and subconjunctival haemorrhage

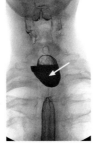
Pharyngeal pouch

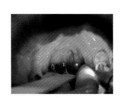
Pharyngitis

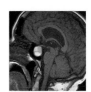
Pituitary apoplexy

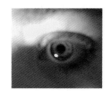

Pituitary tumour

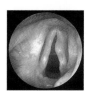

Pupillary reflex

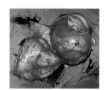

Recurrent laryngeal nerve palsy

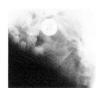

Scalp wounds

Sialectasis

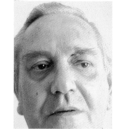

Sinus pathology

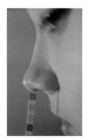

Skull base fracture

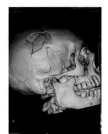

Skull fracture

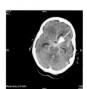

Subarachnoid haemorrhage

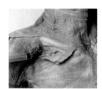

Subclavian vein catheterisation

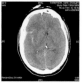

Subdural haemorrhage

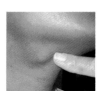

Submandibular tumour

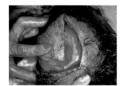

Surgical flaps of scalp

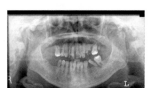

Temporomandibular joint (TMJ) dislocation

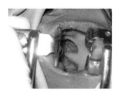

Tongue carcinoma

Tonsillectomy

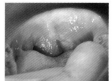

Tonsillitis

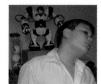

Torticollis

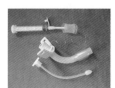

Tracheostomy

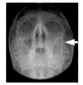

Tripod fracture

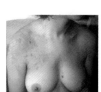

Trochlear nerve palsy

Varicella-zoster virus infection – head and neck

Vertebral column and spinal cord

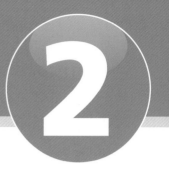

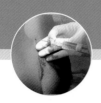 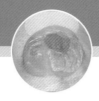 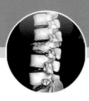

Back and vertebral column
A *surface anatomy* **B** *axial skeleton* **C** *vertebral column*

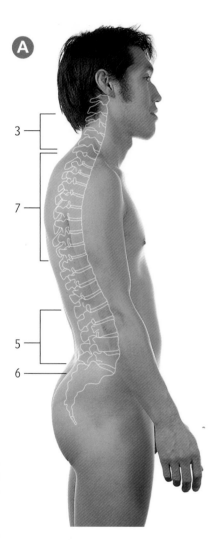

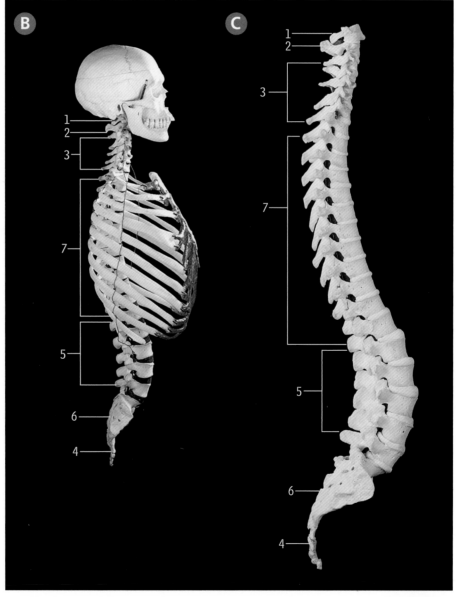

1 Atlas vertebra
2 Axis vertebra
3 Cervical vertebrae, lordosis
4 Coccyx
5 Lumbar vertebrae, lordosis
6 Sacrum
7 Thoracic vertebrae, kyphosis

Back and shoulder
Ⓐ *surface anatomy*   Ⓑ *muscles*

1 Coccyx
2 Deltoid
3 External oblique
4 Gluteus maximus
5 Iliac crest
6 Latissimus dorsi
7 Medial border scapula (dotted)
8 Rhomboid major
9 Rhomboid minor
10 Sacrum
11 Trapezius
12 Thoracolumbar fascia

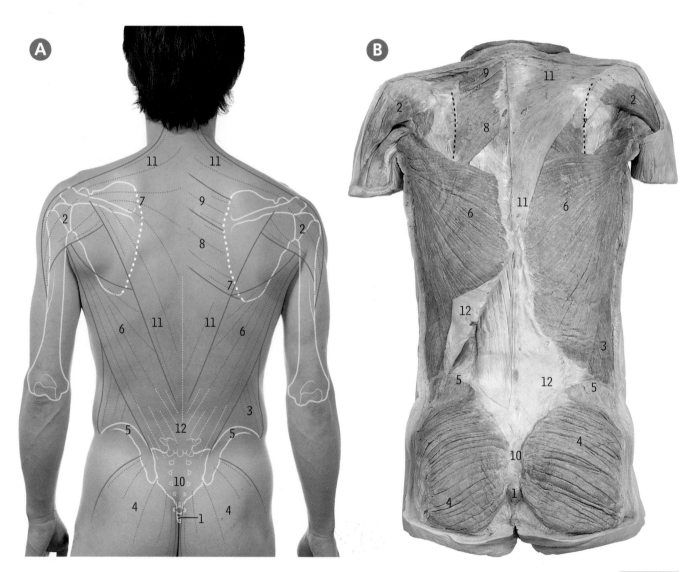

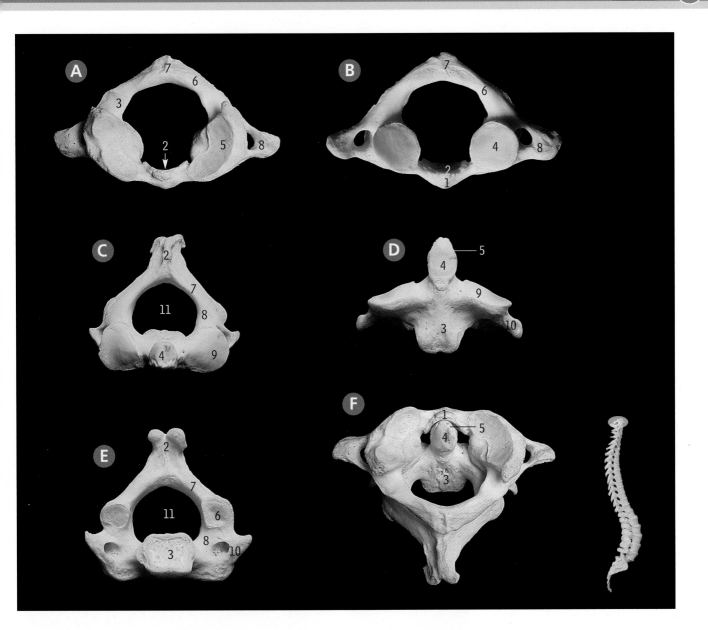

First cervical vertebra *atlas*

A from above

B from below

1 Anterior arch and tubercle	**5** Lateral mass with superior
2 Facet for dens of axis	articular facet
3 Groove for vertebral artery	**6** Posterior arch
4 Lateral mass with inferior	**7** Posterior tubercle
articular facet	**8** Transverse process and foramen

> The superior articular facets (5) are concave and kidney-shaped.
>
> The inferior articular facets (4) are circular and almost flat.
>
> The anterior arch (1) is straighter and shorter than the posterior arch (6) and contains on its posterior surface the facet for the dens of the axis (2).
>
> The atlas is the only vertebra that has no body.

Second cervical vertebra *axis*

C from above

D from the front

E from below

F articulated with the atlas, from above

1 Anterior arch of atlas	**7** Lamina
2 Bifid spinous process	**8** Pedicle
3 Body	**9** Superior articular surface
4 Dens (odontoid peg)	**10** Transverse process and
5 Impression for alar ligament	foramen
6 Inferior articular facet	**11** Vertebral foramen

> The axis is unique in having the dens (4) which projects upwards from the body, representing the body of the atlas.

Odontoid peg fracture, see page 108.

Fifth cervical vertebra
typical cervical vertebra

A from above

B from the front

C from the left

1   Anterior tubercle of transverse process
2   Bifid spinous process
3   Body
4   Foramen of transverse process
5   Inferior articular process
6   Intertubercular lamella of transverse process
7   Lamina
8   Pedicle
9   Posterior tubercle of transverse process
10 Posterolateral lip (uncus)
11 Superior articular process
12 Vertebral foramen

Seventh cervical vertebra
vertebra prominens

D from above

1   Anterior tubercle of transverse process
2   Body
3   Foramen of transverse process
4   Intertubercular lamella of transverse process
5   Lamina
6   Pedicle
7   Posterior tubercle of transverse process
8   Posterolateral lip (uncus)
9   Spinous process with tubercle
10 Superior articular process
11 Vertebral foramen

All cervical vertebrae (first to seventh) have a foramen in each transverse process (as A4).

Typical cervical vertebrae (third to sixth) have superior articular processes that face backwards and upwards (A11, C11), posterolateral lips on the upper surface of the body (A10), a triangular vertebral foramen (A12) and a bifid spinous process (A2).

The anterior tubercle of the transverse process of the sixth cervical vertebra is large and known as the carotid tubercle.

The seventh cervical vertebra (vertebra prominens) has a spinous process that ends in a single tubercle (D9).

The rib element of a cervical vertebra is represented by the anterior root of the transverse process, the anterior tubercle, the intertubercular lamella (with its groove for the ventral ramus of a spinal nerve) and the anterior part of the posterior tubercle (as at D1, 4 and 7).

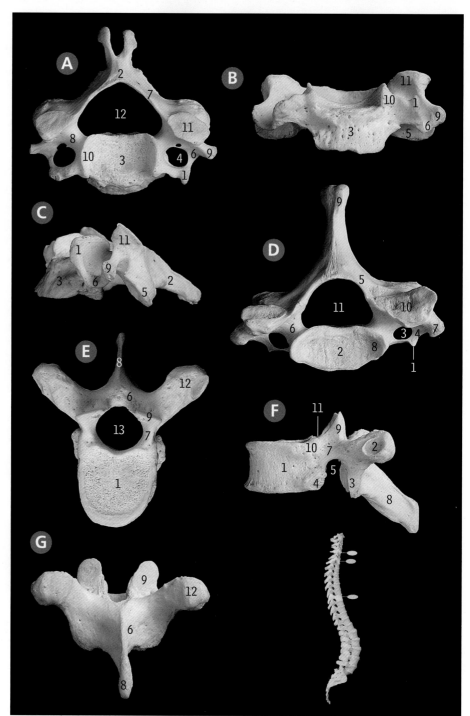

Seventh thoracic vertebra
typical

E from above

F from the left

G from behind

1   Body
2   Costal facet of transverse process
3   Inferior articular process
4   Inferior costal facet
5   Inferior vertebral notch
6   Lamina
7   Pedicle
8   Spinous process
9   Superior articular process
10 Superior costal facet
11 Superior vertebral notch
12 Transverse process
13 Vertebral foramen

Typical thoracic vertebrae (second to ninth) are characterised by costal facets on the bodies (F10, 4), costal facets on the transverse processes (F2), a round vertebral foramen (E13), a spinous process that points downwards as well as backwards (F8, G8) and superior articular processes that are vertical, flat and face backwards and laterally (E9, F9, G9).

 Ankylosing spondylitis, see page 108.

First thoracic vertebra

A from above

B from the front and the left

1 Body
2 Inferior articular process
3 Inferior costal facet
4 Lamina
5 Pedicle
6 Posterolateral lip (uncus)
7 Spinous process
8 Superior articular process
9 Superior costal facet
10 Transverse process with costal facet
11 Vertebral foramen

Tenth and eleventh thoracic vertebrae

C tenth thoracic vertebra, from the left

D eleventh thoracic vertebra, from the left

1 Body
2 Costal facet
3 Inferior articular process
4 Inferior vertebral notch
5 Pedicle
6 Spinous process
7 Superior articular process
8 Transverse process

Twelfth thoracic vertebra

E from the left

F from above

G from behind

1 Body
2 Costal facet
3 Inferior articular process
4 Inferior tubercle
5 Lateral tubercle
6 Pedicle
7 Spinous process
8 Superior articular process
9 Superior tubercle

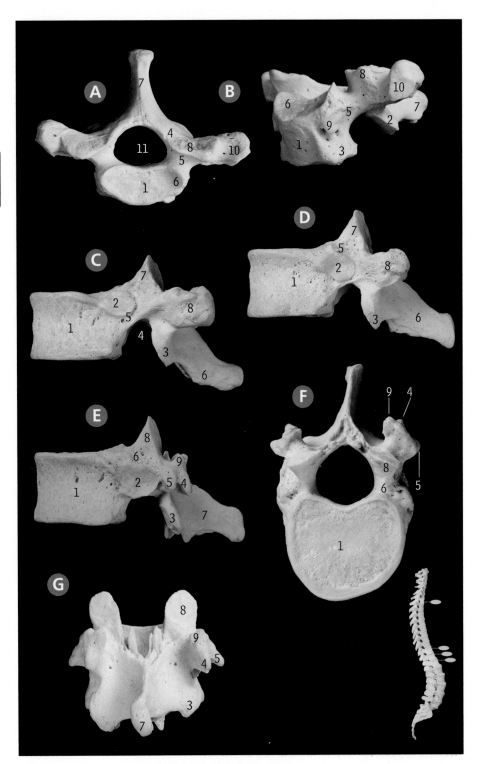

The atypical thoracic vertebrae are the first, tenth, eleventh and twelfth.

The first thoracic vertebra has a posterolateral lip (A6, B6) on each side of the upper surface of the body and a triangular vertebral foramen (features like typical cervical vertebrae), and complete (round) superior costal facets (B9) on the sides of the body.

The tenth, eleventh and twelfth thoracic vertebrae are characterised by a single complete costal facet on each side of the body that in successive vertebrae comes to lie increasingly far from the upper surface of the body and encroaches increasingly onto the pedicle (C2, D2 and E2). There is also no articular facet on the transverse process.

Spondylolisthesis, see page 108.

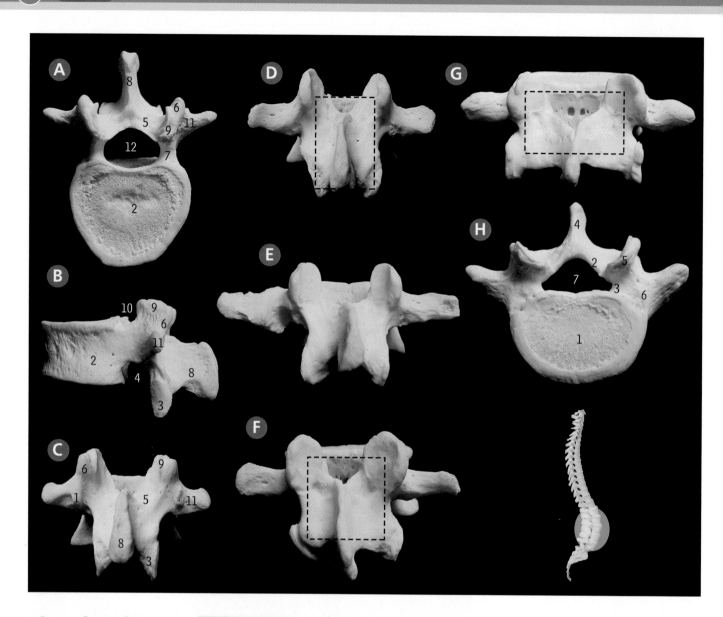

First lumbar vertebra

A from above

B from the left

C from behind

1. Accessory process
2. Body
3. Inferior articular process
4. Inferior vertebral notch
5. Lamina
6. Mammillary process
7. Pedicle
8. Spinous process
9. Superior articular process
10. Superior vertebral notch
11. Transverse process
12. Vertebral foramen

Lumbar vertebrae are characterised by the large size of the bodies, the absence of costal facets on the bodies and the transverse processes, a triangular vertebral foramen (A12), a spinous process that points backwards and is quadrangular or hatchet-shaped (B8) and superior articular processes that are vertical, curved, face backwards and medially (A9) and possess a mamillary process at their posterior rim (A6).

The rib element of a lumbar vertebra is represented by the transverse process (A11).

The level at which facet joint orientation changes between the thoracic and lumbar regions is variable.

Posterior view

D second lumbar vertebra

E third lumbar vertebra

F fourth lumbar vertebra

G fifth lumbar vertebra

View from above

H fifth lumbar vertebra

1. Body
2. Lamina
3. Pedicle
4. Spinous process
5. Superior articular process
6. Transverse process fusing with pedicle and body
7. Vertebral foramen

Viewed from behind, the four articular processes of the first and second lumbar vertebrae make a pattern (indicated by the interrupted line) of a vertical rectangle; those of the third or fourth vertebra make a square, and those of the fifth lumbar vertebra make a horizontal rectangle.

The fifth lumbar vertebra is unique in that the transverse process (H6) unites directly with the side of the body (H1) as well as with the pedicle (H3).

Laminectomy, lumbar stenosis, vertebral fracture, vertebral lumbar fracture, see page 108.

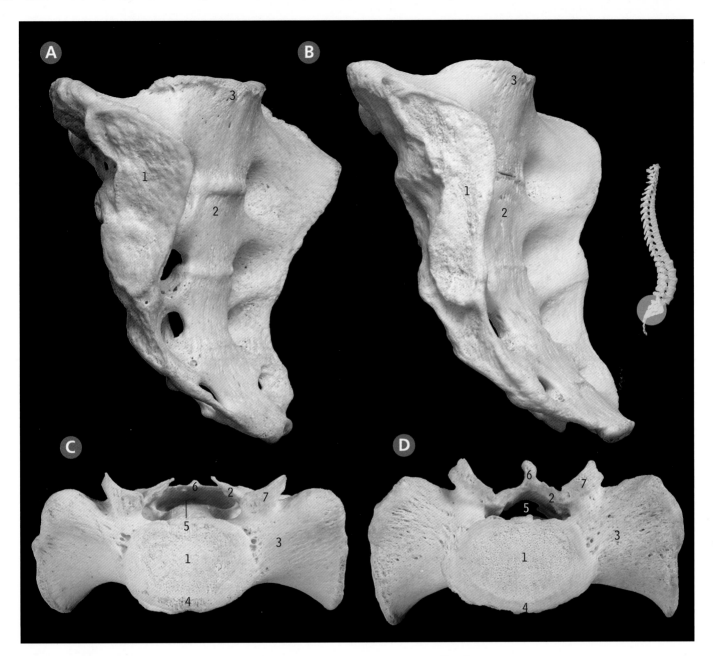

Sacrum *from the front and the right*

A in the female

B in the male

1 Auricular surface
2 Pelvic surface
3 Promontory

In the female, the pelvic surface is relatively straight over the first three sacral vertebrae and becomes more curved below. In the male, the pelvic surface is more uniformly curved.

The capsule of the sacro-iliac joint is attached to the margin of the auricular (articular) surface (A1, B1).

Base of the sacrum *upper surface*

C in the female

D in the male

1 Body of first sacral vertebra
2 Lamina
3 Lateral part (ala)
4 Promontory
5 Sacral canal
6 Spinous tubercle of median sacral crest
7 Superior articular process

In the male, the body of the first sacral vertebra (judged by its transverse diameter) forms a greater part of the base of the sacrum than in the female (compare D1 with C1).

In C, there is some degree of spina bifida (non-fusion of the laminae, 2, in the vertebral arch of the first sacral vertebra). Compare with the complete arch in D.

Sacralisation, see page 108.

Sacrum and coccyx

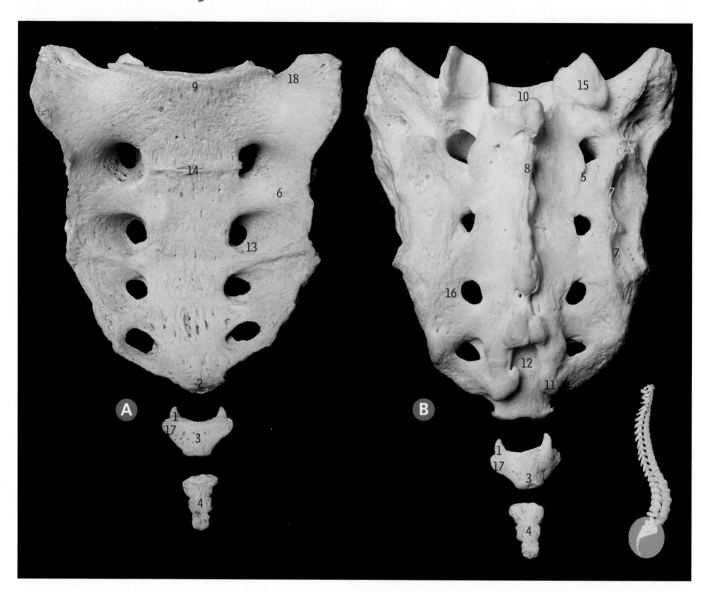

A pelvic surface

1 Coccygeal cornu
2 Facet for coccyx
3 First coccygeal vertebra
4 Fused second to fourth vertebrae
5 Intermediate sacral crest
6 Lateral part
7 Lateral sacral crest
8 Median sacral crest
9 Promontory
10 Sacral canal

B dorsal surface

11 Sacral cornu
12 Sacral hiatus
13 Second pelvic sacral foramen
14 Site of fusion of first and second sacral vertebrae
15 Superior articular process
16 Third dorsal sacral foramen
17 Transverse process
18 Upper surface of lateral part (ala)

The sacrum is formed by the fusion of the five sacral vertebrae. The median sacral crest (B8) represents the fused spinous processes, the intermediate crest (B5) the fused articular processes, and the lateral crest (B7) the fused transverse processes.

The sacral hiatus (B12) is the lower opening of the sacral canal (B10).

The coccyx is usually formed by the fusion of four rudimentary vertebrae but the number varies from three to five. In this specimen, the first piece of the coccyx (3) is not fused with the remainder (4).

Coccydynia, see page 108.

Sacrum *with sacralisation of the fifth lumbar vertebra*

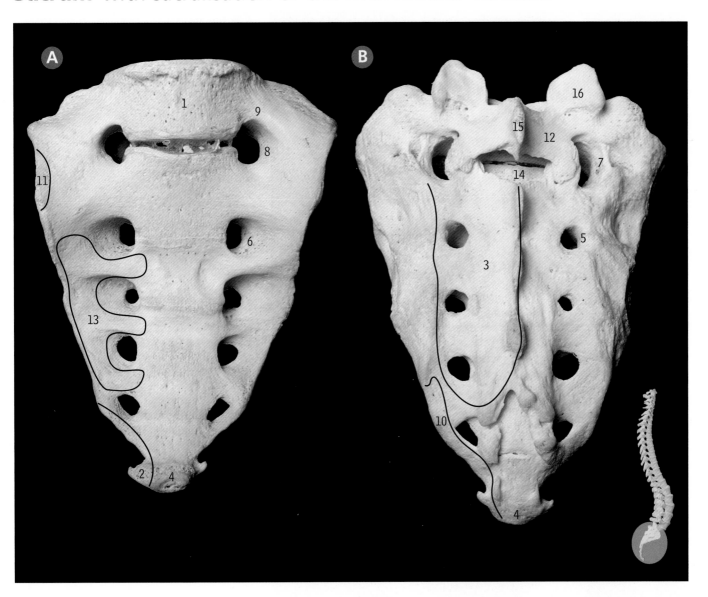

A pelvic surface

B dorsal surface, and sacral muscle attachments

1 Body of fifth lumbar vertebra
2 Coccygeus
3 Erector spinae
4 First coccygeal vertebra fused to apex of sacrum
5 First dorsal sacral foramen
6 First pelvic sacral foramen
7 Foramen for dorsal ramus of fifth lumbar nerve
8 Foramen for ventral ramus of fifth lumbar nerve
9 Fusion of transverse process and lateral part of sacrum
10 Gluteus maximus
11 Iliacus
12 Lamina
13 Piriformis
14 Sacral canal
15 Spinous process of fifth lumbar vertebra
16 Superior articular process of fifth lumbar vertebra

In sacralisation of the fifth lumbar vertebra, that vertebra (A1) is (usually incompletely) fused with the sacrum. In the more rare condition of lumbarization of the first sacral vertebra (not illustrated) the first piece of the sacrum is incompletely fused with the remainder.

In this specimen, as well as fusion of the fifth lumbar vertebra with the top of the sacrum, the body of the first coccygeal vertebra (4) is fused with the apex of the sacrum.

Caudal anaesthesia, see page 108.

Bony pelvis *from in front and above*

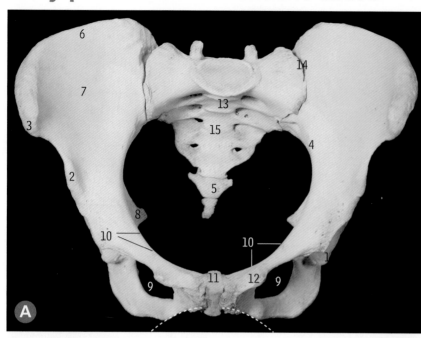

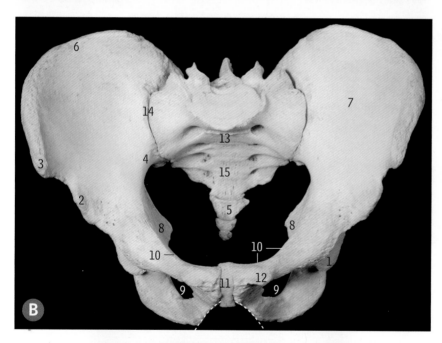

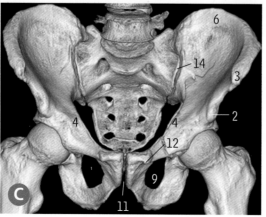

A female

B male

C from the front

1 Acetabulum
2 Anterior inferior iliac spine
3 Anterior superior iliac spine
4 Arcuate line
5 Coccyx
6 Iliac crest
7 Iliac fossa
8 Ischial spine
9 Obturator foramen
10 Pectineal line
11 Pubic symphysis
12 Pubic tubercle
13 Sacral promontory
14 Sacro-iliac joint
15 Sacrum

The pelvic inlet (brim) is bounded by the sacral promontory (13), arcuate and pectineal lines (4 and 10), the crest of the pubic bones and anteriorly the pubic symphysis (11).

The female brim is more circular, the male more heart-shaped.

The female sacrum (15) is wider, shorter and less curved.

The female ischial spines (8) are further apart.

The female subpubic angle (white dotted line on A) is wide (90–120°) and the male subpubic angle (white dotted line on B) only 60–90°.

Vertebrae, ribs and sternum
ossification

A typical vertebra in a 6-month fetus

F axis, primary and secondary centres

B at 4 years of age

G typical rib, secondary centres

C **D** during puberty

H sternum at birth, with primary centres

E atlas at 4 years of age

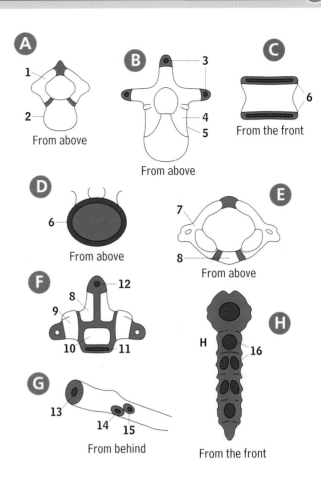

A   From above
B
C   From the front
From above
D   From above
E   From above
F   From behind
G   From behind
H   From the front

A typical vertebra, which is first cartilaginous, ossifies in early fetal life from three primary centres – one for most of the body (the centrum, A2) and one for each half of the neural arch (A1). The part of the adult body to which the pedicle is attached (B4) is part of the centre for the arch; the site in the developing vertebra where they meet is the neurocentral junction (B5). The two halves of the arch and the neurocentral junctions unite at variable times between birth and 6 years. Ossification spreads into the transverse processes and spine which grow out from the arch, but secondary centres (B3) appear at their tips during puberty and become fused at about 25 years of age. (Lumbar vertebrae have similar additional secondary centres for the mamillary processes.) There are also ring-like epiphyses on the periphery of the upper and lower surfaces of the vertebral bodies (C6 and D6).

The atlas has a primary centre (E7) for each lateral mass and the adjacent half of the posterior arch, and one for the anterior arch (E8). Fusion is complete by about 8 years.

The axis has five primary centres – one for most of the body (F10), one for each lateral mass (F9), and one for each half of the dens and adjacent part of the body (F8). They should all fuse by about 3 years. There are secondary centres for the tip of the dens (F12, appearing by about 2 years and fusing at 12 years) and the lower surface of the body (F11, appearing during puberty and fusing at about 25 years).

The sacrum, representing five fused sacral vertebrae, has many ossification centres, corresponding to the centrum, neural arch halves and costal elements of each vertebra, as well as ring epiphyses for the vertebral bodies and for the auricular surfaces. Most have fused by about 20 years, but some not until middle-age or later.

A typical rib has a primary centre for the body with secondary centres for the head (G13) and the articular and non-articular parts of the tubercle (G14 and 15), appearing during puberty and uniting at about 20 years.

The sternum has a variable number of primary centres (H16), one or two in the manubrium and in each of the four pieces of the body. Fusion occurs between puberty and 25 years of age. 'Bullet holes' in the sternum (sternal foramina) may occur when fusion is incomplete.

I Vertebrae *developmental origins*

Red, costal elements; green, centrum; yellow, neural arch

Parts of the cervical, lumbar and sacral vertebrae represent the ribs that articulate with thoracic vertebrae. These costal elements are indicated here in red.

Cervical: anterior and posterior tubercles and the intertubercular lamella.

Thoracic: the true rib articulates with the vertebra.

Lumbar: the anterior part of the transverse process.

Sacral: the lateral part, including the auricular surface.

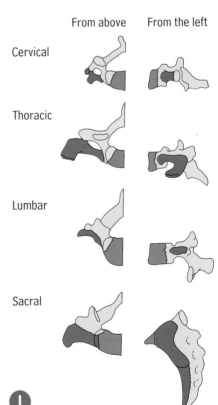

From above   From the left

Cervical

Thoracic

Lumbar

Sacral

I

Vertebral column and spinal cord

Ⓐ cervical region, from the front Ⓑ cervical region, from behind

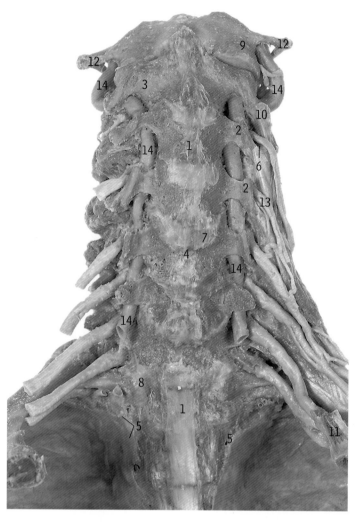

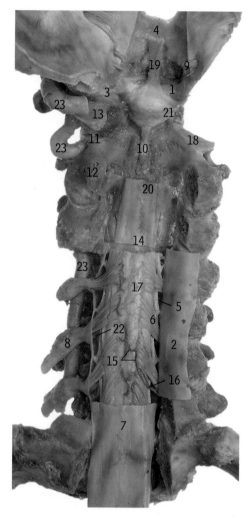

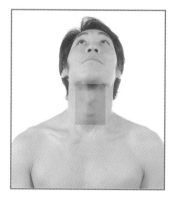

The vertebral artery (14) is seen within foramina of cervical transverse processes.

1 Anterior longitudinal ligament
2 Anterior tubercle of transverse process
3 Axis
4 Body of the fifth cervical vertebra
5 Cut edge of the pleura
6 Intertubercular lamella of transverse process
7 Intervertebral disc
8 Joint of head of first rib
9 Lateral mass of atlas
10 Posterior tubercle of transverse process
11 Scalenus anterior muscle
12 Transverse process of atlas
13 Ventral ramus of fourth cervical nerve
14 Vertebral artery

Much of the skull, the vertebral arches, brainstem and the upper part of the spinal cord have been removed to show the cruciform, transverse and alar ligaments (19, 10, 21 and 1). Lower down, the arachnoid and dura mater (2) have been reflected to show dorsal and ventral nerve roots (as at 6 and 22).

1 Alar ligament
2 Arachnoid and dura mater (reflected)
3 Atlanto-occipital joint
4 Basilar part of occipital bone and position of attachment of tectorial membrane
5 Denticulate ligament
6 Dorsal rootlets of spinal nerve
7 Dura mater
8 Dural sheath over dorsal root ganglion
9 Hypoglossal nerve and canal
10 Inferior longitudinal band of cruciform ligament
11 Lateral atlanto-axial joint
12 Pedicle of axis
13 Posterior arch of atlas
14 Posterior longitudinal ligament
15 Posterior spinal arteries
16 Radicular artery
17 Spinal cord
18 Superior articular surface of axis
19 Superior longitudinal band of cruciform ligament
20 Tectorial membrane
21 Transverse ligament of atlas (transverse part of cruciform ligament)
22 Ventral rootlets of spinal nerve
23 Vertebral artery

Vertebral column and spinal cord

C cervical and upper thoracic regions, from the right

Ventral and dorsal rami of spinal nerves (as at 16 and 4) are seen emerging from intervertebral foramina (as at 7).

1 Anterior tubercle of transverse process of fifth cervical vertebra
2 Body of first thoracic vertebra
3 Body of seventh cervical vertebra
4 Dorsal ramus of first cervical nerve
5 First cervical nerve
6 First rib
7 Intervertebral foramen
8 Lateral atlanto-axial joint
9 Lateral mass of atlas
10 Posterior arch of atlas
11 Eighth cervical nerve
12 Spinous process of second cervical vertebra
13 Spinous process of seventh cervical vertebra
14 Transverse process of atlas
15 Tubercle of first rib
16 Ventral ramus of sixth cervical nerve
17 Vertebral artery
18 Zygapophyseal joint

> The first and second spinal nerves pass, respectively, above and below the posterior arch of the atlas.

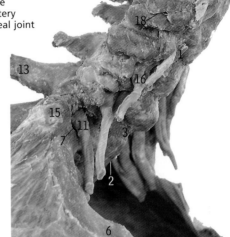

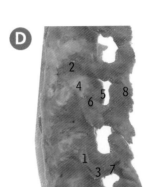

D Cervical region, from the left

Soft tissue has been removed to show the boundaries of intervertebral foramina (as at 5). Compare with the cleared specimens of thoracic vertebrae on page 98, A.

1 Anterior tubercle of transverse process of fifth cervical vertebra
2 Body of third cervical vertebra
3 Intertubercular lamella of transverse process of fifth cervical vertebra
4 Intervertebral disc
5 Intervertebral foramen
6 Pedicle
7 Posterior tubercle of transverse process of fifth cervical vertebra
8 Zygapophyseal joint

> Each intervertebral foramen (as at D5) is bounded in front by a vertebral body and intervertebral disc (D2 and 4), above and below by pedicles (D6), and behind by a zygapophyseal joint (D8).
>
> In the thoracic and lumbar regions there are the same number of pairs of spinal nerves as there are vertebrae (twelve thoracic and five lumbar), and spinal nerves are numbered from the vertebra beneath whose pedicles they emerge. In the cervical region, there are seven cervical vertebrae and eight cervical nerves. The first nerve emerges between the occipital bone of the skull and the atlas, and the eighth below the pedicle of the seventh cervical vertebra.

E Lower cervical and upper thoracic regions, from behind

The vertebral arches and most of the dura mater and arachnoid have been removed, to show dorsal nerve rootlets (5) emerging from the spinal cord (9) to unite as a dorsal nerve root and enter the dural sheath (as at 7). Ventral nerve roots do the same from the ventral aspect of the cord but are not seen in this view as they are obscured by the dorsal roots.

1 Angulation of nerve roots entering dural sheath
2 Dorsal ramus of fifth thoracic nerve
3 Dorsal root ganglion of eighth cervical nerve
4 Dorsal root ganglion of second thoracic nerve
5 Dorsal rootlets of eighth cervical nerve
6 Dura mater
7 Dural sheath of second thoracic nerve
8 Pedicle of first thoracic vertebra
9 Spinal cord and posterior spinal vessels
10 Ventral ramus of fifth thoracic nerve

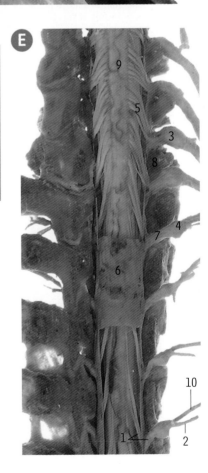

A Vertebral column and spinal cord
cervical and upper thoracic regions, from the left

1 Arachnoid mater
2 Body of first thoracic vertebra
3 Denticulate ligament
4 Dorsal ramus of fifth cervical nerve
5 Dorsal root ganglion of eighth cervical nerve
6 Dorsal root ganglion of fifth cervical nerve
7 Dorsal rootlets of fifth cervical nerve
8 Dura mater
9 Foramen magnum
10 Medulla oblongata

11 Occipital bone
12 Posterior arch of atlas
13 Spinal cord
14 Spinal part of accessory nerve
15 Spinous process of axis (abnormally large)
16 Spinous process of seventh cervical vertebra
17 Sympathetic trunk
18 Ventral ramus of fifth cervical nerve
19 Ventral rootlets of fifth cervical nerve

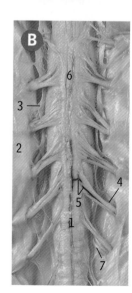

Parts of the vertebral arches and meninges have been removed to show the denticulate ligament (3). Dorsal nerve rootlets lie behind it (as at 7) and ventral nerve rootlets in front of it (as at 19 but largely hidden in this view).

Each spinal nerve is formed by the union of ventral and dorsal nerve roots.

Each nerve root is formed by the union of several rootlets (as at A7).

The union of ventral and dorsal nerve roots to form a spinal nerve occurs immediately distal to the ganglion on the dorsal root (as at A6), within the intervertebral foramen, and the nerve at once divides into a ventral and a dorsal ramus (formerly called ventral and dorsal primary rami) (as at A18 and 4). The spinal nerve proper is thus only 1–2 mm in length, but is often so short that the rami appear to be branches of the ganglion itself.

The lowest cervical and upper thoracic nerve roots become acutely angled in order to enter their dural sheaths.

B Spinal cord
cervical region, from the front

For this ventral view of the upper part of the spinal cord (6), the dura and arachnoid mater have been incised longitudinally and turned aside (2) to show the ventral nerve rootlets and roots (as at 7) passing laterally in front of the denticulate ligament (3) to enter meningeal nerve sheaths with dorsal roots (as at 4) and form a spinal nerve. On some roots, branches of radicular vessels (as at 5) are seen anastomosing with anterior spinal vessels (1).

1 Anterior spinal vessels
2 Arachnoid and dura mater
3 Denticulate ligament
4 Dorsal root of sixth cervical nerve
5 Radicular vessels
6 Spinal cord
7 Ventral root of seventh cervical nerve entering dural sheath

The denticulate ligament (B3) is composed of pia mater. The ventral and dorsal nerve roots pass, respectively, ventral and dorsal to the ligament, which extends laterally from the side of the cord and is attached by its spiky denticulations (as at B3) to the arachnoid and dura mater in the intervals between dural nerve sheaths. The highest denticulation is above the first cervical nerve and the lowest below the twelfth thoracic nerve.

Transverse myelitis, see page 108.

Vertebral column and spinal cord
C Lumbar and sacral regions, from behind

Parts of the vertebral arches and meninges have been removed, to show the cauda equina (1) and nerve roots entering their meningeal sheaths (as at 11), outlined as linear bands by contrast medium in the radiculogram (D).

1 Cauda equina
2 Conus medullaris of spinal cord
3 Dorsal root ganglion of fifth lumbar nerve
4 Dura mater
5 Dural sheath of first sacral nerve roots
6 Fifth lumbar (lumbosacral) intervertebral disc
7 Filum terminale
8 Fourth lumbar intervertebral disc

9 Lateral part of sacrum
10 Pedicle of fifth lumbar vertebra
11 Roots of fifth lumbar nerve
12 Second sacral vertebra
13 Superior articular process of third lumbar vertebra
14 Thecal sac

D Lumbar radiculogram

See label list above for D.

E Lower thoracic and upper lumbar regions

The specimen is seen from the left with parts of the vertebral arches and meninges removed, to show (at the front) part of the sympathetic trunk (13) on the vertebral bodies and (at the back) the spinous ligaments (7 and 11).

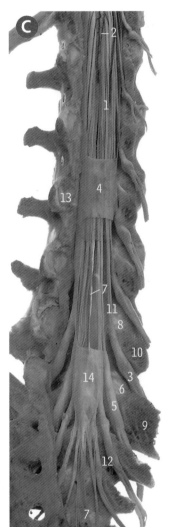

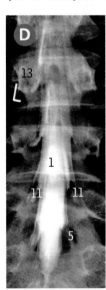

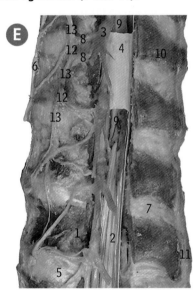

1 Body of first lumbar vertebra
2 Cauda equina
3 Dorsal root ganglion of tenth thoracic nerve
4 Dura mater
5 First lumbar intervertebral disc
6 Greater splanchnic nerve
7 Interspinous ligament
8 Rami communicantes
9 Spinal cord
10 Spinous process of tenth thoracic vertebra
11 Supraspinous ligament
12 Sympathetic ganglion
13 Sympathetic trunk

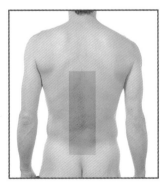

The spinal cord usually ends at the level of the first lumbar vertebra.

The subarachnoid space ends at the level of the second sacral vertebra.

The conus medullaris (C2) is the lower, pointed end of the spinal cord.

The cauda equina (C1) consists of the dorsal and ventral roots of the lumbar, sacral and coccygeal nerves. Note that it is nerve roots which form the cauda, not the spinal nerves themselves; these are not formed until ventral and dorsal roots unite at the level of an intervertebral foramen, immediately distal to the dorsal root ganglion (as at C3).

Epidural anaesthesia, spinal anaesthesia, see page 108.

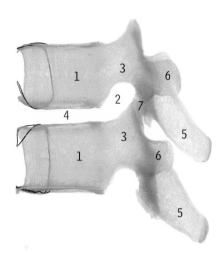

Ⓐ Thoracic vertebrae *cleared specimens*

The pairs of vertebrae are seen from the side and articulated to show the boundaries of an intervertebral foramen (2).

1 Body
2 Intervertebral foramen
3 Pedicle
4 Space for intervertebral disc
5 Spinous process
6 Transverse process
7 Zygapophyseal joint

> The intervertebral foramen (A2) is bounded in front by the lower part of the vertebral body (A1) and the intervertebral disc (A4), above and below by the pedicles (A3), and behind by the zygapophyseal joint (A7).
>
> The posterior longitudinal ligament is broad where it is firmly attached to the intervertebral discs, but narrow and less firmly attached to the vertebral bodies, leaving vascular foramina patent and allowing the basivertebral veins which emerge from them to enter the internal vertebral venous plexus.
>
> The anterior longitudinal ligament (B1) is uniformly broad and firmly attached to discs and vertebral bodies.

Ⓑ Vertebral column *lower lumbar region, from the front*

At the top the anterior longitudinal ligament (1) has a marker behind it, and part of it lower down has been reflected off an intervertebral disc (4) and vertebral bodies (2 and 3).

1 Anterior longitudinal ligament
2 Body of fifth lumbar vertebra
3 Body of fourth lumbar vertebra
4 Fourth lumbar intervertebral disc
5 Lateral part of sacrum
6 Ventral ramus of fifth lumbar nerve

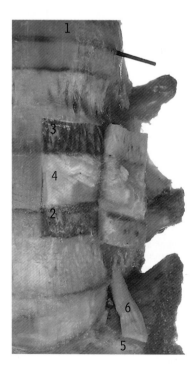

Ⓒ Vertebral column *upper lumbar region, from the right*

The side view shows lumbar nerves emerging from intervertebral foramina (as at 5).

1 Anterior longitudinal ligament
2 Dorsal ramus of first lumbar nerve
3 Dorsal ramus of second lumbar nerve
4 First lumbar intervertebral disc
5 First lumbar nerve emerging from intervertebral foramen
6 First lumbar vertebra
7 Interspinous ligament
8 Rami communicantes
9 Spinous process of second lumbar vertebra
10 Supraspinous ligament
11 Sympathetic trunk ganglion
12 Twelfth rib
13 Ventral ramus of first lumbar nerve
14 Ventral ramus of second lumbar nerve
15 Zygapophyseal joint

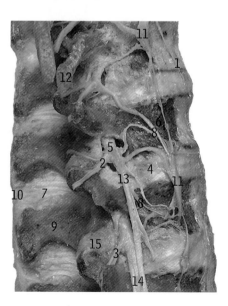

 Compression of spinal nerve, vertebral venous plexus, see page 108.

Ⓐ Vertebral column
lumbar region, from the right and behind

This posterolateral view of the right side of some lumbar vertebrae shows ligamenta flava (as at 4), which pass between the laminae of adjacent vertebrae (as at 2 and 3).

1 Interspinous ligament
2 Lamina of second lumbar vertebra
3 Lamina of third lumbar vertebra
4 Ligamentum flavum
5 Spinous process of second lumbar vertebra
6 Supraspinous ligament
7 Transverse process of third lumbar vertebra
8 Zygapophyseal joint

Ⓑ Lumbar intervertebral disc
from above, in situ

1 Annulus fibrosus
2 Aorta
3 Extraperitoneal fat
4 Inferior vena cava
5 Laminations of annulus
6 Nucleus pulposus
7 Gonadal artery
8 Gonadal vein
9 Peritoneum, posterior abdominal wall
10 Psoas major muscle
11 Thoracolumbar fascia, anterior layer
12 Ureter

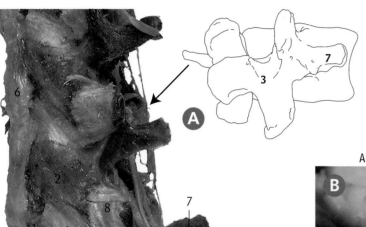

The nucleus pulposus of an intervertebral disc represents the remains of the notochord.

The annulus fibrosus of an intervertebral disc is derived from the mesenchyme between adjacent vertebral bodies.

ANTERIOR

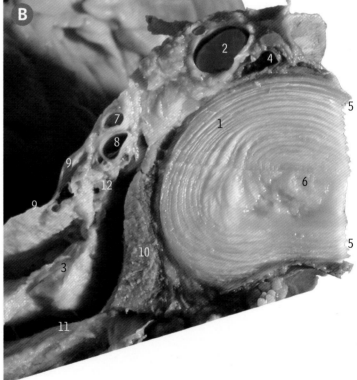

POSTERIOR

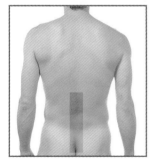

Lumbar puncture, spinal malformations (meningocoele), see page 108.

Back *surface anatomy*

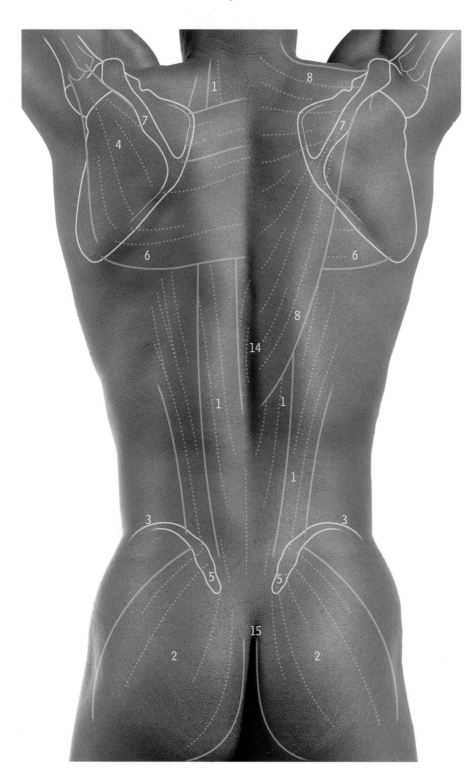

1 Erector spinae
2 Gluteus maximus
3 Iliac crest
4 Infraspinatus
5 Posterior superior iliac spine
6 Rhomboids
7 Spine of scapula
8 Trapezius

Back

Superficial musculature on left, deeper dissection on right.

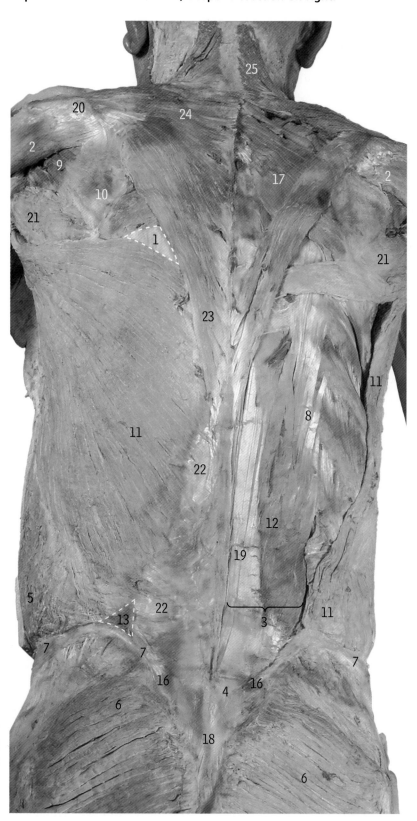

1 Auscultation triangle
2 Deltoid
3 Erector spinae
4 Erector spinae, tendon
5 External oblique muscle of the abdomen
6 Gluteus maximus
7 Iliac crest
8 Iliocostalis
9 Infraspinatus
10 Infraspinatus fascia
11 Latissimus dorsi
12 Longissimus
13 Lumbar triangle (of Petit)
14 Median furrow – see surface
15 Natal cleft – see surface
16 Posterior superior iliac spine
17 Rhomboid major
18 Sacrum
19 Spinalis
20 Spine of scapula
21 Teres major
22 Thoracolumbar fascia
23 Trapezius, lower fibres
24 Trapezius, middle fibres
25 Trapezius, upper fibres

Back

A *close up left side*

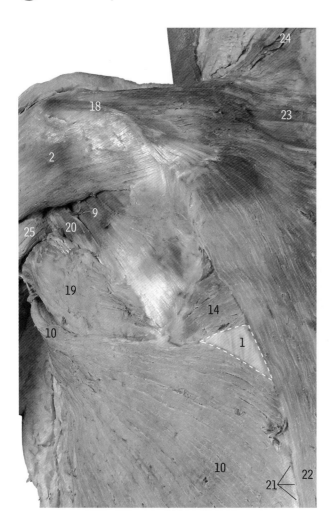

B *close up right side*

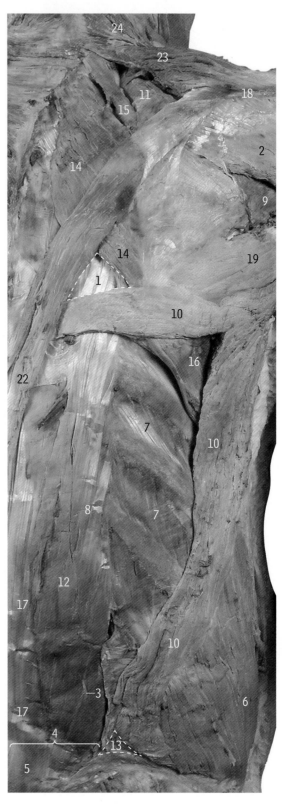

Windows cut in latissimus dorsi and trapezius muscles to reveal deeper layer of back musculature.

1	Auscultation triangle	**13**	Lumbar triangle
2	Deltoid	**14**	Rhomboid major
3	Dorsal ramus, lumbar spinal nerve	**15**	Rhomboid minor
		16	Serratus anterior
4	Erector spinae	**17**	Spinalis
5	Erector spinae, tendon	**18**	Spine of scapula
6	External oblique muscle of the abdomen	**19**	Teres major
		20	Teres minor
7	External intercostal	**21**	Thoracolumbar fascia
8	Iliocostalis	**22**	Trapezius, lower fibres
9	Infraspinatus	**23**	Trapezius, middle fibres
10	Latissimus dorsi	**24**	Trapezius, upper fibres
11	Levator scapulae	**25**	Triceps, long head
12	Longissimus		

Back

A *close up right side*

Note windows cut in latissimus dorsi and trapezius.

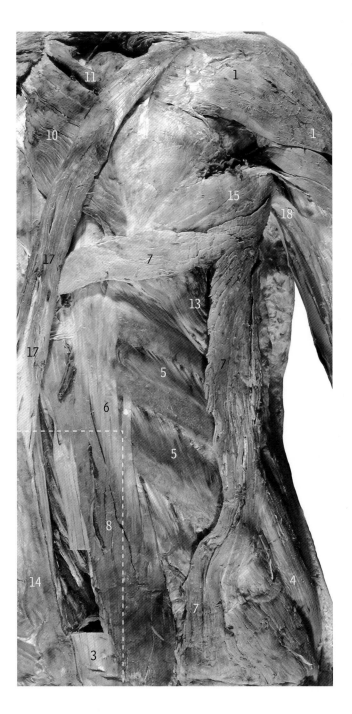

B *close up right side*

Note resection of upper lumbar and lower thoracic spinalis and part of longissimus muscles to reveal the transversospinalis group of muscles – the deepest components of erector spinae.

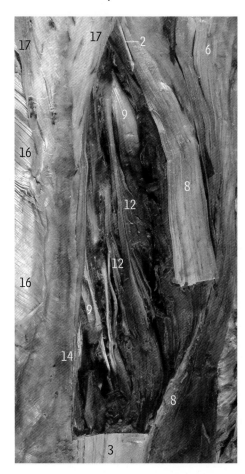

1	Deltoid	**9**	Multifidus
2	Dorsal ramus, thoracic spinal nerve	**10**	Rhomboid major
		11	Rhomboid minor
3	Erector spinae, tendon	**12**	Semispinalis
4	External oblique muscle of the abdomen	**13**	Serratus anterior
		14	Spinalis
5	External intercostal	**15**	Teres major
6	Iliocostalis	**16**	Thoracolumbar fascia
7	Latissimus dorsi	**17**	Trapezius, lower fibres
8	Longissimus	**18**	Triceps, long head

Sub-occipital triangle *superficial dissection*

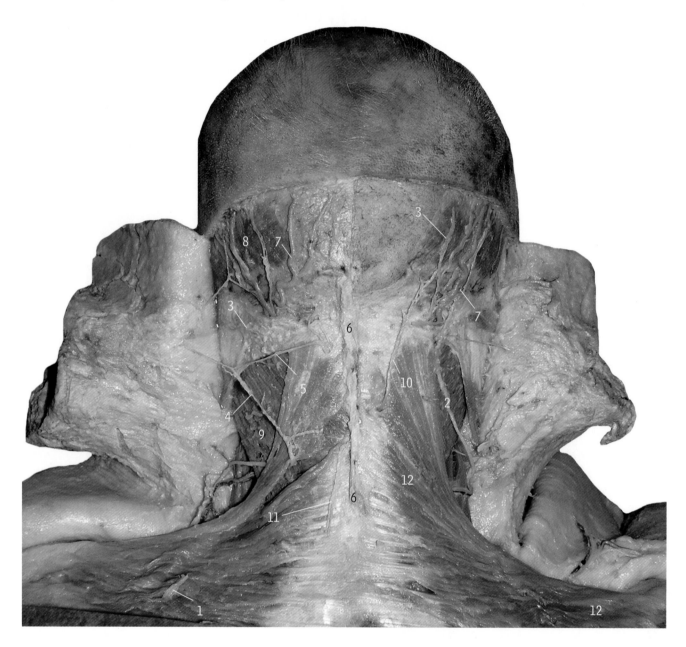

1. Dorsal cutaneous branch, spinal nerve
2. Great auricular nerve
3. Greater occipital nerve
4. Lesser occipital nerve
5. Lesser occipital nerve anastomosis with third occipital nerve
6. Ligamentum nuchae
7. Occipital artery
8. Occipital belly (occipitalis) of occipitofrontalis muscle
9. Splenius capitis muscle
10. Third occipital nerve
11. Third occipital nerve reflected
12. Trapezius muscle

Sub-occipital triangle *deep dissection*

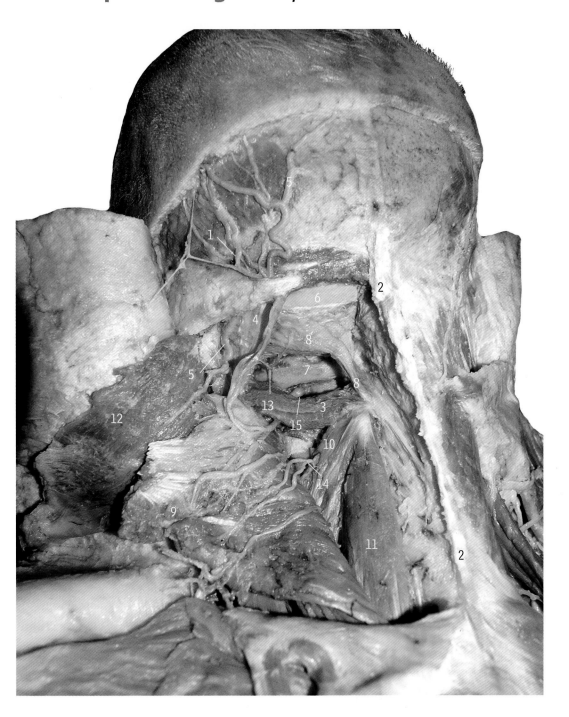

1 Greater occipital nerve	**9** Semispinalis capitis muscle reflected
2 Ligamentum nuchae	**10** Semispinalis cervicis muscle
3 Obliquus capitis inferior muscle	**11** Spinalis cervicis muscle
4 Obliquus capitis superior muscle	**12** Splenius capitis muscle reflected
5 Occipital artery	**13** Suboccipital nerve
6 Occipital bone	**14** Third occipital nerve
7 Posterior arch of C1 vertebra	**15** Vertebral artery
8 Rectus capitis posterior major muscle	

Upper cervical vertebrae *intraoral view*

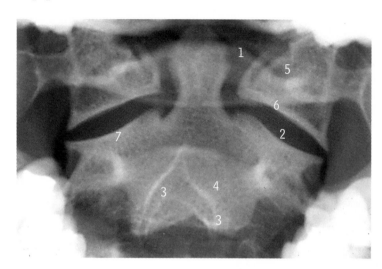

This is a standard radiographic view of the axis and its dens. The correct angle must be chosen with the mouth open to avoid overlying shadows of the teeth and jaws. The surfaces of the lateral atlanto-axial joints (5 and 7) do not make bony contact because the hyaline cartilage which covers the bony surfaces is not radio-opaque (this applies to any synovial joint). The outlines of the arches of the atlas are seen faintly between the sides of the shadow of the dens and the lateral masses of the atlas (5).

1 Arch of atlas
2 Atlanto-axial joint
3 Bifid spinous process
4 Body of axis
5 Lateral mass of atlas
6 Inferior articular process of atlas
7 Superior articular process of axis

Lower cervical and upper thoracic vertebrae

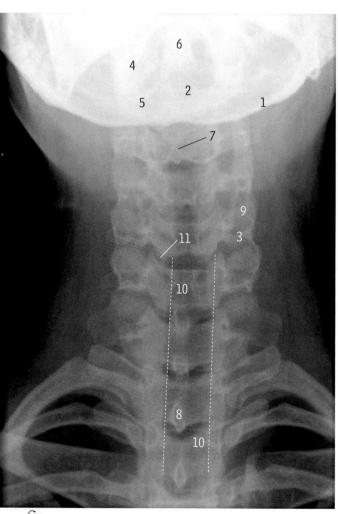

Note the tracheal shadow produced by the translucency of its contained air.

1 Basi-occiput
2 Body of axis
3 Inferior articular process
4 Lateral mass of atlas
5 Lateral mass of axis
6 Odontoid peg (dens)
7 Spinous process of third cervical vertebra
8 Spinous process of first thoracic vertebra
9 Superior articular process
10 Trachea
11 Uncovertebral joint

Atlanto-axial instability, cervical spinal immobilisation, see page 108.

Spine

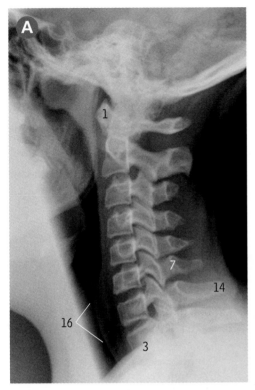

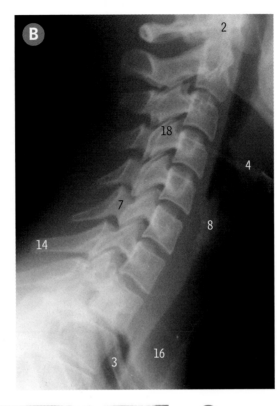

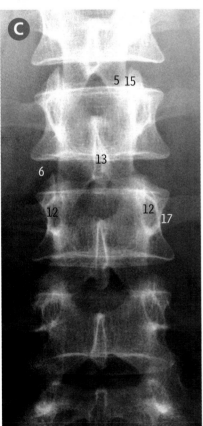

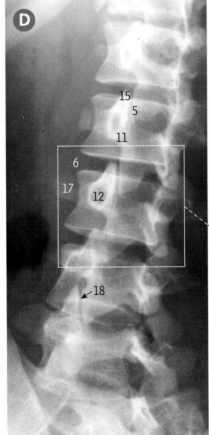

1 Anterior arch of axis
2 Dens of axis
3 First rib
4 Hyoid bone
5 Inferior articular process of first lumbar vertebra
6 Intervertebral disc space L2/3 level
7 Lamina of sixth cervical vertebra
8 Larynx
9 Lateral atlanto-axial joint
10 Lateral mass of atlas
11 Pars interarticularis of second lumbar vertebra
12 Pedicle of third lumbar vertebra
13 Spinous process of second lumbar vertebra
14 Spinous process of seventh cervical vertebra
15 Superior articular process of second lumbar vertebra
16 Trachea
17 Transverse process of third lumbar vertebra
18 Zygapophyseal joint

A cervical spine, lateral projection

B cervical spine, lateral projection

C lumbar spine, anteroposterior projection

D lumbar spine, oblique projection

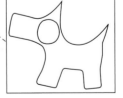

The Scottie dog is seen on the oblique projection lumbar spine. The nose (17) is the transverse process, the ear (15) is the superior articular process, the eye (12) is the pedicle and the neck (11) is the pars interarticularis which may be incomplete in spondylolysis.

Vertebral fractures, see page 108.

Vertebral column and spinal cord

Clinical thumbnails, see website for details and further clinical images to download into your own notes.

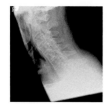

Ankylosing spondylitis

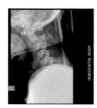

Atlanto-axial instability

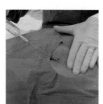

Caudal anaesthesia

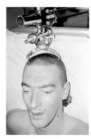

Cervical spinal immobilisation

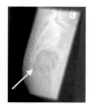

Coccydynia

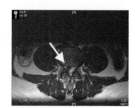

Compression of spinal nerve

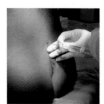

Epidural anaesthesia

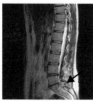

Laminectomy

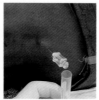

Lumbar puncture

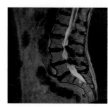

Lumbar stenosis

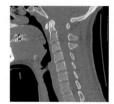

Odontoid peg fracture

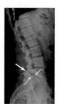

Sacralisation

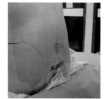

Spinal anaesthesia

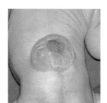

Spinal malformations (meningocoele)

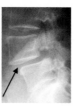

Spondylolisthesis

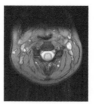

Transverse myelitis

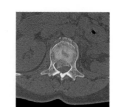

Vertebral fracture

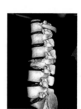

Vertebral lumbar fracture

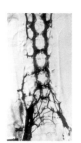

Vertebral venous plexus

Upper limb

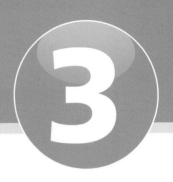

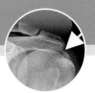

Upper limb

A *surface anatomy* **B** *muscles* **C** *bones*

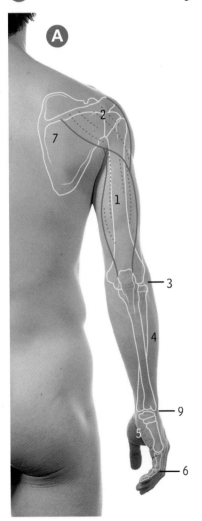

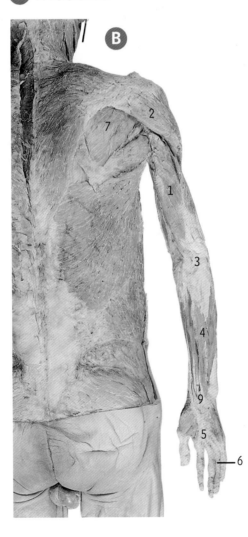

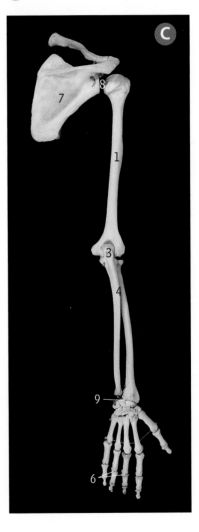

1 Arm	**6** Interphalangeal joint
2 Deltoid	**7** Scapula
3 Elbow joint	**8** Shoulder joint
4 Forearm	**9** Wrist joint
5 Hand	

Accessory ossicles, see pages 170–172.

Left scapula

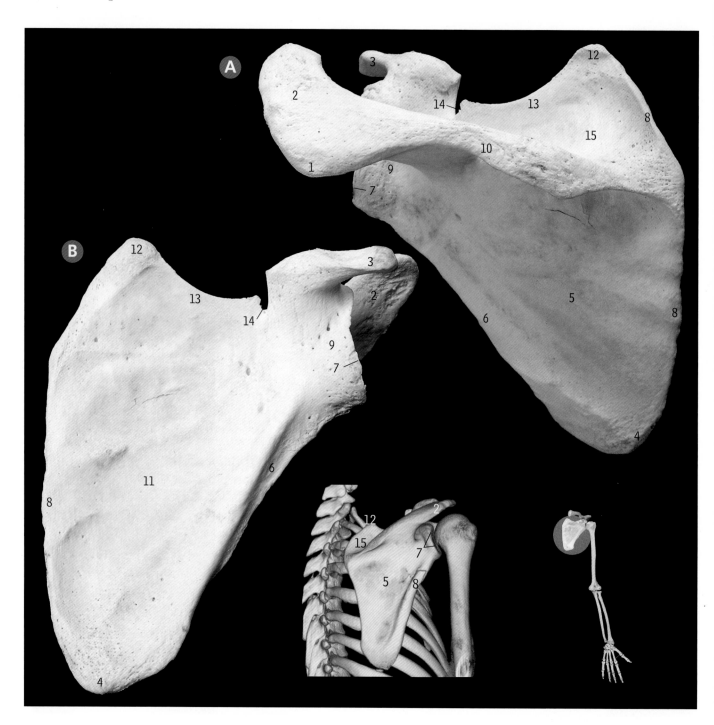

A dorsal surface

B costal surface

1 Acromial angle	**9** Neck (and spinoglenoid notch on dorsal surface)
2 Acromion	**10** Spine
3 Coracoid process	**11** Subscapular fossa
4 Inferior angle	**12** Superior angle
5 Infraspinous fossa	**13** Superior border
6 Lateral border	**14** Suprascapular notch
7 Margin of glenoid cavity	**15** Supraspinous fossa
8 Medial border	

The spine (A10) of the scapula projects from its dorsal surface with the acromion (A2) at the lateral end of the spine.

Left scapula *attachments*

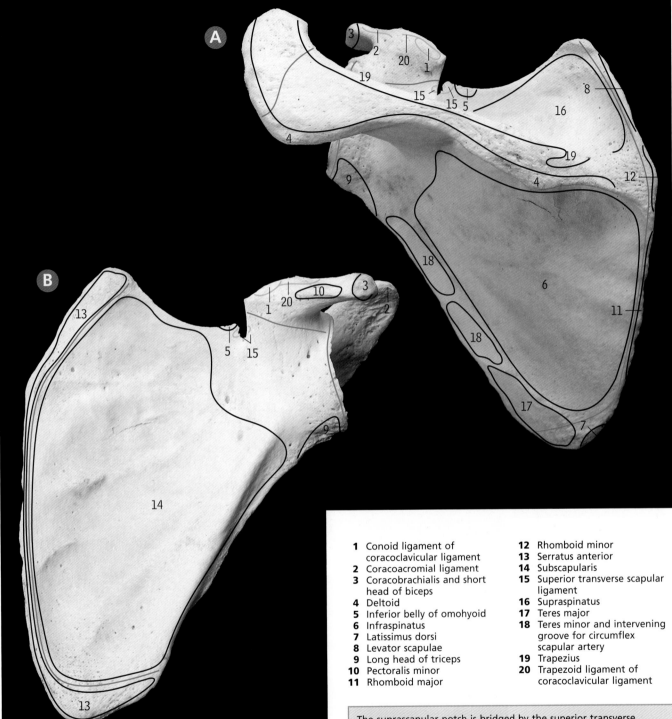

A dorsal surface **B** costal surface

Blue lines, epiphysial lines; green lines, capsular attachments of shoulder joint; pale green lines, ligament attachments

1 Conoid ligament of coracoclavicular ligament
2 Coracoacromial ligament
3 Coracobrachialis and short head of biceps
4 Deltoid
5 Inferior belly of omohyoid
6 Infraspinatus
7 Latissimus dorsi
8 Levator scapulae
9 Long head of triceps
10 Pectoralis minor
11 Rhomboid major
12 Rhomboid minor
13 Serratus anterior
14 Subscapularis
15 Superior transverse scapular ligament
16 Supraspinatus
17 Teres major
18 Teres minor and intervening groove for circumflex scapular artery
19 Trapezius
20 Trapezoid ligament of coracoclavicular ligament

The suprascapular notch is bridged by the superior transverse scapular ligament (15).

The conoid (1) and trapezoid (20) ligaments together form the coracoclavicular ligament, which attaches the coracoid process of the scapula to the under-surface of the lateral end of the clavicle.

The coracoacromial ligament (2) passes between the coracoid process and the acromion, forming with these bony processes an arch above the shoulder joint.

Ⓐ **Left scapula** *from the lateral side*

1	Acromion	**6**	Infraspinous fossa
2	Coracoid process	**7**	Lateral border
3	Glenoid cavity	**8**	Spine
4	Inferior angle	**9**	Supraglenoid tubercle
5	Infraglenoid tubercle	**10**	Supraspinous fossa

Ⓑ **Left scapula and clavicle** *articulation, from above*

1	Acromial end of clavicle	**5**	Shaft of clavicle
2	Acromioclavicular joint	**6**	Spine of scapula
3	Acromion	**7**	Sternal end of clavicle
4	Coracoid process	**8**	Supraspinous fossa

Ⓒ **Left clavicle** *from below*

1 Acromial end with articular surface (arrow)
2 Conoid tubercle
3 Groove for subclavius muscle
4 Impression for costoclavicular ligament
5 Sternal end with articular surface (arrow)
6 Trapezoid line

The sternal end of the clavicle (B7, C5) is bulbous; the acromial end (B1, C1) is flattened. The shaft is convex towards the front in its medial two-thirds, and the groove for the subclavius muscle is on the inferior surface (C3).

Acromioclavicular separation, see pages 170–172.

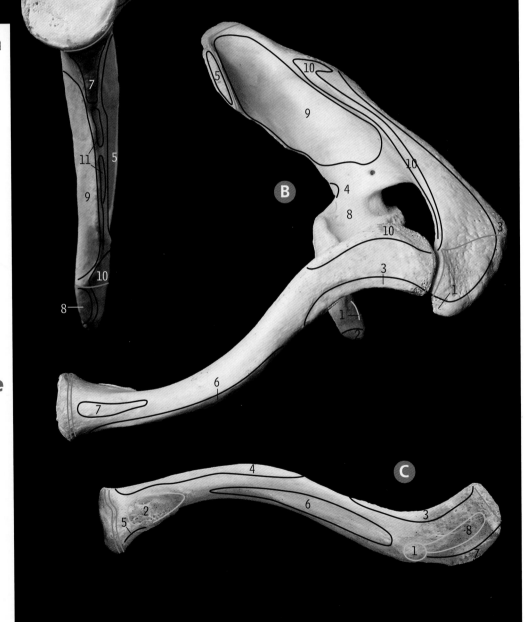

A Left scapula *attachments, from the lateral side*

Blue lines, epiphysial lines; green lines, capsular attachments of shoulder joint; pale green lines, ligament attachments

1 Coracoacromial ligament
2 Coracobrachialis and short head of biceps
3 Coracohumeral ligament
4 Deltoid
5 Infraspinatus
6 Long head of biceps
7 Long head of triceps
8 Serratus anterior
9 Subscapularis
10 Teres major
11 Teres minor (with intervening groove for circumflex scapular artery)

B Left scapula and clavicle *articulation, from above*

Blue lines, epiphysial lines; green lines, capsular attachments of sternoclavicular and acromioclavicular joints; pale green lines, ligament attachments

1 Coracoacromial ligament
2 Coracobrachialis and short head of biceps
3 Deltoid
4 Inferior belly of omohyoid
5 Levator scapulae
6 Pectoralis major
7 Sternocleidomastoid
8 Superior transverse scapular ligament
9 Supraspinatus
10 Trapezius

C Left clavicle *attachments, from below*

Blue lines, epiphysial lines; green lines, capsular attachments of sternoclavicular and acromioclavicular joints; pale green lines, ligament attachments

1 Conoid ligament
2 Costoclavicular ligament
3 Deltoid
4 Pectoralis major
5 Sternohyoid
6 Subclavius and clavipectoral fascia
7 Trapezius
8 Trapezoid ligament

Fractured clavicle, fractured scapula, see pages 170–172.

Right humerus *upper end*

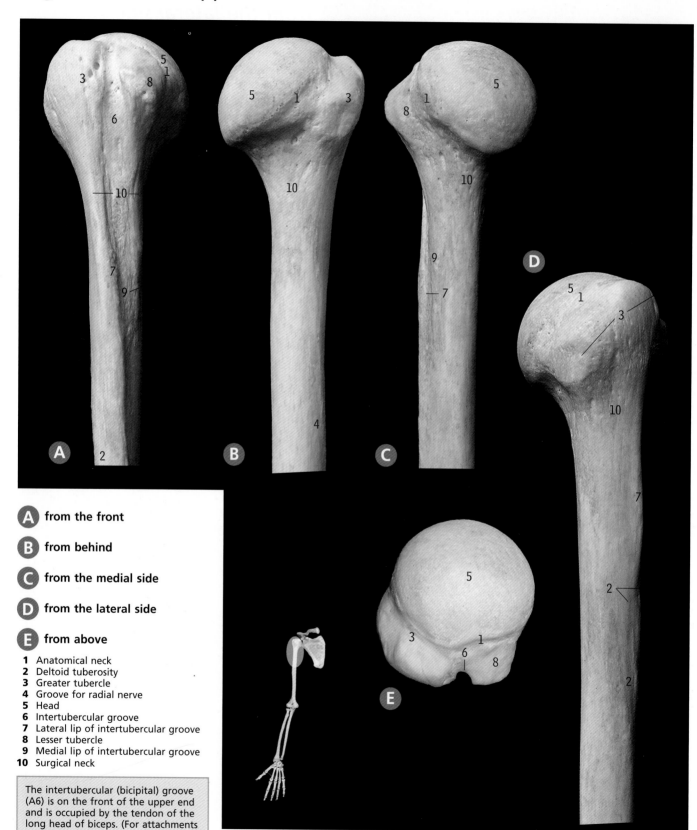

A from the front

B from behind

C from the medial side

D from the lateral side

E from above

1 Anatomical neck
2 Deltoid tuberosity
3 Greater tubercle
4 Groove for radial nerve
5 Head
6 Intertubercular groove
7 Lateral lip of intertubercular groove
8 Lesser tubercle
9 Medial lip of intertubercular groove
10 Surgical neck

The intertubercular (bicipital) groove (A6) is on the front of the upper end and is occupied by the tendon of the long head of biceps. (For attachments see page 115.)

Dislocation of the humerus, see pages 170–172.

Right humerus *attachments, upper end*

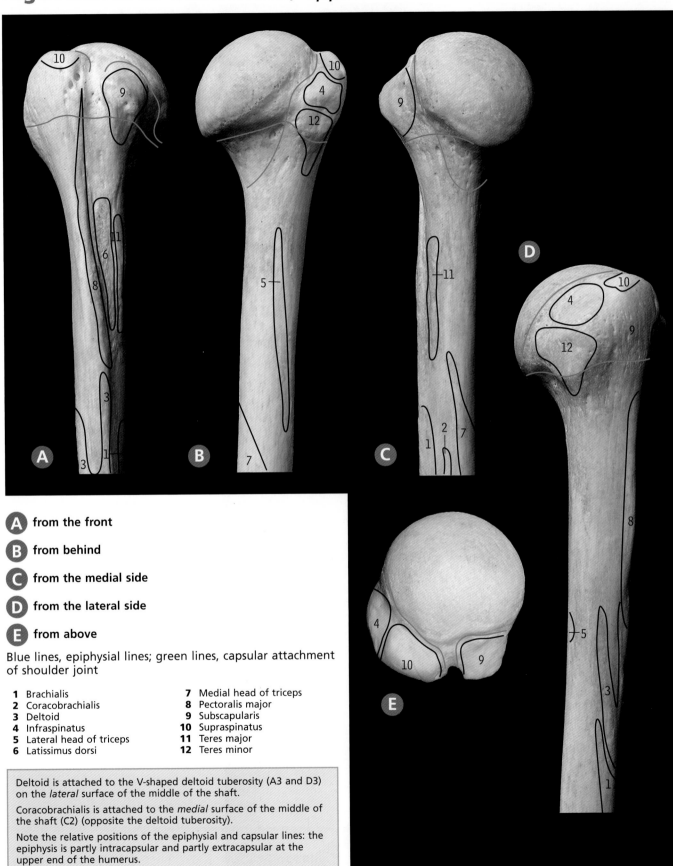

A from the front

B from behind

C from the medial side

D from the lateral side

E from above

Blue lines, epiphysial lines; green lines, capsular attachment of shoulder joint

1 Brachialis
2 Coracobrachialis
3 Deltoid
4 Infraspinatus
5 Lateral head of triceps
6 Latissimus dorsi
7 Medial head of triceps
8 Pectoralis major
9 Subscapularis
10 Supraspinatus
11 Teres major
12 Teres minor

Deltoid is attached to the V-shaped deltoid tuberosity (A3 and D3) on the *lateral* surface of the middle of the shaft.

Coracobrachialis is attached to the *medial* surface of the middle of the shaft (C2) (opposite the deltoid tuberosity).

Note the relative positions of the epiphysial and capsular lines: the epiphysis is partly intracapsular and partly extracapsular at the upper end of the humerus.

Right humerus *lower end*

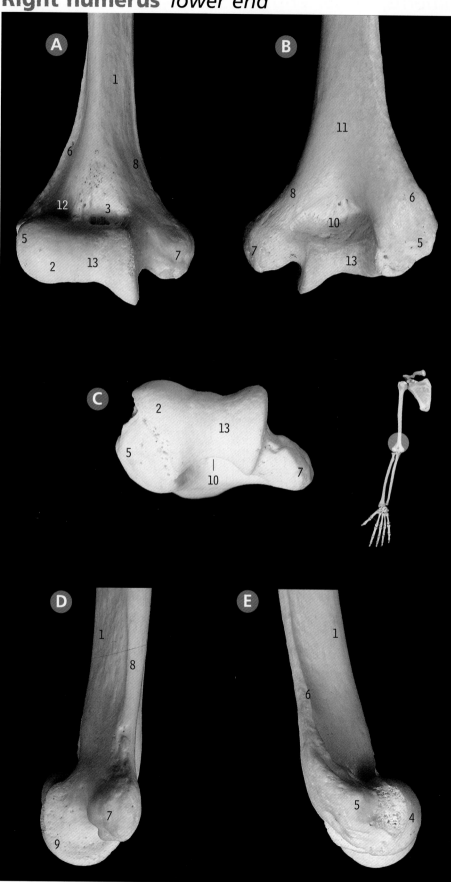

A **from the front**

B **from behind**

C **from below**

D **from the medial side**

E **from the lateral side**

1 Anterior surface
2 Capitulum
3 Coronoid fossa
4 Lateral edge of capitulum
5 Lateral epicondyle
6 Lateral supracondylar ridge
7 Medial epicondyle
8 Medial supracondylar ridge
9 Medial surface of trochlea
10 Olecranon fossa
11 Posterior surface
12 Radial fossa
13 Trochlea

The medial epicondyle (7) is more prominent than the lateral (5).

The medial part of the trochlea (13) is more prominent than the lateral part.

The olecranon fossa (10) on the posterior surface is deeper than the radial and coronoid fossae on the anterior surface (12 and 3).

Avulsion medial epicondyle, supracondylar spur, see pages 170–172.

Right humerus *attachments, lower end*

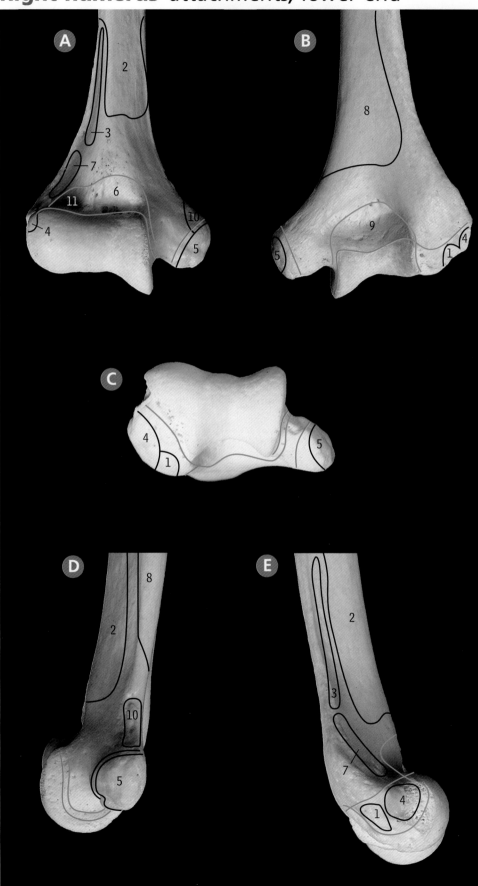

A from the front

B from behind

C from below

D from the medial side

E from the lateral side

Blue lines, epiphysial lines; green lines, capsular attachments of elbow joint

1 Anconeus
2 Brachialis
3 Brachioradialis
4 Common extensor origin
5 Common flexor origin
6 Coronoid fossa
7 Extensor carpi radialis longus
8 Medial head of triceps
9 Olecranon fossa
10 Pronator teres, humeral head
11 Radial fossa

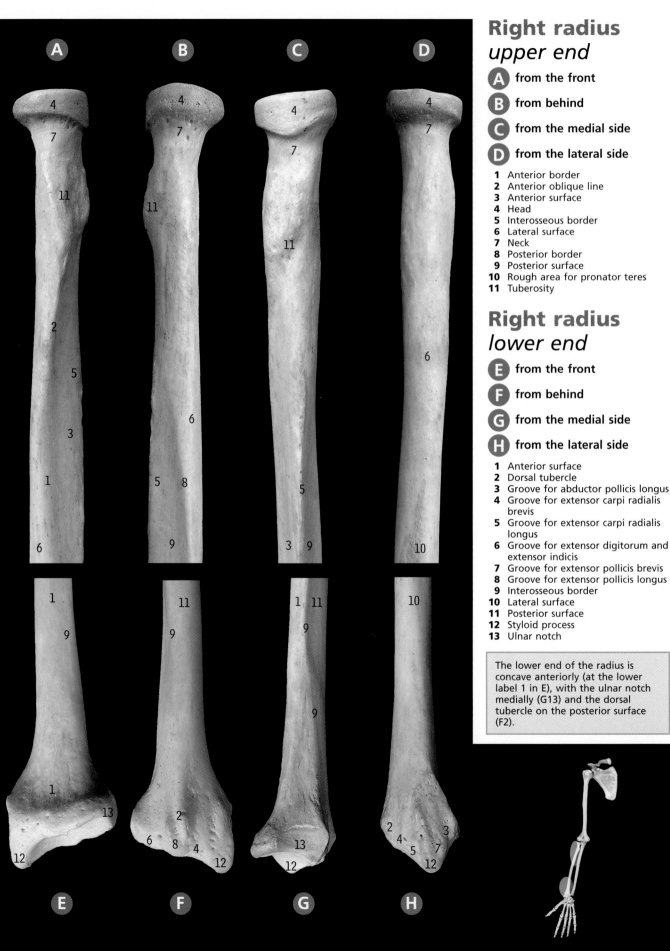

Right radius
upper end

A from the front

B from behind

C from the medial side

D from the lateral side

1 Anterior border
2 Anterior oblique line
3 Anterior surface
4 Head
5 Interosseous border
6 Lateral surface
7 Neck
8 Posterior border
9 Posterior surface
10 Rough area for pronator teres
11 Tuberosity

Right radius
lower end

E from the front

F from behind

G from the medial side

H from the lateral side

1 Anterior surface
2 Dorsal tubercle
3 Groove for abductor pollicis longus
4 Groove for extensor carpi radialis brevis
5 Groove for extensor carpi radialis longus
6 Groove for extensor digitorum and extensor indicis
7 Groove for extensor pollicis brevis
8 Groove for extensor pollicis longus
9 Interosseous border
10 Lateral surface
11 Posterior surface
12 Styloid process
13 Ulnar notch

The lower end of the radius is concave anteriorly (at the lower label 1 in E), with the ulnar notch medially (G13) and the dorsal tubercle on the posterior surface (F2).

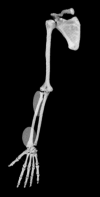

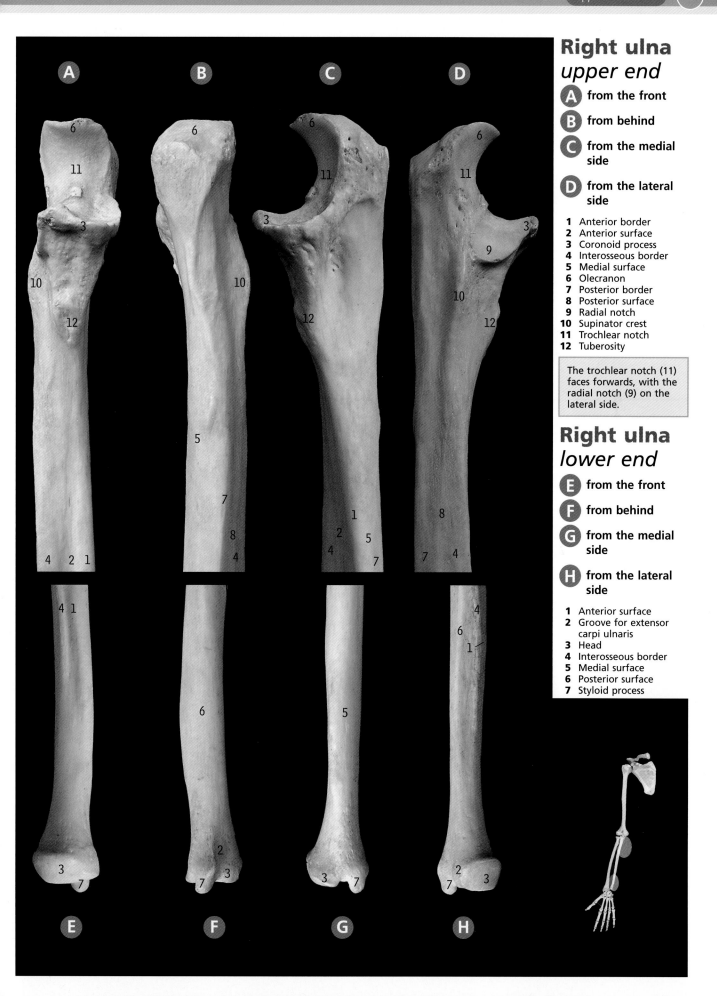

Right ulna
upper end

A from the front

B from behind

C from the medial side

D from the lateral side

1 Anterior border
2 Anterior surface
3 Coronoid process
4 Interosseous border
5 Medial surface
6 Olecranon
7 Posterior border
8 Posterior surface
9 Radial notch
10 Supinator crest
11 Trochlear notch
12 Tuberosity

The trochlear notch (11) faces forwards, with the radial notch (9) on the lateral side.

Right ulna
lower end

E from the front

F from behind

G from the medial side

H from the lateral side

1 Anterior surface
2 Groove for extensor carpi ulnaris
3 Head
4 Interosseous border
5 Medial surface
6 Posterior surface
7 Styloid process

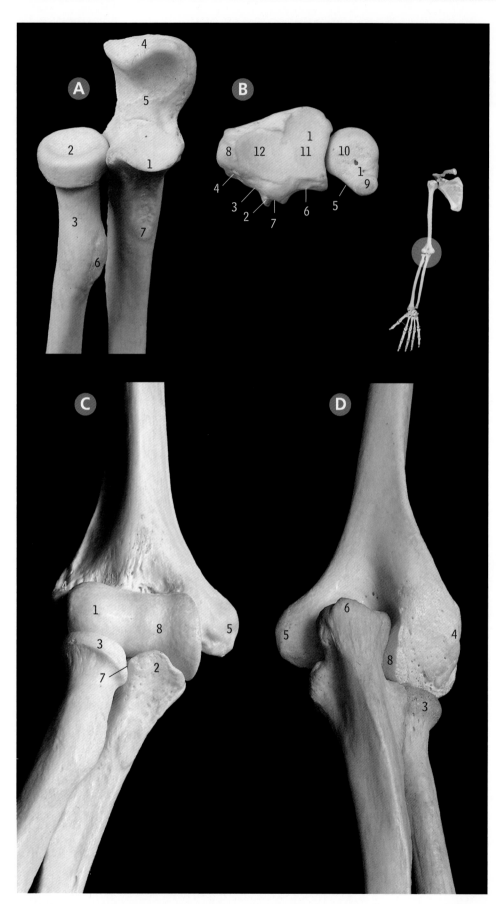

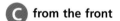

A Right radius and ulna
upper ends, from above and in front

1 Coronoid process of ulna
2 Head of radius
3 Neck of radius
4 Olecranon of ulna
5 Trochlear notch of ulna
6 Tuberosity of radius
7 Tuberosity of ulna

B Right radius and ulna
lower ends, from below

1 Attachment of articular disc
2 Dorsal tubercle
3 Groove for extensor carpi radialis brevis
4 Groove for extensor carpi radialis longus
5 Groove for extensor carpi ulnaris
6 Groove for extensor digitorum and extensor indicis
7 Groove for extensor pollicis longus
8 Styloid process of radius
9 Styloid process of ulna
10 Surface for disc
11 Surface for lunate
12 Surface for scaphoid

Right humerus, radius and ulna
articulation

C from the front

D from behind

1 Capitulum of humerus
2 Coronoid process of ulna
3 Head of radius
4 Lateral epicondyle of humerus
5 Medial epicondyle of humerus
6 Olecranon of ulna
7 Radial notch of ulna
8 Trochlea of humerus

The elbow joint and the proximal radio-ulnar joint share a common synovial cavity.

Dislocation of the elbow, supracondylar fracture of the humerus, see pages 170–172.

Right radius and ulna *attachments*

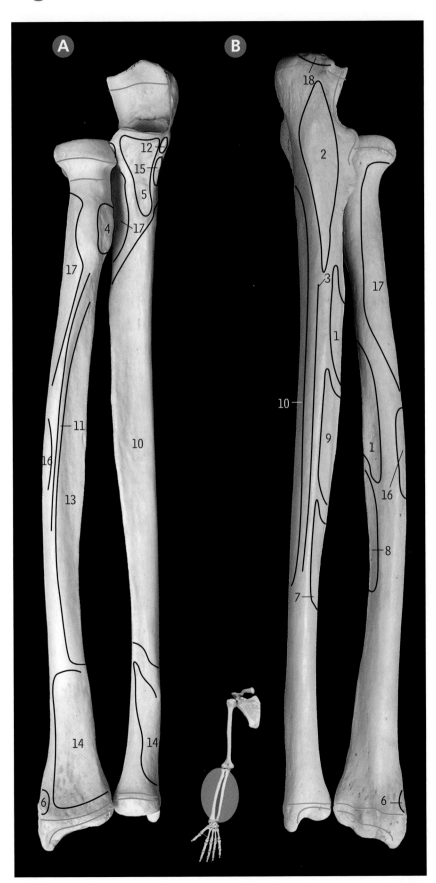

A from the front

B from behind

Blue lines, epiphysial lines; green lines, capsular attachments of elbow and wrist joints

1. Abductor pollicis longus
2. Anconeus
3. Aponeurotic attachment of flexor digitorum profundus, flexor carpi ulnaris and extensor carpi ulnaris
4. Biceps
5. Brachialis
6. Brachioradialis
7. Extensor indicis
8. Extensor pollicis brevis
9. Extensor pollicis longus
10. Flexor digitorum profundus
11. Flexor digitorum superficialis, radial head
12. Flexor digitorum superficialis, ulnar head
13. Flexor pollicis longus
14. Pronator quadratus
15. Pronator teres, ulnar head
16. Pronator teres
17. Supinator
18. Triceps

Abductor pollicis longus (1) and extensor pollicis brevis (8) are the only two muscles to have an origin from the posterior surface of the radius (although both extend on to the interosseous membrane and the abductor also has an origin from the posterior surface of the ulna). These muscles remain companions as they wind round the lateral side of the radius (page 152) and form the radial boundary of the anatomical snuffbox (pages 153 and 166).

In the young subject, the radius sometimes fractures across the lower epiphysis following an injury to the wrist. In the adult the term "Colles' fracture" (page 123) refers to a transverse break across the lower radius within about 2.5 cm of the lower end of the bone. The ulnar styloid process is also often fractured.

Traction of forearm fractures, see pages 170–172.

Bones of the right hand

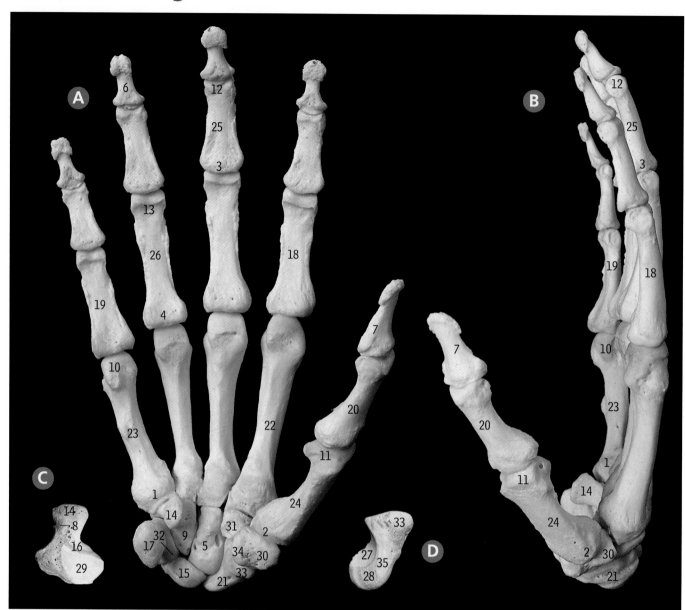

A palmar surface

B from the lateral side

C hamate from the medial side

D scaphoid, palmar surface

The scaphoid, lunate, triquetral and pisiform bones form the proximal row of carpal bones.

The trapezium, trapezoid, capitate and hamate bones form the distal row of carpal bones.

The tubercle (33) and waist (35) are the non-articular parts of the scaphoid and therefore contain nutrient foramina. A fracture across the waist may therefore interfere with the blood supply of the proximal pole of the bone and lead to avascular necrosis (see page 167). The waist of the scaphoid lies in the anatomical snuffbox; the tubercle may be palpated in front of the radial boundary of the snuffbox.

1 Base of fifth metacarpal
2 Base of first metacarpal
3 Base of middle phalanx of middle finger
4 Base of proximal phalanx of ring finger
5 Capitate
6 Distal phalanx of ring finger
7 Distal phalanx of thumb
8 Groove for deep branch of ulnar nerve
9 Hamate
10 Head of fifth metacarpal
11 Head of first metacarpal
12 Head of middle phalanx of middle finger
13 Head of proximal phalanx of ring finger
14 Hook of hamate
15 Lunate
16 Palmar surface, hamate
17 Pisiform
18 Proximal phalanx of index finger
19 Proximal phalanx of little finger
20 Proximal phalanx of thumb
21 Scaphoid
22 Shaft of second metacarpal
23 Shaft of fifth metacarpal
24 Shaft of first metacarpal
25 Shaft of middle phalanx of middle finger
26 Shaft of proximal phalanx of ring finger
27 Surface for capitate
28 Surface for lunate
29 Surface for triquetral
30 Trapezium
31 Trapezoid
32 Triquetral
33 Tubercle of scaphoid
34 Tubercle of trapezium
35 Waist of scaphoid

Bones of the right hand *dorsal surface*

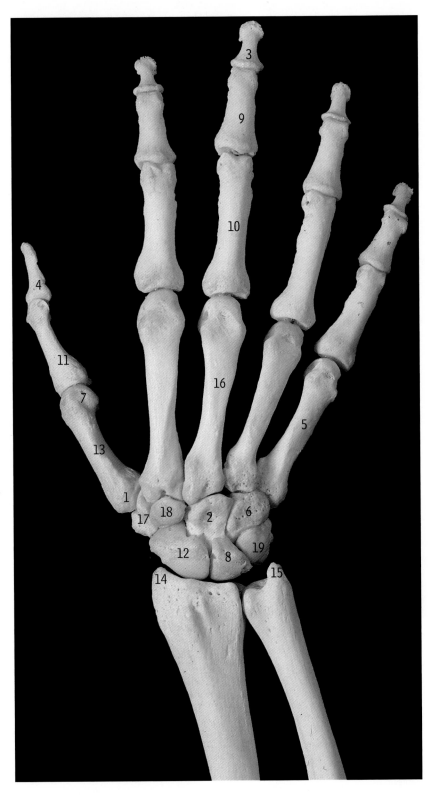

1 Base of first metacarpal
2 Capitate
3 Distal phalanx of middle finger
4 Distal phalanx of thumb
5 Fifth metacarpal
6 Hamate
7 Head of first metacarpal
8 Lunate
9 Middle phalanx of middle finger
10 Proximal phalanx of middle finger
11 Proximal phalanx of thumb
12 Scaphoid
13 Shaft of first metacarpal
14 Styloid process of radius
15 Styloid process of ulna
16 Third metacarpal
17 Trapezium
18 Trapezoid
19 Triquetral

The wrist joint (properly called the radiocarpal joint) is the joint between (proximally) the lower end of the radius and the interarticular disc which holds the lower ends of the radius and the ulna together, and (distally) the scaphoid, lunate and triquetral bones.

The midcarpal joint is the joint between the proximal and distal rows of carpal bones (see pages 163 and 168).

The carpometacarpal joint of the thumb is the joint between the trapezium and the base of the first metacarpal.

Bar room fracture, Colles' fracture, dislocation of the finger, Smith's fracture, see pages 170–172.

Bones of the right hand *attachments*

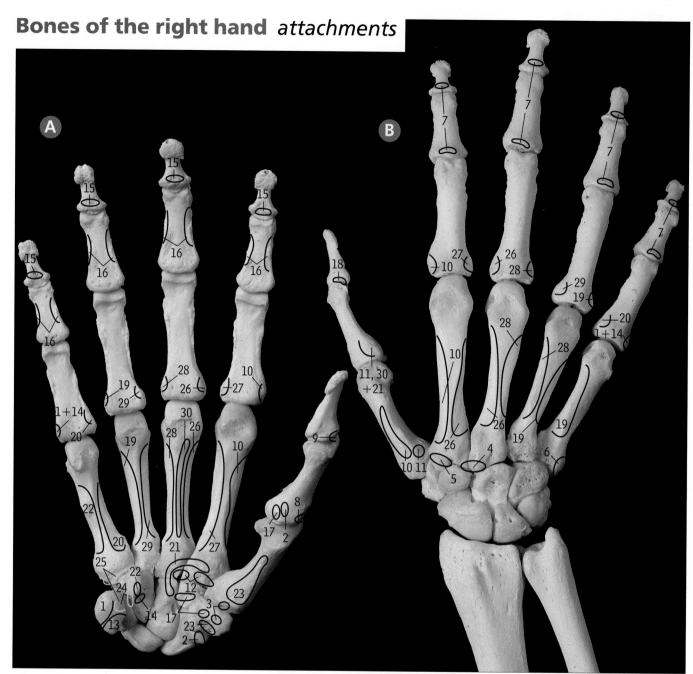

A **palmar surface**

B **dorsal surface**

Pale green lines, ligament attachments

1 Abductor digiti minimi	**17** Flexor pollicis brevis
2 Abductor pollicis brevis	**18** Flexor pollicis longus
3 Abductor pollicis longus	**19** Fourth dorsal interosseous
4 Extensor carpi radialis brevis	**20** Fourth palmar interosseous
5 Extensor carpi radialis longus	**21** Oblique head of adductor
6 Extensor carpi ulnaris	pollicis
7 Extensor expansion	**22** Opponens digiti minimi
8 Extensor pollicis brevis	**23** Opponens pollicis
9 Extensor pollicis longus	**24** Pisohamate ligament
10 First dorsal interosseous	**25** Pisometacarpal ligament
11 First palmar interosseous	**26** Second dorsal interosseous
12 Flexor carpi radialis	**27** Second palmar interosseous
13 Flexor carpi ulnaris	**28** Third dorsal interosseous
14 Flexor digiti minimi brevis	**29** Third palmar interosseous
15 Flexor digitorum profundus	**30** Transverse head of adductor
16 Flexor digitorum superficialis	pollicis

The metacarpophalangeal joints are the joints between the heads of the metacarpals and the bases of the proximal phalanges.

The interphalangeal joints are the joints between the head of one phalanx and the base of the adjoining phalanx.

The pisiform is a sesamoid bone in the tendon of flexor carpi ulnaris and is anchored by the pisohamate and pisometacarpal ligaments (24 and 25).

Dorsal interossei arise from the sides of two adjacent metacarpal bones (as at 26, from the sides of the second and third metacarpals); palmar interossei arise only from the metacarpal of their own finger (as at 27, from the second metacarpal). Compare with dissection B on page 166 and note that when looking at the palm, parts of the dorsal interossei can be seen as well as the palmar interossei, but when looking at the dorsum of the hand (as on page 166) only dorsal interossei are seen.

Digital development abnormality, fractured hamate, see pages 170–172.

Right upper limb bones *secondary centres of ossification*

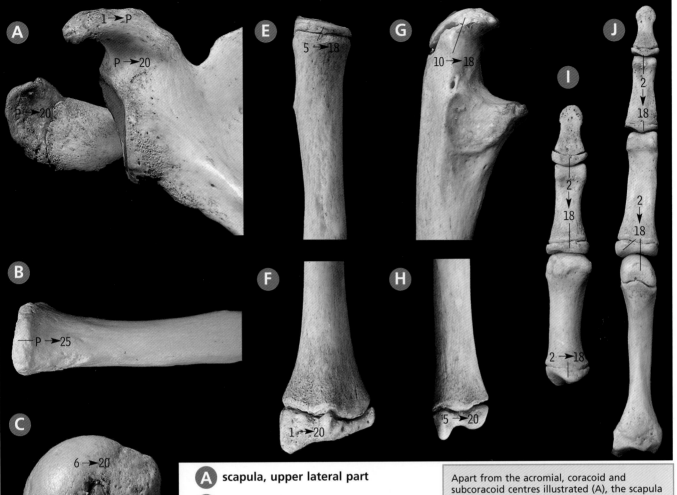

A scapula, upper lateral part

B clavicle, sternal end

C **D** humerus, upper and lower ends

E **F** radius, upper and lower ends

G **H** ulna, upper and lower ends

I first metacarpal and phalanges of thumb

J second metacarpal and phalanges of index finger

Figures in years after birth, commencement of ossification → fusion. (P, puberty)

The first figure indicates the approximate date when ossification begins in the secondary centre, and the second figure (beyond the arrowhead) when the centre finally becomes fused with the rest of the bone. Single average dates have been given (both here and for the lower limb bone centres on pages 314 and 315) and although there may be considerable individual variations, the 'growing end' of the bone (when fusion occurs last) is constant. The dates in females are often a year or more earlier than in males.

Apart from the acromial, coracoid and subcoracoid centres illustrated (A), the scapula usually has other centres for the inferior angle, medial border, and the lower part of the rim of the glenoid cavity (all P → 20; see pages 137 and 169).

The clavicle is the first bone in the body to start to ossify (fifth week of gestation). It ossifies in membrane, but the ends of the bone have a cartilaginous phase of ossification; a secondary centre appearing at the sternal end (B) unites with the body at about the 25th year.

The centre illustrated at the upper end of the humerus (C) is the result of the union at 6 years of centres for the head (1 year), greater tubercle (3 years) and lesser tubercle (5 years).

At the lower end of the humerus (D) the centres for the capitulum, trochlea and lateral epicondyle fuse together before uniting with the shaft.

All the phalanges (as in J), and the first metacarpal (I) have a secondary centre at their proximal ends; the other metacarpals (as in J) have one at their distal ends.

All the carpal bones are cartilaginous at birth and none has a secondary centre. The largest, the capitate, is the first to begin to ossify (in the second month after birth), followed in a month or so by the hamate, with the triquetral at 3 years, lunate at 4 years, scaphoid, trapezoid and trapezium at 5 years and the pisiform last at 9 years or later. There are often variations in the above common pattern.

Right shoulder

surface markings, from the front

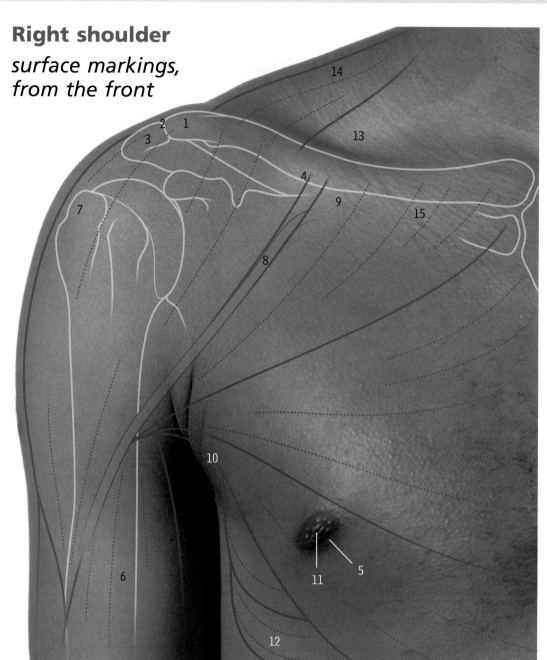

1 Acromial end of clavicle
2 Acromioclavicular joint
3 Acromion
4 Anterior margin of deltoid
5 Areola
6 Biceps
7 Deltoid overlying greater tubercle of humerus
8 Deltopectoral groove and cephalic vein
9 Infraclavicular fossa
10 Lower margin of pectoralis major
11 Nipple
12 Serratus anterior
13 Supraclavicular fossa
14 Trapezius
15 Upper margin of pectoralis major

The nipple in the male (11) normally lies at the level of the fourth intercostal space.

The lower border of pectoralis major (10) forms the anterior axillary fold.

Note that the most lateral bony point in the shoulder is the greater tubercle (7).

The clavicle is subcutaneous throughout its length. Its acromial end (1) at the acromioclavicular joint (2) lies at a slightly higher level than the acromion of the scapula (3). At the most lateral part of the shoulder, the deltoid overlies the humerus; the acromion of the scapula does not extend so far laterally. Compare the positions of the features noted here with the dissection on the next page.

Dislocation of humerus, sternoclavicular dislocation, see pages 170–172.

Right shoulder *superficial dissection*

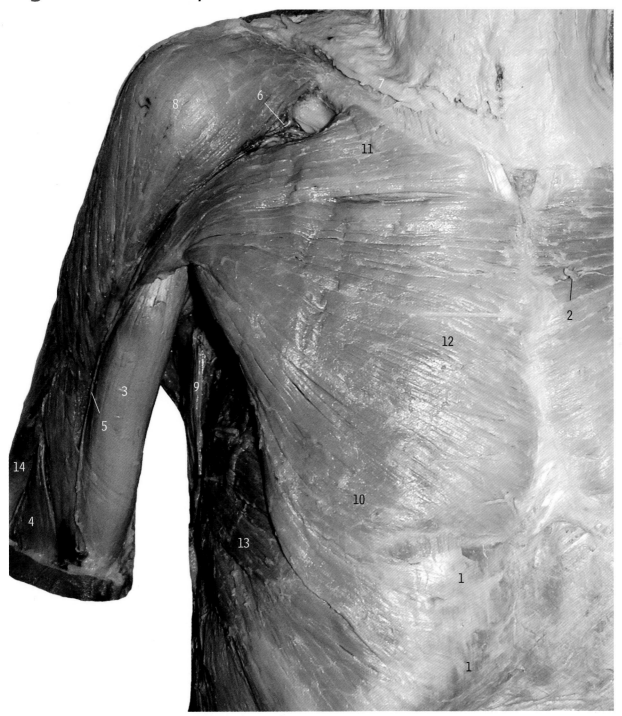

Removal of skin and fascia displays the anterior musculature of the shoulder and thoracic wall.

1 Anterior layer of rectus
  sheath
2 Anterior perforating branches
  of intercostal neurovascular
  bundle
3 Biceps brachii muscle (long
  head)
4 Brachioradialis muscle
5 Cephalic vein
6 Cephalic vein in deltopectoral
  groove
7 Clavicle

8 Deltoid muscle
9 Latissimus dorsi muscle
10 Pectoralis major muscle,
  abdominal head
11 Pectoralis major muscle,
  clavicular head
12 Pectoralis major muscle,
  sternal head
13 Serratus anterior muscle
14 Triceps brachii muscle (lateral
  head)

Right shoulder
superficial dissection, from the front

**Removal of skin and fascia displays branches of the supraclavicular nerve
(6) crossing the clavicle (9), and the cephalic vein (7) lying in the
deltopectoral groove between deltoid (13) and pectoralis major (11).**

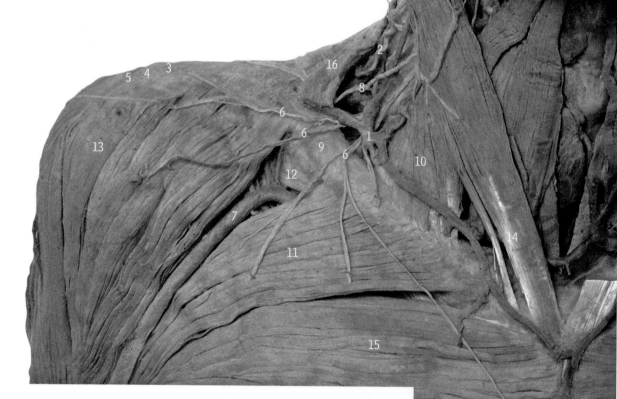

1 A superficial venous plexus
2 Accessory nerve
3 Acromial end of clavicle
4 Acromioclavicular joint
5 Acromion of scapula
6 Branches of supraclavicular nerves
7 Cephalic vein
8 Cervical nerve to trapezius
9 Clavicle
10 Clavicular head of sternocleidomastoid
11 Clavicular part of pectoralis major
12 Clavipectoral fascia
13 Deltoid
14 Sternal head of sternocleidomastoid
15 Sternocostal part of pectoralis major
16 Trapezius

The position of the acromioclavicular joint (4)
is indicated by the small 'step down' between
the acromial end of the clavicle (3) and the
acromion (5); compare with the surface feature
2 on page 126. This is the normal appearance;
when the joint is dislocated, with the acromion
being forced below the end of the clavicle, the
'step' is much exaggerated.

The cephalic vein (7) runs in the deltopectoral
groove between deltoid (13) and pectoralis
major (11) and pierces the clavipectoral fascia
(12) to drain into the axillary vein.

Right shoulder *deeper dissection, from the front*

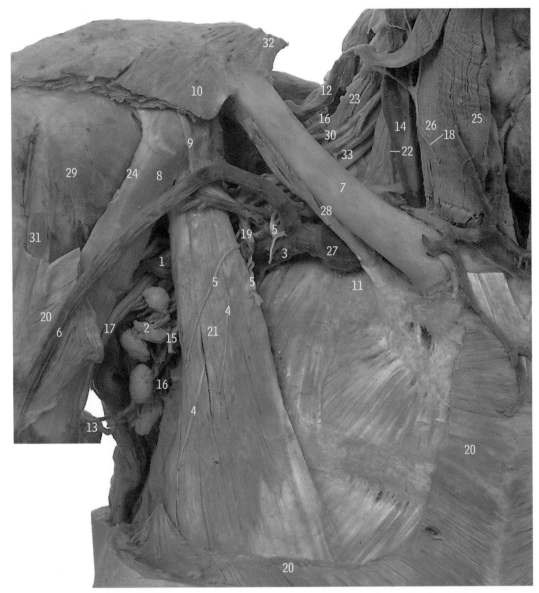

1 Anterior circumflex humeral artery and musculocutaneous nerve
2 Axillary lymph nodes (enlarged)
3 Axillary vein
4 Branches of medial pectoral nerve
5 Branches of lateral pectoral nerve
6 Cephalic vein
7 Clavicle
8 Coracobrachialis
9 Coracoid process and acromial branch of thoracoacromial artery
10 Deltoid
11 First rib
12 Inferior belly of omohyoid (displaced upwards)
13 Intercostobrachial nerve
14 Internal jugular vein
15 Lateral thoracic artery
16 Long thoracic nerve (to serratus anterior)
17 Median nerve
18 Nerve to sternothyroid
19 Pectoral branch of thoracoacromial artery
20 Pectoralis major
21 Pectoralis minor
22 Phrenic nerve overlying scalenus anterior
23 Scalenus medius
24 Short head of biceps
25 Sternohyoid
26 Sternothyroid
27 Subclavian vein
28 Subclavius
29 Subscapularis
30 Suprascapular nerve
31 Tendon of long head of biceps
32 Trapezius
33 Trunks of brachial plexus

Most of deltoid (10) and pectoralis major (20) have been removed to show the underlying pectoralis minor (21) and its associated vessels and nerves. The clavipectoral fascia which passes between the clavicle (7) and the upper (medial) border of the pectoralis minor (21) has also been removed to show the axillary vein (3) receiving the cephalic vein (6) and continuing as the subclavian vein (27) as it crosses the first rib (11).

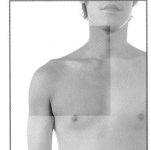

Shoulder arthroscopy

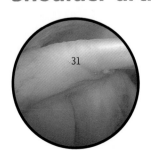

This shows the arthroscopic view of the right shoulder seen from behind. The supraspinatus tendon and the long head of biceps is in pristine condition. The anterior edge of the glenoid labrum shows some wear.

Klumpke's paralysis, see pages 170–172.

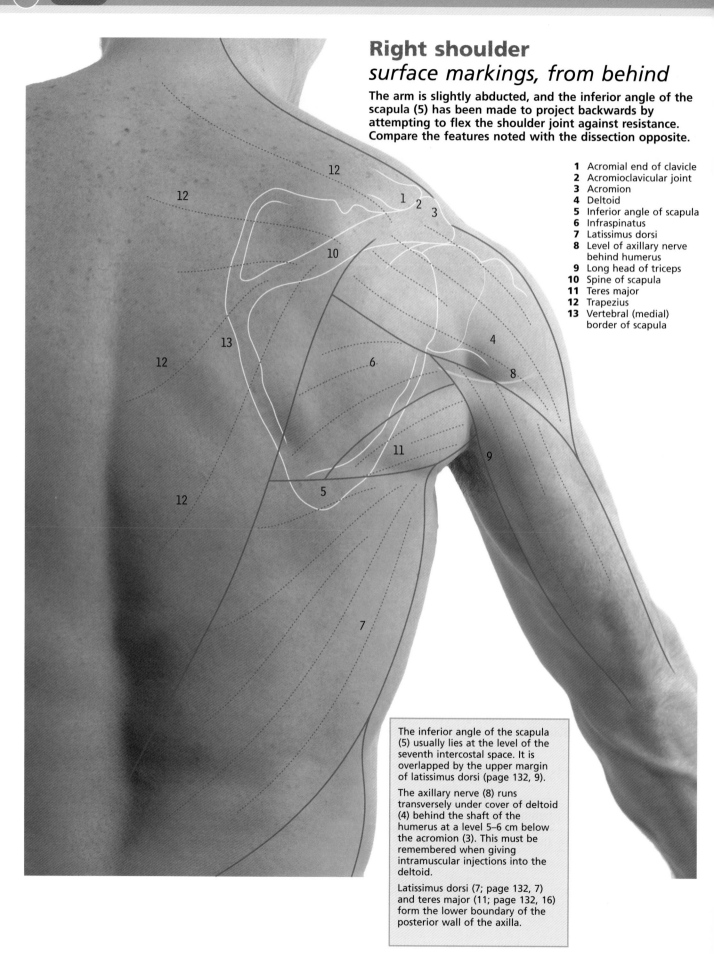

Right shoulder
surface markings, from behind

The arm is slightly abducted, and the inferior angle of the scapula (5) has been made to project backwards by attempting to flex the shoulder joint against resistance. Compare the features noted with the dissection opposite.

1 Acromial end of clavicle
2 Acromioclavicular joint
3 Acromion
4 Deltoid
5 Inferior angle of scapula
6 Infraspinatus
7 Latissimus dorsi
8 Level of axillary nerve behind humerus
9 Long head of triceps
10 Spine of scapula
11 Teres major
12 Trapezius
13 Vertebral (medial) border of scapula

The inferior angle of the scapula (5) usually lies at the level of the seventh intercostal space. It is overlapped by the upper margin of latissimus dorsi (page 132, 9).

The axillary nerve (8) runs transversely under cover of deltoid (4) behind the shaft of the humerus at a level 5–6 cm below the acromion (3). This must be remembered when giving intramuscular injections into the deltoid.

Latissimus dorsi (7; page 132, 7) and teres major (11; page 132, 16) form the lower boundary of the posterior wall of the axilla.

Right shoulder *superficial dissection, from behind*

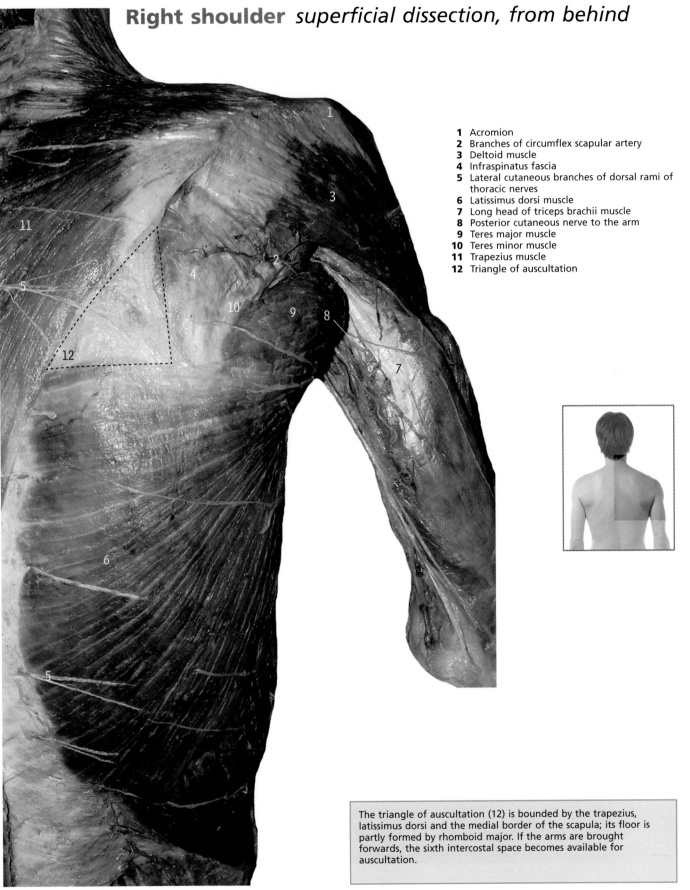

1 Acromion
2 Branches of circumflex scapular artery
3 Deltoid muscle
4 Infraspinatus fascia
5 Lateral cutaneous branches of dorsal rami of thoracic nerves
6 Latissimus dorsi muscle
7 Long head of triceps brachii muscle
8 Posterior cutaneous nerve to the arm
9 Teres major muscle
10 Teres minor muscle
11 Trapezius muscle
12 Triangle of auscultation

The triangle of auscultation (12) is bounded by the trapezius, latissimus dorsi and the medial border of the scapula; its floor is partly formed by rhomboid major. If the arms are brought forwards, the sixth intercostal space becomes available for auscultation.

Intramuscular injections, see pages 170–172.

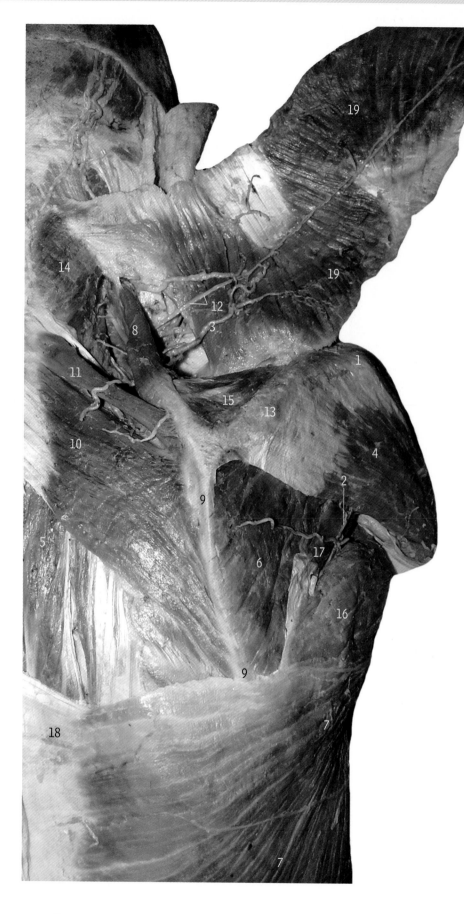

Right shoulder
from behind, trapezius reflected

1 Acromion
2 Branches of circumflex scapular artery
3 Deep branch of transverse cervical artery
4 Deltoid muscle
5 Erector spinae muscle
6 Infraspinatus muscle
7 Latissimus dorsi muscle
8 Levator scapulae muscle
9 Medial border of scapula
10 Rhomboid major muscle
11 Rhomboid minor muscle
12 Spinal accessory nerve
13 Spine of scapula
14 Splenius capitis muscle
15 Supraspinatus muscle
16 Teres major muscle
17 Teres minor muscle
18 Thoracic part of thoracolumbar fascia
19 Trapezius muscle (cut and reflected)

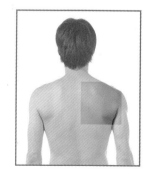

Shoulder joint injection, see pages 170–172.

A Right shoulder *from above and behind*

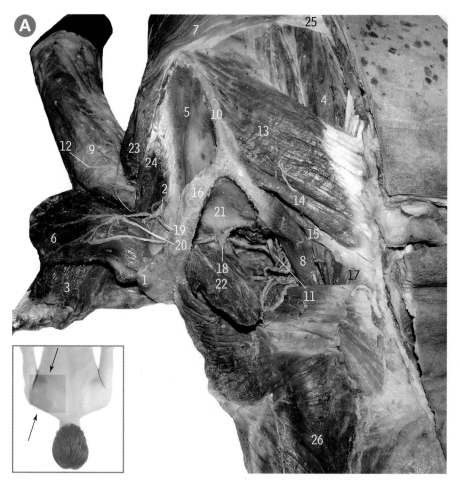

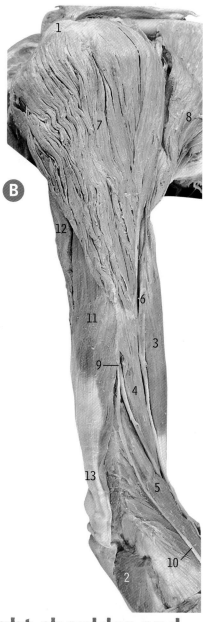

1 Acromion
2 Branches of circumflex scapular artery anastomosing with suprascapular artery
3 Deltoid muscle (cut and reflected)
4 Erector spinae muscle
5 Infraspinous fossa
6 Infraspinatus muscle (cut and reflected)
7 Latissimus dorsi muscle
8 Levator scapulae muscle
9 Long head of triceps brachii muscle
10 Medial border of scapula
11 Omohyoid muscle
12 Posterior cutaneous nerve to the arm
13 Rhomboid major muscle
14 Rhomboid minor muscle
15 Serratus posterior superior muscle
16 Spine of the scapula
17 Splenius capitis muscle
18 Superior transverse scapular ligament
19 Suprascapular artery
20 Suprascapular nerve
21 Supraspinous fossa
22 Supraspinatus muscle (cut and reflected)
23 Teres major muscle
24 Teres minor muscle
25 Thoracic part of thoracolumbar fascia
26 Trapezius muscle (cut and reflected)

B Right shoulder and upper arm *from the right*

Deltoid (7) extends over the tip of the shoulder to its attachment halfway down the lateral side of the shaft of the humerus. Biceps brachii (3) is on the front of the arm below pectoralis major (8) and triceps (11 and 12) is at the back.

1 Acromion
2 Anconeus
3 Biceps brachii
4 Brachialis
5 Brachioradialis
6 Cephalic vein
7 Deltoid
8 Pectoralis major
9 Radial nerve
10 Radial nerve, posterior cutaneous branch to the forearm
11 Triceps, lateral head
12 Triceps, long head
13 Triceps, tendon

Posterior dislocation of the shoulder, see pages 170–172.

Right shoulder *deep dissection of scapular region*

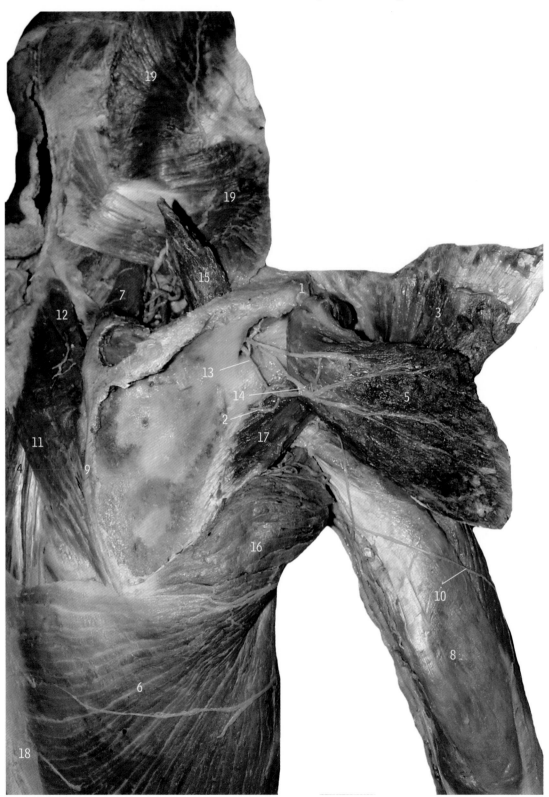

1 Acromion	**11** Rhomboid major muscle
2 Branches of circumflex scapular artery	**12** Rhomboid minor muscle
3 Deltoid muscle (cut and reflected)	**13** Suprascapular artery
4 Erector spinae muscle	**14** Suprascapular nerve
5 Infraspinatus muscle (cut and reflected)	**15** Supraspinatus muscle (cut and reflected)
6 Latissimus dorsi muscle	**16** Teres major muscle
7 Levator scapulae muscle	**17** Teres minor muscle
8 Long head of triceps brachii muscle	**18** Thoracic part of thoracolumbar fascia
9 Medial border of scapula	**19** Trapezius muscle (cut and reflected)
10 Posterior cutaneous nerve to the arm	

Right shoulder deep dissection of scapular region
as seen from above and behind

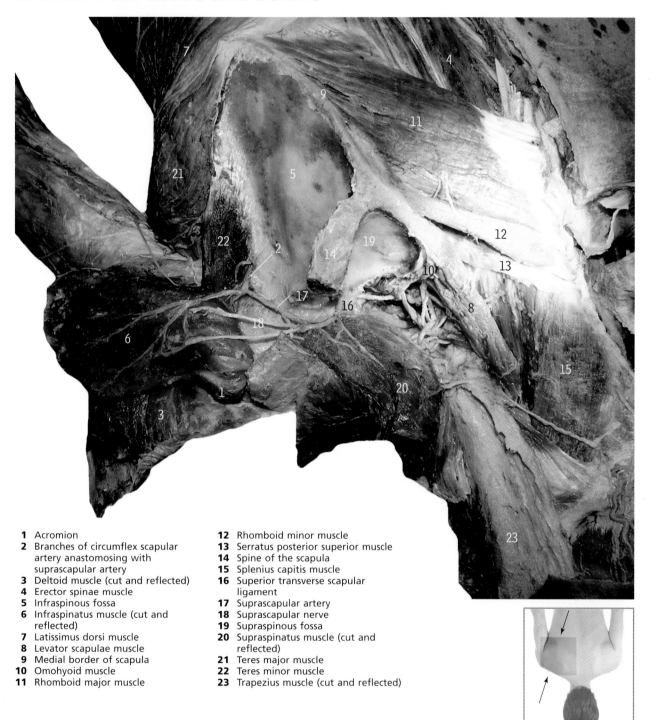

1 Acromion
2 Branches of circumflex scapular artery anastomosing with suprascapular artery
3 Deltoid muscle (cut and reflected)
4 Erector spinae muscle
5 Infraspinous fossa
6 Infraspinatus muscle (cut and reflected)
7 Latissimus dorsi muscle
8 Levator scapulae muscle
9 Medial border of scapula
10 Omohyoid muscle
11 Rhomboid major muscle
12 Rhomboid minor muscle
13 Serratus posterior superior muscle
14 Spine of the scapula
15 Splenius capitis muscle
16 Superior transverse scapular ligament
17 Suprascapular artery
18 Suprascapular nerve
19 Supraspinous fossa
20 Supraspinatus muscle (cut and reflected)
21 Teres major muscle
22 Teres minor muscle
23 Trapezius muscle (cut and reflected)

Scapular arterial anastomoses, see pages 170–172.

Right shoulder joint Ⓐ cross section Ⓑ axial MR image

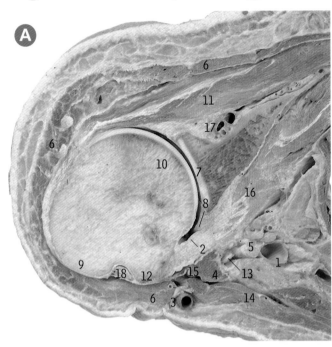

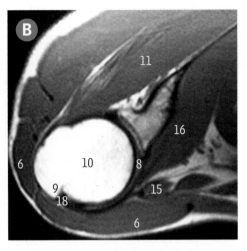

Viewed from below, this cadaveric section shows the articulation of the head of the humerus (10) with the glenoid cavity of the scapula (7). The tendon of the long head of biceps (18) lies in the groove between the greater and lesser tubercles of the humerus (9 and 12). Subscapularis (16) passes immediately in front of the joint, and infraspinatus (11) behind it. Compare the MR image in B with features in A.

1 Axillary artery
2 Capsule
3 Cephalic vein
4 Coracobrachialis
5 Cords of brachial plexus
6 Deltoid
7 Glenoid cavity
8 Glenoid labrum
9 Greater tubercle
10 Head of humerus
11 Infraspinatus
12 Lesser tubercle
13 Musculocutaneous nerve
14 Pectoralis major
15 Short head of biceps
16 Subscapularis
17 Suprascapular nerve and vessels
18 Tendon of long head of biceps in intertubercular groove

Right shoulder joint Ⓒ from the front

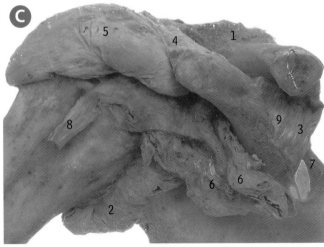

The synovial joint cavity inside the capsule (2) and the subacromial bursa (5) have been injected separately with green resin.

1 Acromioclavicular joint
2 Capsule of shoulder joint
3 Conoid ligament
4 Coracoacromial ligament
5 Subacromial bursa
6 Subscapularis bursa
7 Superior transverse scapular (suprascapular) ligament
8 Tendon of long head of biceps
9 Trapezoid ligament

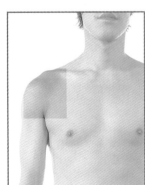

Ⓓ Shoulder coronal oblique MR arthrogram

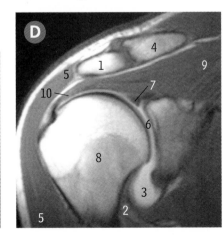

1 Acromion
2 Axillary nerve and circumflex humeral vessels
3 Axillary recess of shoulder joint
4 Clavicle
5 Deltoid
6 Glenoid cavity
7 Glenoid labrum
8 Humerus
9 Supraspinatus muscle
10 Supraspinatus tendon

E Right Shoulder *dissection, coronal section*

E

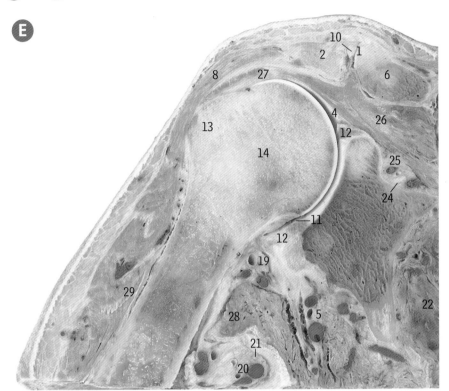

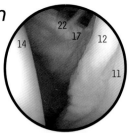

This is the first view of the shoulder on entering the joint from the posterior aspect with an arthroscope. The humerus head is on the left, the subscapularis tendon is in the middle and the glenoid and the surrounding labrum is on the right. The joint is slightly distracted with the aid of traction and also the fluid in the joint used in the arthroscopy.

G Right shoulder joint *opened from behind*

In this view, after removing all the posterior part of the capsule, the inner surface of the front of the capsule (4) is seen, with its reinforcing glenohumeral ligaments (15, 17 and 23).

F Right shoulder *radiograph*

anteroposterior projection in a 9-year-old child

F

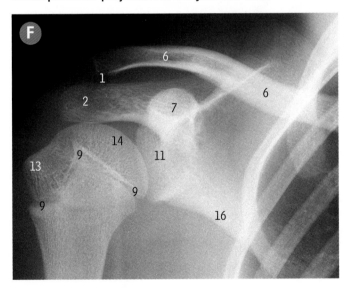

G

The joint cavity communicates with the subscapularis bursa through an opening between the superior and middle glenohumeral ligaments.

The tendon of the long head of biceps is continuous with the glenoid labrum.

1 Acromioclavicular joint	**10** Fibrocartilaginous disc	**18** Opening into subscapularis bursa	**24** Suprascapular nerve
2 Acromion	**11** Glenoid cavity	**19** Posterior circumflex humeral vessels	**25** Suprascapular vessels
3 Biceps, long head	**12** Glenoid labrum	**20** Profunda brachii vessels	**26** Supraspinatus
4 Capsule	**13** Greater tubercle	**21** Radial nerve	**27** Supraspinatus tendon
5 Circumflex scapular vessels	**14** Head of humerus	**22** Subscapularis	**28** Teres major
6 Clavicle	**15** Inferior glenohumeral ligament	**23** Superior glenohumeral ligament	**29** Triceps, lateral head
7 Coracoid process	**16** Lateral border of scapula		
8 Deltoid	**17** Middle glenohumeral ligament		
9 Epiphysial line			

Bicipital tendinitis and rupture, calcific tendinitis, painful arc syndrome/rotator cuff tear, see pages 170–172.

Right axilla *anterior chest wall*

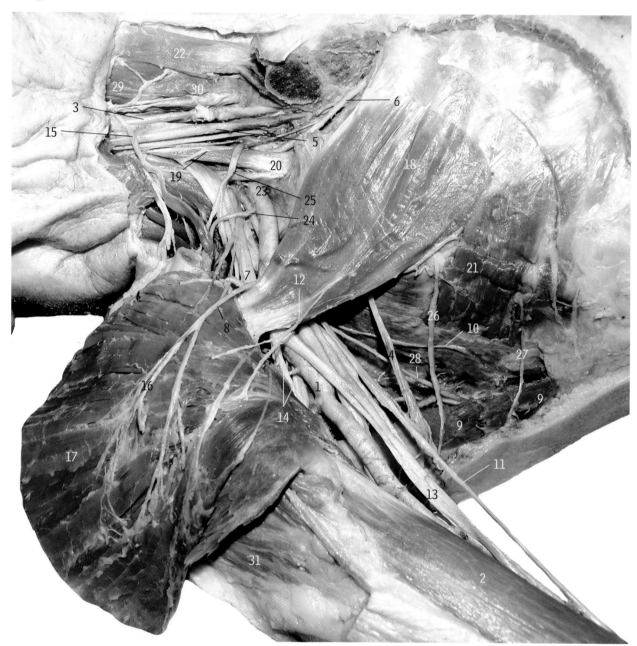

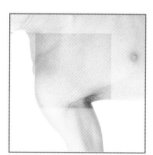

1 Axillary artery	**17** Pectoralis major muscle (reflected)
2 Biceps brachii muscle	**18** Pectoralis minor muscle
3 Common carotid artery	**19** Phrenic nerve
4 Intercostobrachial nerve	**20** Scalenus anterior muscle
5 Internal jugular vein	**21** Serratus anterior muscle
6 Internal thoracic artery	**22** Sternohyoid muscle
7 Lateral cord of brachial plexus	**23** Subclavian artery
8 Lateral pectoral nerve	**24** Suprascapular artery
9 Latissimus dorsi muscle	**25** Suprsascapular nerve
10 Long thoracic nerve	**26** T3 spinal nerve
11 Medial cutaneous nerve to the forearm	**27** T4 spinal nerve
12 Medial pectoral nerve	**28** Thoracodorsal nerve
13 Median nerve	**29** Thyrohyoid muscle
14 Musculocutaneous nerve	**30** Thyroid gland
15 Omohyoid tendon	**31** Triceps brachii muscle
16 Pectoral branch of thoracoacromial trunk	

Axillary-subclavian vein thrombosis, cervical rib, see pages 170–172.

Right axilla and brachial plexus *from the front*

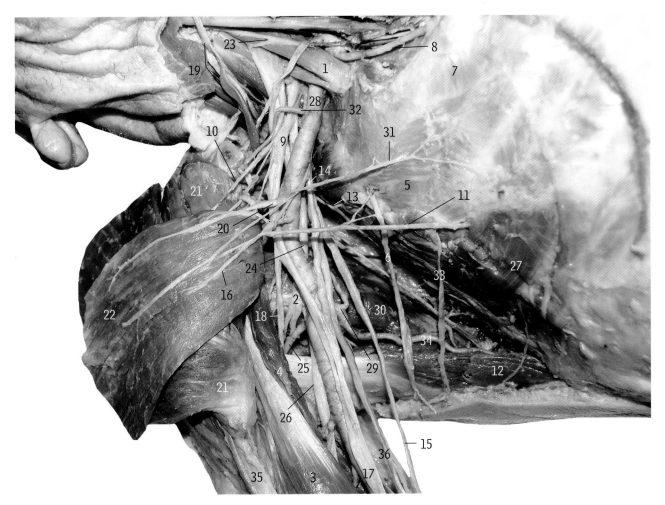

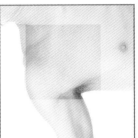

1 Anterior scalene muscle	**20** Pectoral branch of thoracoacromial trunk
2 Axillary nerve	**21** Pectoralis major muscle (reflected)
3 Biceps brachii muscle	**22** Pectoralis minor muscle (reflected)
4 Coracobrachialis	**23** Phrenic nerve
5 External intercostal muscle	**24** Posterior cord of brachial plexus
6 Intercostobrachial nerve	**25** Posterior circumflex humeral artery
7 Internal intercostal muscle	**26** Radial nerve
8 Internal thoracic artery	**27** Serratus anterior muscle
9 Lateral cord of brachial plexus	**28** Subclavian artery
10 Lateral pectoral nerve	**29** Subscapular trunk
11 Lateral thoracic artery	**30** Subscapularis muscle
12 Latissimus dorsi muscle	**31** Superior thoracic artery
13 Long thoracic nerve	**32** Suprascapular artery
14 Medial cord of brachial plexus	**33** T3 spinal nerve
15 Medial cutaneous nerve to the forearm	**34** Thoracodorsal artery
16 Medial pectoral nerve	**35** Triceps brachii muscle
17 Median nerve	**36** Ulnar nerve
18 Musculocutaneous nerve	
19 Omohyoid muscle	

Erb's palsy, winging of the scapula, see pages 170–172.

Right brachial plexus *reflected to reveal arterial branches*

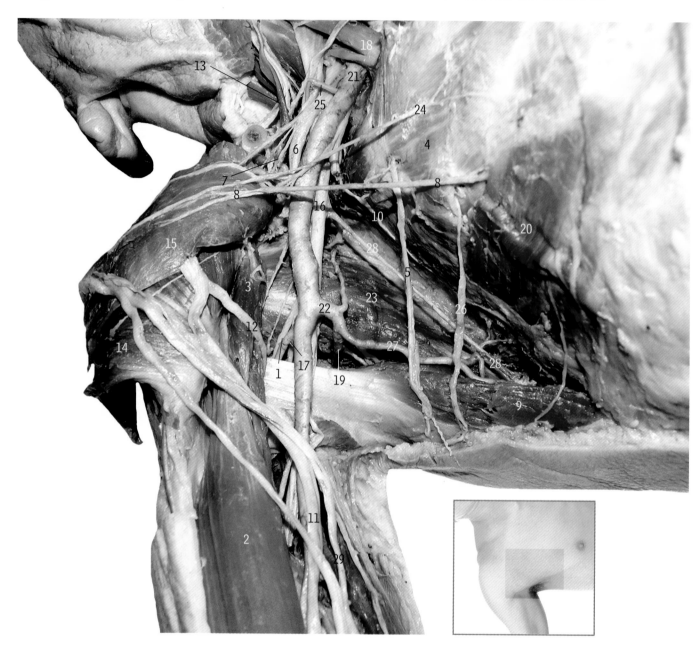

1 Axillary nerve	**9** Latissimus dorsi muscle	**16** Posterior cord of brachial plexus	**23** Subscapularis muscle
2 Biceps brachii muscle	**10** Long thoracic nerve		**24** Superior thoracic artery
3 Coracobrachialis muscle	**11** Median nerve	**17** Posterior circumflex humeral artery	**25** Suprascapular artery
4 External intercostal muscle	**12** Musculocutaneous nerve		**26** T3 spinal nerve
5 Intercostobrachial nerve	**13** Omohyoid muscle	**18** Scalenus anterior muscle	**27** Thoracodorsal artery
6 Lateral cord of brachial plexus	**14** Pectoralis major muscle (reflected)	**19** Scapular circumflex artery	**28** Thoracodorsal nerve
7 Lateral pectoral nerve	**15** Pectoralis minor muscle (reflected)	**20** Serratus anterior muscle	**29** Ulnar nerve
8 Lateral thoracic artery		**21** Subclavian artery	
		22 Subscapular trunk	

Axillary artery aneurysm, vascular abnormalities, winging of the scapula, see pages 170–172.

Left brachial plexus and branches *from the front*

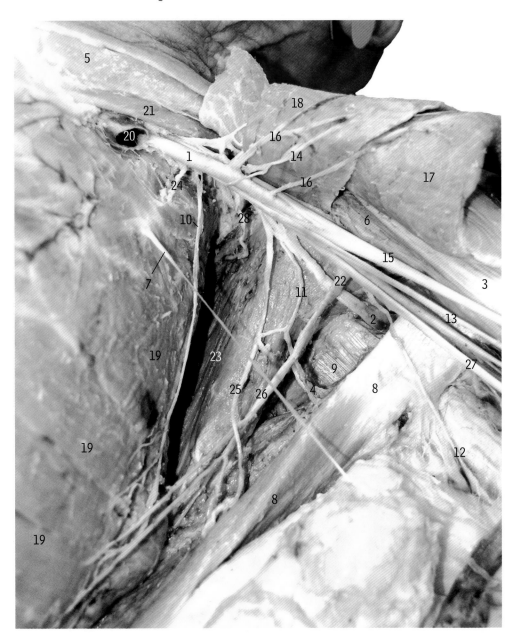

1	Axillary artery	**15**	Median nerve
2	Axillary nerve (passing through the quadrangular space)	**16**	Pectoral arteries
		17	Pectoralis major muscle (reflected)
3	Biceps brachii muscle	**18**	Pectoralis minor muscle (reflected)
4	Circumflex scapular artery	**19**	Serratus anterior muscle
5	Clavicle	**20**	Subclavian vein (cut)
6	Coracobrachialis muscle	**21**	Subclavius muscle
7	Intercostobrachial nerve	**22**	Subscapular trunk
8	Latissimus dorsi muscle	**23**	Subscapularis muscle
9	Long head of triceps brachii muscle	**24**	Superior thoracic artery
10	Long thoracic nerve	**25**	Thoracodorsal (middle subscapular) nerve
11	Lower subscapular nerve	**26**	Thoracodorsal artery
12	Medial cutaneous nerve to the arm	**27**	Ulnar nerve
13	Medial cutaneous nerve to the forearm	**28**	Upper subscapular nerve
14	Medial pectoral nerve		

Brachial plexus block, see pages 170–172.

Right brachial plexus and branches

In this front view of the plexus, all the blood vessels have been removed to show the cords of the plexus and their branches more clearly. Note the 'capital M' pattern formed by the musculocutaneous nerve (18), the lateral root of the median nerve (8), the median nerve itself (17), the medial root of the median nerve (16) and the ulnar nerve (26). In this specimen, the tendon of latissimus dorsi (9) is unusually broad and has become blended with the long head of triceps (10).

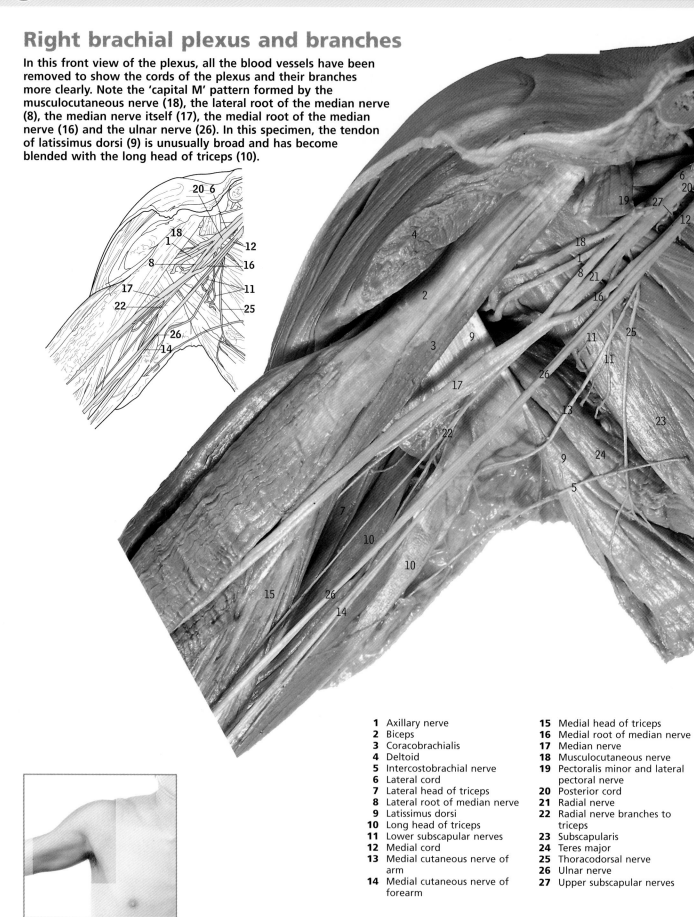

1	Axillary nerve	15	Medial head of triceps
2	Biceps	16	Medial root of median nerve
3	Coracobrachialis	17	Median nerve
4	Deltoid	18	Musculocutaneous nerve
5	Intercostobrachial nerve	19	Pectoralis minor and lateral
6	Lateral cord		pectoral nerve
7	Lateral head of triceps	20	Posterior cord
8	Lateral root of median nerve	21	Radial nerve
9	Latissimus dorsi	22	Radial nerve branches to
10	Long head of triceps		triceps
11	Lower subscapular nerves	23	Subscapularis
12	Medial cord	24	Teres major
13	Medial cutaneous nerve of	25	Thoracodorsal nerve
	arm	26	Ulnar nerve
14	Medial cutaneous nerve of	27	Upper subscapular nerves
	forearm		

Dislocation of the shoulder, see pages 170–172.

A Right arm *vessels and nerves, from the front*

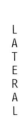

Biceps (16 and 8) has been turned laterally to show the musculocutaneous nerve (12) emerging from coracobrachialis (6), giving branches to biceps and brachialis (14 and 13) and becoming the lateral cutaneous nerve of the forearm (7) on the lateral side of the biceps tendon (17).

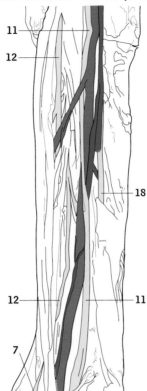

The median nerve (11) gradually crosses over in front of the brachial artery (2) from the lateral to the medial side. The ulnar nerve (18) passes behind the medial intermuscular septum (10), and the end of the basilic vein (1) is seen joining a vena comitans (19) of the brachial artery to form the brachial vein (3).

1	Basilic vein (cut end)	**11**	Median nerve
2	Brachial artery	**12**	Musculocutaneous nerve
3	Brachial vein	**13**	Nerve to brachialis
4	Brachialis	**14**	Nerve to short head of
5	Brachioradialis		biceps
6	Coracobrachialis	**15**	Pronator teres
7	Lateral cutaneous nerve	**16**	Short head of biceps
	of forearm	**17**	Tendon of biceps
8	Long head of biceps	**18**	Ulnar nerve
9	Long head of triceps	**19**	Vena comitans of
10	Medial intermuscular		brachial artery
	septum		

The musculocutaneous nerve (A12) supplies coracobrachialis (A6), biceps (A16 and 8) and brachialis (A4), and at the level where the muscle fibres of biceps become tendinous (A17) it pierces the deep fascia to become the lateral cutaneous nerve of the forearm (A7).

The median nerve does not give off any muscular branches in the arm.

The ulnar nerve (A18) leaves the anterior compartment of the arm by piercing the medial intermuscular septum (A10), and does not give off any muscular branches in the arm.

B Right arm *cross-section, from below*

Looking from the elbow towards the shoulder, the section is taken through the middle of the arm. The musculocutaneous nerve (9) lies between brachialis (4) and biceps (2), and the median nerve (8) is on the medial side of the brachial artery (3) which has several venae comitantes adjacent (unlabelled). The ulnar nerve (13), with the superior ulnar collateral artery (11) beside it, is behind the median nerve (8) and the basilic vein (1). The radial nerve and the profunda brachii vessels (10) are in the posterior compartment at the lateral side of the humerus (6).

FRONT

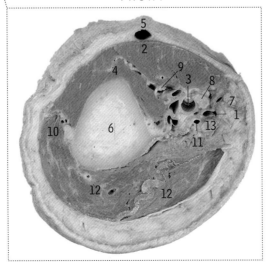

1	Basilic vein
2	Biceps
3	Brachial artery
4	Brachialis
5	Cephalic vein
6	Humerus
7	Medial cutaneous nerve of forearm
8	Median nerve
9	Musculocutaneous nerve
10	Radial nerve and profunda brachii vessels
11	Superior ulnar collateral artery
12	Triceps
13	Ulnar nerve

Volkmann's ischaemic contracture, see pages 170–172.

Right arm *posterior view*

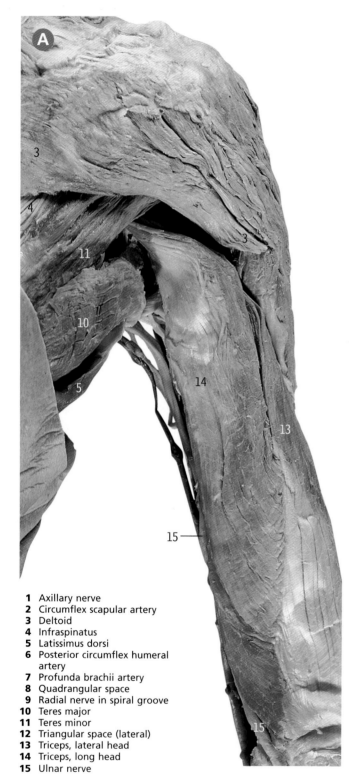

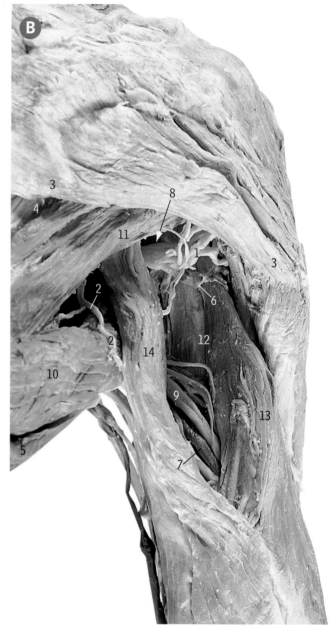

1 Axillary nerve
2 Circumflex scapular artery
3 Deltoid
4 Infraspinatus
5 Latissimus dorsi
6 Posterior circumflex humeral
artery
7 Profunda brachii artery
8 Quadrangular space
9 Radial nerve in spiral groove
10 Teres major
11 Teres minor
12 Triangular space (lateral)
13 Triceps, lateral head
14 Triceps, long head
15 Ulnar nerve

A after removal of skin and
subcutaneous fat

B after muscle separation to
demonstrate spaces and
neurovascular bundle

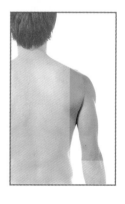

Radial nerve palsy, see pages 170–172.

C Left elbow *surface markings, from behind*

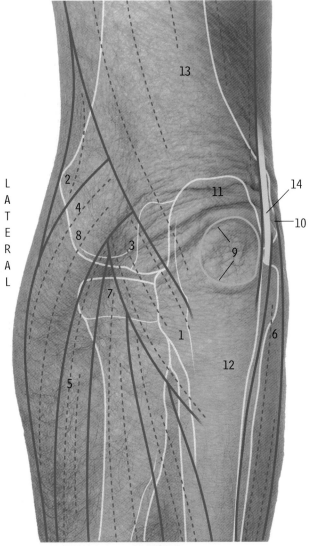

D Right elbow *medial view from behind*

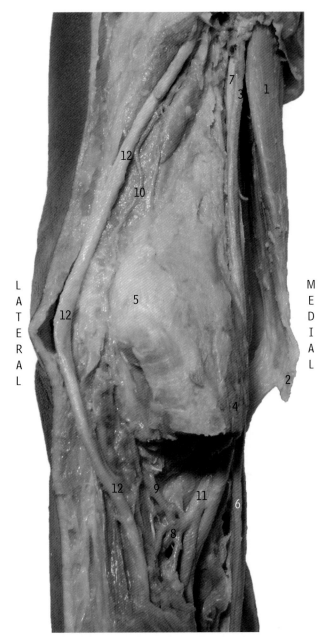

With the elbow fully extended, the extensor muscles (5, 4) form a bulge on the lateral side. In the adjacent hollow can be felt the head of the radius (7) and the capitulum of the humerus (3) which indicate the line of the humeroradial part of the elbow joint. The lateral and medial epicondyles of the humerus (8 and 10) are palpable on each side. Wrinkled skin lies at the back of the prominent olecranon of the ulna (11), and in this arm the margin of the olecranon bursa (9) is outlined. The most important structure in this region is the ulnar nerve (14) which is palpable as it lies in contact with the humerus behind the medial epicondyle (10). The posterior border of the ulna (12) is subcutaneous throughout its whole length.

1 Anconeus	9 Margin of olecranon bursa
2 Brachioradialis	10 Medial epicondyle of
3 Capitulum of humerus	humerus
4 Extensor carpi radialis longus	11 Olecranon of ulna
5 Extensor muscles	12 Posterior border of ulna
6 Flexor carpi ulnaris	13 Triceps
7 Head of radius	14 Ulnar nerve
8 Lateral epicondyle of humerus	

1 Biceps muscle
2 Bicipital aponeurosis
3 Brachial artery
4 Common flexor origin
5 Medial epicondyle
6 Median artery
7 Median nerve
8 Muscular arterial branches to flexors of forearm
9 Posterior ulnar recurrent artery
10 Superior ulnar collateral artery
11 Ulnar artery
12 Ulnar nerve

Note: high division and persistent median artery.

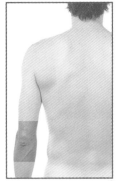

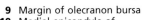

Olecranon bursitis, triceps tendon reflex, ulnar nerve palsy, see pages 170–172.

Left elbow and radioulnar joint

A from the medial side　　**B** from the lateral side

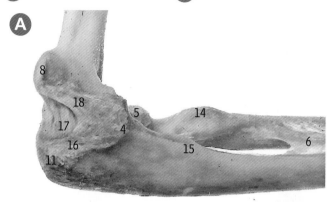

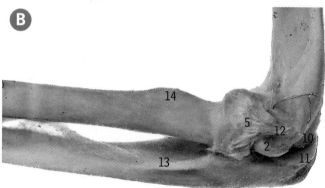

Right elbow and radioulnar joint

D from the medial side　　**E** from the lateral side

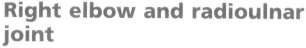

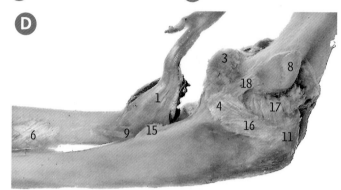

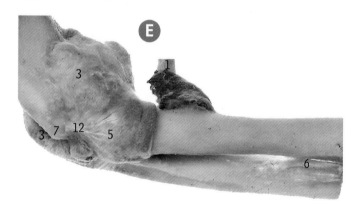

In A and B the forearm is flexed to a right angle. In D and E the forearm is partially flexed, and the synovial cavity within the capsule (3) and the bursa beneath the biceps tendon (1) have been injected with green resin.

1	Biceps tendon and underlying bursa	**11**	Olecranon process of ulna
2	Capitulum	**12**	Radial collateral ligament
3	Capsule (distended)	**13**	Supinator crest of ulna
4	Coronoid process of ulna	**14**	Tuberosity of radius
5	Head and neck of radius covered by annular ligament	**15**	Tuberosity of ulna
6	Interosseous membrane	**16**	Ulnar collateral ligament: oblique band
7	Lateral epicondyle	**17**	Ulnar collateral ligament: posterior band
8	Medial epicondyle	**18**	Ulnar collateral ligament: upper band
9	Oblique cord		
10	Olecranon fossa		

Elbow *radiographs*

C lateral projection

F AP projection

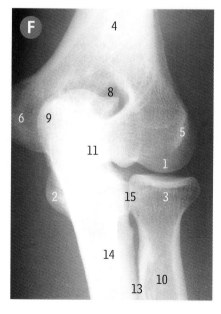

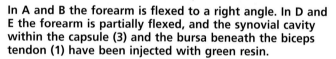

1	Capitulum of humerus
2	Coronoid process of ulna
3	Head of radius
4	Humerus
5	Lateral epicondyle of humerus
6	Medial epicondyle of humerus
7	Neck of radius
8	Olecranon fossa of humerus
9	Olecranon process of ulna
10	Radius
11	Trochlea of humerus
12	Trochlear notch of ulna
13	Tuberosity of radius
14	Ulna
15	Radioulnar joint

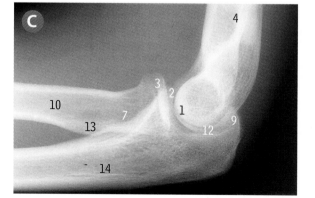

Dislocation of the radial head, see pages 170–172.

Left elbow joint

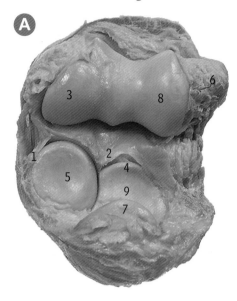

A

opened from behind

The joint has been 'forced open' from behind: the capitulum (3) and trochlea (8) of the lower end of the humerus are seen from below with the forearm in forced flexion to show the upper ends of the radius and ulna (5 and 9) from above.

1 Annular ligament
2 Anterior part of capsule
3 Capitulum of humerus
4 Coronoid process of ulna
5 Head of radius
6 Medial epicondyle of humerus
7 Olecranon process of ulna
8 Trochlea of humerus
9 Trochlear notch of ulna

Left elbow

B

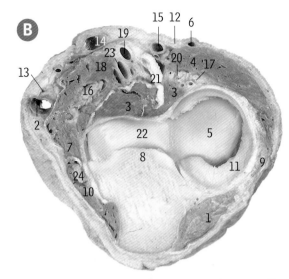

D Right elbow *coronal section*

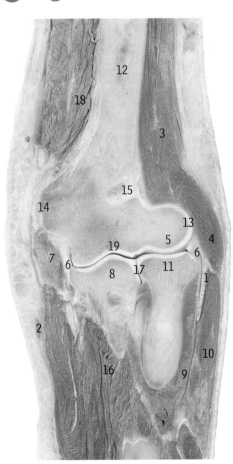

1 Annular ligament
2 Basilic vein
3 Brachialis
4 Brachioradialis
5 Capitulum of humerus
6 Capsule
7 Common flexor origin
8 Coronoid process of ulna
9 Extensor carpi radialis brevis
10 Extensor carpi radialis longus
11 Head of radius
12 Humerus
13 Lateral epicondyle
14 Medial epicondyle
15 Olecranon fossa
16 Pronator teres
17 Radio-ulnar joint, proximal
18 Triceps, medial head
19 Trochlea of humerus

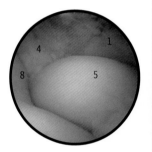

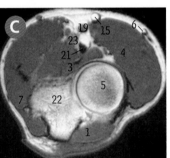

This is the arthroscopic view of an elbow joint. The view is from the superior aspect showing the orientation and the articulation of the radio-capitellar joint. Just distal to the radial head is the proximal edge of the annular ligament. The radial head is seen articulating with the coronoid process of the ulna.

B cross-section   ## C axial MR image

The section is viewed from below, looking towards the shoulder, and is just below the point where the brachial artery has divided into radial and ulnar arteries (19 and 23). The cut has passed immediately below the trochlea (22) and capitulum (5) of the humerus, and has gone through the coronoid process of the ulna (8). The radial nerve (20) and its posterior interosseous branch (17) lie between brachioradialis (4) and brachialis (3). The median nerve (16) is under the main part of pronator teres (18), and the ulnar nerve (24) is passing under flexor carpi ulnaris (10).

1 Anconeus
2 Basilic vein
3 Brachialis
4 Brachioradialis
5 Capitulum of humerus
6 Cephalic vein
7 Common flexor origin
8 Coronoid process of ulna
9 Extensor carpi radialis longus and brevis
10 Flexor carpi ulnaris
11 Fringe of synovial membrane
12 Lateral cutaneous nerve of forearm
13 Medial cutaneous nerve of forearm
14 Median basilic vein
15 Median cephalic vein
16 Median nerve
17 Posterior interosseous nerve
18 Pronator teres
19 Radial artery
20 Radial nerve
21 Tendon of biceps brachii
22 Trochlea of humerus
23 Ulnar artery
24 Ulnar nerve

Elbow arthroscopy, wrist arthroscopy, see pages 170–172.

Left cubital fossa (A) *surface markings* (B) *superficial veins*

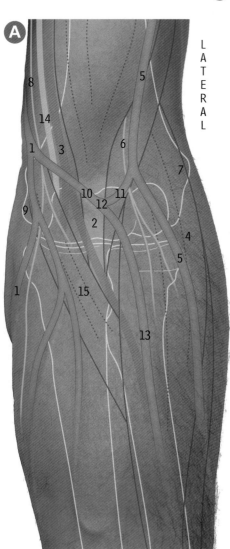

L
A
T
E
R
A
L

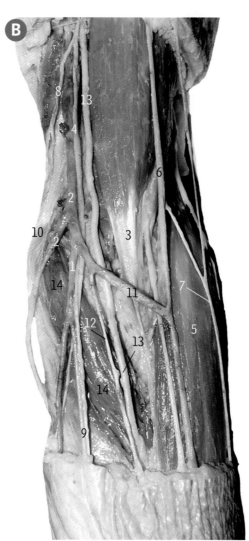

The superficial veins on the front of the elbow such as the cephalic (5) and basilic (1) and their intercommunicating tributaries are those most commonly used for intravenous injections and obtaining specimens of venous blood. The pattern of veins is typically M-shaped (as in A) or H-shaped (as in B), but there is much variation and it is not always possible or necessary to name every vessel.

The order of the structures in the cubital fossa from lateral to medial is: biceps tendon (2), brachial artery (3) and median nerve (14).

A

1 Basilic vein
2 Biceps tendon
3 Brachial artery
4 Brachioradialis
5 Cephalic vein
6 Lateral cutaneous nerve of forearm
7 Lateral epicondyle
8 Medial cutaneous nerve of forearm
9 Medial epicondyle
10 Median basilic vein
11 Median cephalic vein
12 Median cubital vein
13 Median forearm vein
14 Median nerve
15 Pronator teres

B

1 Accessory basilic vein
2 Basilic vein
3 Biceps brachii tendon
4 Brachial artery
5 Brachioradialis muscle
6 Cephalic vein
7 Lateral cutaneous nerve of forearm
8 Medial cutaneous nerve of arm
9 Medial cutaneous nerve of forearm
10 Medial epicondyle
11 Median cubital vein
12 Median forearm vein
13 Median nerve
14 Pronator teres muscle

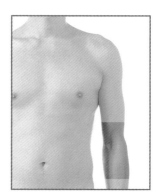

Auscultation of the brachial pulse, biceps tendon reflex, golfer's elbow, tennis elbow, see pages 170–172.

Left elbow and upper forearm
C *deeper dissection* **D** *deeper dissection of nerves and arteries*

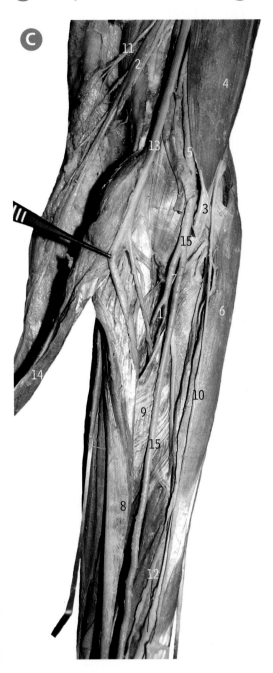

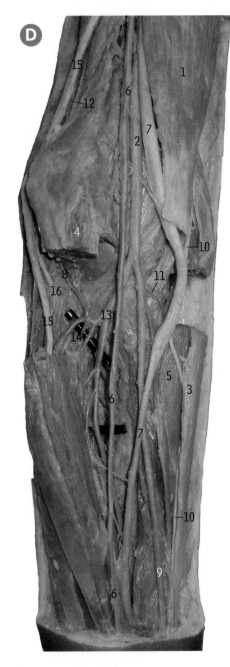

1	Anterior interosseous artery	**10**	Lateral cutaneous nerve of forearm
2	Basilic vein	**11**	Medial cutaneous nerve of arm
3	Biceps brachii aponeurosis, reflected	**12**	Median nerve
4	Biceps brachii muscle	**13**	Median nerve, reflected medially
5	Brachial artery	**14**	Pronator teres muscle, reflected
6	Brachioradialis muscle	**15**	Ulnar artery
7	Common interosseous artery		
8	Flexor carpi ulnaris muscle		
9	Flexor digitorum profundus muscle		

1	Biceps	**11**	Radial recurrent artery
2	Brachial artery	**12**	Superior ulnar collateral artery
3	Brachioradialis	**13**	Ulnar artery
4	Common flexor origin	**14**	Ulnar artery, branches to forearm flexors
5	Extensor carpi radialis longus	**15**	Ulnar nerve
6	Median artery	**16**	Ulnar nerve, branch to flexor carpi ulnaris
7	Median nerve, pulled laterally		
8	Posterior ulnar recurrent artery		
9	Radial artery		
10	Radial nerve, superficial branch		

Note: high division and persistent median artery

Anterior interosseous nerve entrapment, arterial puncture at the elbow, see pages 170–172.

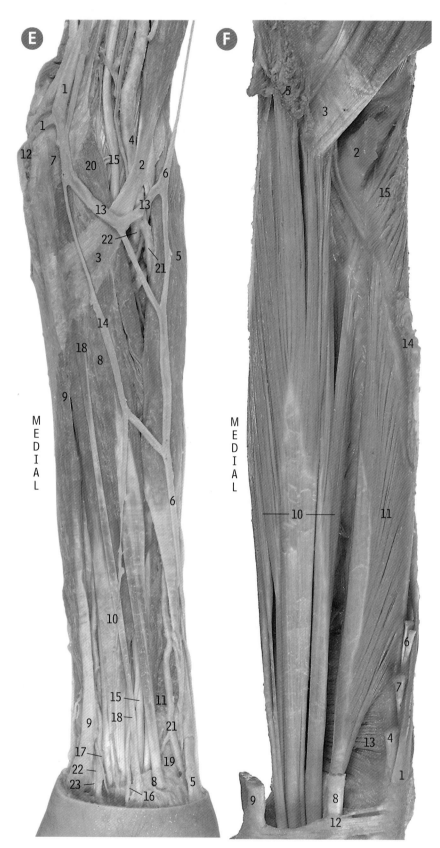

E Left forearm superficial muscles, from the front

Skin and fascia have been removed, but the larger superficial veins (1, 6 and 13) have been preserved. On the lateral side, the radial artery (21) is largely covered by brachioradialis (5). At the wrist the tendon of flexor carpi radialis (8) has the radial artery (21) on its lateral side; on its medial side is the median nerve (15), slightly overlapped from the medial side by the tendon of palmaris longus (18) (if present; it is absent in 13% of forearms).

1	Basilic vein	13	Median cubital vein
2	Biceps tendon	14	Median forearm
3	Bicipital aponeurosis		vein
4	Brachial artery	15	Median nerve
5	Brachioradialis	16	Palmar branch of
6	Cephalic vein		median nerve
7	Common flexor	17	Palmar branch of
	origin		ulnar nerve
8	Flexor carpi radialis	18	Palmaris longus
9	Flexor carpi ulnaris	19	Pronator quadratus
10	Flexor digitorum	20	Pronator teres
	superficialis	21	Radial artery
11	Flexor pollicis	22	Ulnar artery
	longus	23	Ulnar nerve
12	Medial epicondyle		

F Left forearm deep muscles, from the front

All vessels and nerves have been removed, together with the superficial muscles, to show the deep flexor group – flexor digitorum profundus (10), flexor pollicis longus (11) and pronator quadratus (13).

1	Abductor pollicis longus
2	Biceps
3	Brachialis
4	Brachioradialis
5	Common flexor origin
6	Extensor carpi radialis brevis
7	Extensor carpi radialis longus
8	Flexor carpi radialis
9	Flexor carpi ulnaris
10	Flexor digitorum profundus
11	Flexor pollicis longus
12	Flexor retinaculum
13	Pronator quadratus
14	Pronator teres
15	Supinator

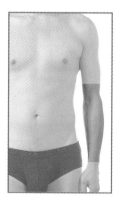

Venepuncture of the upper limb, venous cutdown, see pages 170–172.

A Right cubital fossa and forearm *arteries*

The arteries have been injected, and after removal of most of the superficial muscles, the brachial artery (4) is seen dividing into the radial artery (18) and the ulnar artery (20). The radial artery gives off the radial recurrent (19) which runs upwards in front of supinator, giving branches to the carpal extensor muscles (10 and 9). The ulnar artery gives off the anterior and posterior ulnar recurrent vessels (2 and 15), and its common interosseous branch (8) is seen giving off the anterior interosseous (1) which passes down in front of the interosseous membrane between flexor pollicis longus (13) and flexor digitorum profundus (12).

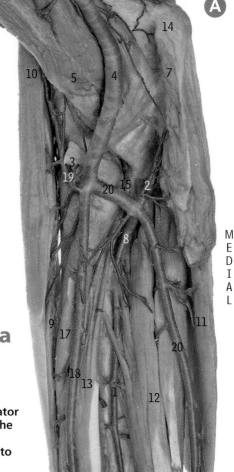

1 Anterior interosseous artery overlying interosseous membrane
2 Anterior ulnar recurrent artery
3 Biceps tendon
4 Brachial artery
5 Brachialis
6 Brachioradialis
7 Common flexor origin

8 Common interosseous artery
9 Extensor carpi radialis brevis
10 Extensor carpi radialis longus
11 Flexor carpi ulnaris
12 Flexor digitorum profundus
13 Flexor pollicis longus

14 Medial epicondyle of humerus
15 Posterior ulnar recurrent artery
16 Pronator quadratus
17 Pronator teres
18 Radial artery
19 Radial recurrent artery overlying supinator
20 Ulnar artery

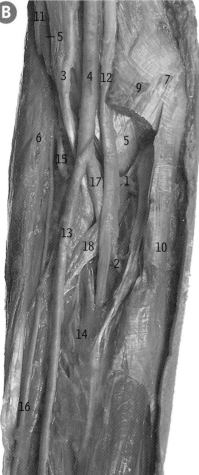

B Right cubital fossa and forearm *arteries and nerves*

Most of the humeral origins of pronator teres and flexor carpi radialis (from the common flexor origin, 9 and 7) and palmaris longus have been removed to show the median nerve (12) passing superficial to the deep head of pronator teres (18) and then deep to the upper border of the radial head of flexor digitorum superficialis (14).

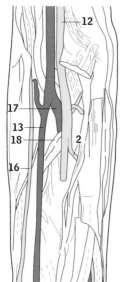

1 A muscular branch of median nerve
2 Anterior interosseous nerve
3 Biceps
4 Brachial artery
5 Brachialis
6 Brachioradialis (displaced laterally)
7 Common flexor origin
8 Flexor carpi ulnaris (displaced medially)
9 Humeral head of pronator teres
10 Humero-ulnar head of flexor digitorum superficialis
11 Lateral cutaneous nerve of forearm
12 Median nerve
13 Radial artery
14 Radial head of flexor digitorum superficialis
15 Radial recurrent artery
16 Superficial terminal branch of radial nerve overlying extensor carpi radialis longus
17 Ulnar artery
18 Ulnar head of pronator teres
19 Ulnar nerve and artery

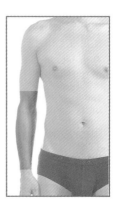

Anterior interosseous nerve entrapment, Volkmann's ischaemic contracture, see pages 170–172.

Ⓐ Left elbow from the lateral side

With the forearm in mid-pronation and seen from the lateral side so that the radius (7) lies in front of the ulna, all muscles have been removed except supinator (8) to show its humeral and ulnar origins (see notes).

1 Annular ligament
2 Capitulum of humerus
3 Interosseous membrane
4 Lateral epicondyle
5 Posterior interosseous nerve
6 Radial collateral ligament
7 Radius
8 Supinator
9 Supinator crest of ulna

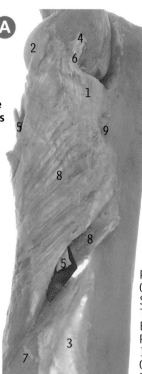

Ⓑ Left forearm *deep muscles, from the lateral side*

1 Abductor pollicis longus
2 Biceps brachii
3 Extensor carpi radialis brevis
4 Ext ensor carpi radialis longus (double)
5 Extensor indicis
6 Extensor pollicis brevis
7 Extensor pollicis longus
8 Extensor retinaculum
9 Flexor pollicis longus
10 Pronator teres
11 Supinator

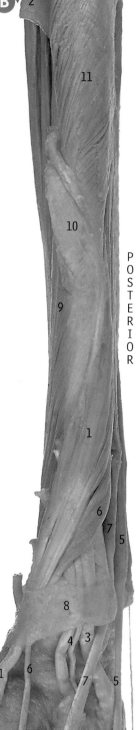

Ⓒ Left forearm *posterior interosseous nerve, from behind*

1 Abductor pollicis longus
2 Branch of posterior interosseous artery
3 Extensor carpi radialis brevis
4 Extensor carpi radialis longus
5 Extensor carpi ulnaris
6 Extensor digitorum
7 Extensor indicis
8 Extensor pollicis brevis
9 Extensor pollicis longus
10 Extensor retinaculum
11 Posterior interosseous nerve
12 Supinator

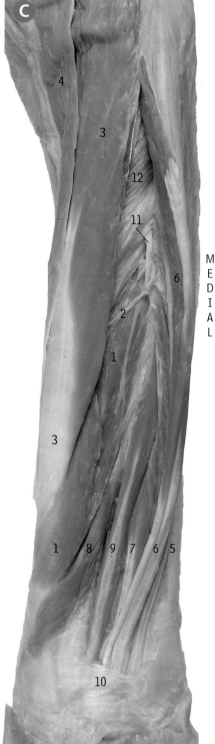

The fibres of the interosseous membrane (A3) pass obliquely downwards from the radius (A7) to the ulna, so transmitting weight from the hand and radius to the ulna.

The supinator muscle (A8) arises from the lateral epicondyle of the humerus (A4), radial collateral ligament (A6), annular ligament (A1), supinator crest of the ulna (A9) and bone in front of the crest (page 119, D10), and an aponeurosis overlying the muscle. From these origins, the fibres wrap themselves round the upper end of the radius above the pronator teres attachment, to be attached to the lateral surface of the radius and extending anteriorly and posteriorly as far as the tuberosity of the radius.

Posterior interosseous nerve entrapment, see pages 170–172.

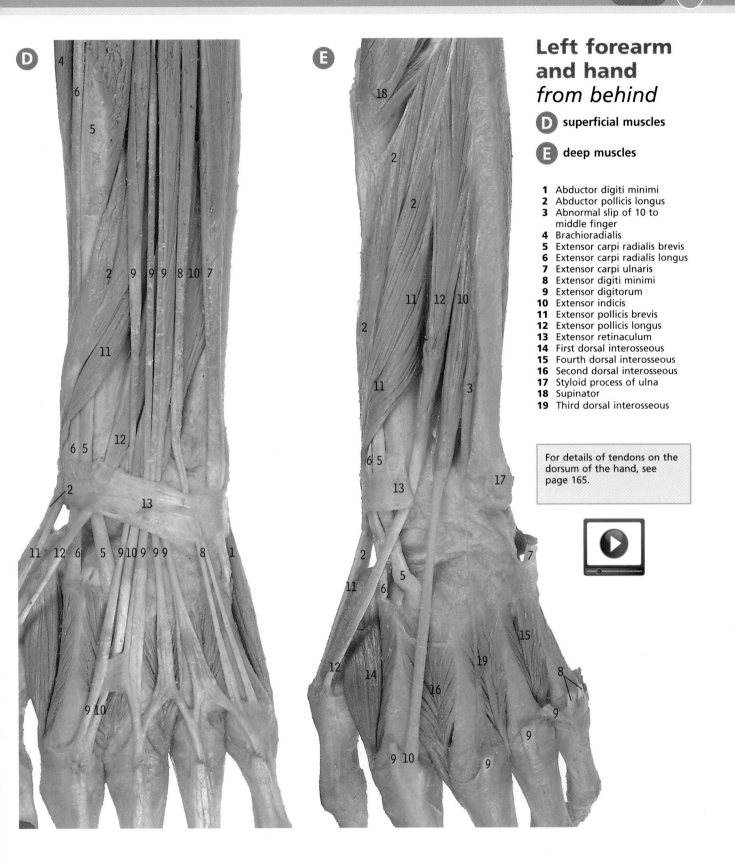

D

E

Left forearm and hand
from behind

D superficial muscles

E deep muscles

1 Abductor digiti minimi
2 Abductor pollicis longus
3 Abnormal slip of 10 to middle finger
4 Brachioradialis
5 Extensor carpi radialis brevis
6 Extensor carpi radialis longus
7 Extensor carpi ulnaris
8 Extensor digiti minimi
9 Extensor digitorum
10 Extensor indicis
11 Extensor pollicis brevis
12 Extensor pollicis longus
13 Extensor retinaculum
14 First dorsal interosseous
15 Fourth dorsal interosseous
16 Second dorsal interosseous
17 Styloid process of ulna
18 Supinator
19 Third dorsal interosseous

For details of tendons on the dorsum of the hand, see page 165.

De Quervain's disease, wrist drop, see pages 170–172.

A Palm of left hand

1 Abductor digiti minimi
2 Abductor pollicis brevis
3 Adductor pollicis
4 Distal transverse crease
5 Distal wrist crease
6 Flexor carpi radialis
7 Flexor carpi ulnaris
8 Flexor digiti minimi brevis
9 Flexor pollicis brevis
10 Head of metacarpal
11 Hook of hamate
12 Level of deep palmar arch
13 Level of superficial palmar arch
14 Longitudinal crease
15 Median nerve
16 Middle wrist crease
17 Palmaris brevis
18 Palmaris longus
19 Pisiform
20 Proximal transverse crease
21 Proximal wrist crease
22 Radial artery
23 Thenar eminence
24 Ulnar artery and nerve

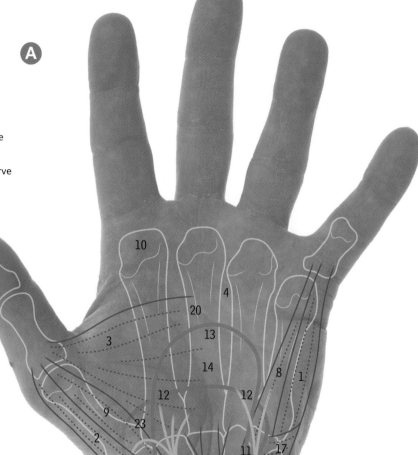

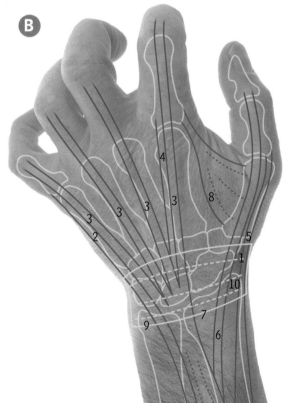

B Dorsum of left hand

The fingers are extended at the metacarpophalangeal joints, causing the extensor tendons of the fingers (2, 3 and 4) to stand out, and partially flexed at the interphalangeal joints. The thumb is extended at the carpometacarpal joint and partially flexed at the metacarpophalangeal and interphalangeal joints. The lines proximal to the bases of the fingers indicate the ends of the heads of the metacarpals and the level of the metacarpophalangeal joints. The anatomical snuffbox (1) is the hollow between the tendons of abductor pollicis longus and extensor pollicis brevis (5) laterally and extensor pollicis longus (6) medially.

1 Anatomical snuffbox
2 Extensor digiti minimi
3 Extensor digitorum
4 Extensor indicis
5 Extensor pollicis brevis and abductor pollicis longus
6 Extensor pollicis longus
7 Extensor retinaculum
8 First dorsal interosseous
9 Head of ulna
10 Styloid process of radius

Fingers *movements*

A flexion of the metacarpophalangeal joints and flexion of the interphalangeal joints

B extension of the metacarpophalangeal joints and flexion of the interphalangeal joints

C extension of the metacarpophalangeal and interphalangeal joints

When 'making a fist' with all finger joints flexed (A), the heads of the metacarpals (6) form the knuckles. To extend the metacarpophalangeal joints (B9) requires the activity of the long extensor tendons of the fingers, but to extend the interphalangeal joints (C10 and 5) as well requires the activity of the interossei and lumbricals, pulling on the dorsal extensor expansions. Only if the metacarpophalangeal joints remain flexed can the long extensors extend the interphalangeal joints.

1 Base of distal phalanx
2 Base of metacarpal
3 Base of middle phalanx
4 Base of proximal phalanx
5 Distal interphalangeal joint
6 Head of metacarpal
7 Head of middle phalanx
8 Head of proximal phalanx
9 Metacarpophalangeal joint
10 Proximal interphalangeal joint

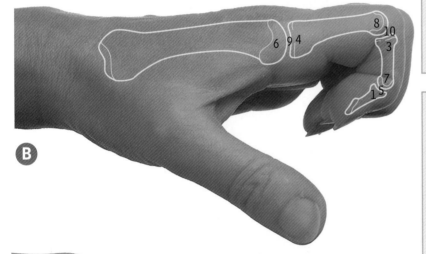

A Muscles producing movements at the metacarpophalangeal joints

Flexion: flexor digitorum profundus, flexor digitorum superficialis, lumbricals, interossei, with flexor digiti minimi brevis for the little finger and flexor pollicis longus, flexor pollicis brevis and the first palmar interosseous for the thumb.

Extension: extensor digitorum, extensor indicis (index finger) and extensor digiti minimi (little finger), with extensor pollicis longus and extensor pollicis brevis for the thumb.

Adduction: palmar interossei; when flexed, the long flexors assist.

Abduction: dorsal interossei and the long extensors, with abductor digiti minimi for the little finger.

B Muscles producing movements at the interphalangeal joints

Flexion: at the proximal joints, flexor digitorum superficialis and flexor digitorum profundus; at the distal joints, flexor digitorum profundus. For the thumb, flexor pollicis longus.

Extension: with the metacarpophalangeal joints flexed, extensor digitorum, extensor indicis and extensor digiti minimi; with the metacarpophalangeal joints extended, interossei and lumbricals. For the thumb, extensor pollicis longus.

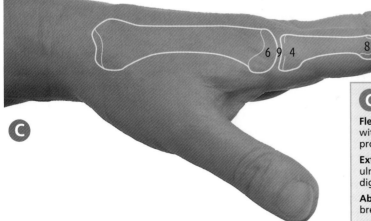

C Muscles producing movements at the wrist joint

Flexion: flexor carpi radialis, flexor carpi ulnaris, palmaris longus, with assistance from flexor digitorum superficialis, flexor digitorum profundus, flexor pollicis longus and abductor pollicis longus.

Extension: extensor carpi radialis longus and brevis, extensor carpi ulnaris, assisted by extensor digitorum, extensor indicis, extensor digiti minimi and extensor pollicis longus.

Abduction: flexor carpi radialis, extensor carpi radialis longus and brevis, abductor pollicis longus and extensor pollicis brevis.

Adduction: flexor carpi ulnaris, extensor carpi ulnaris.

Thumb *movements*

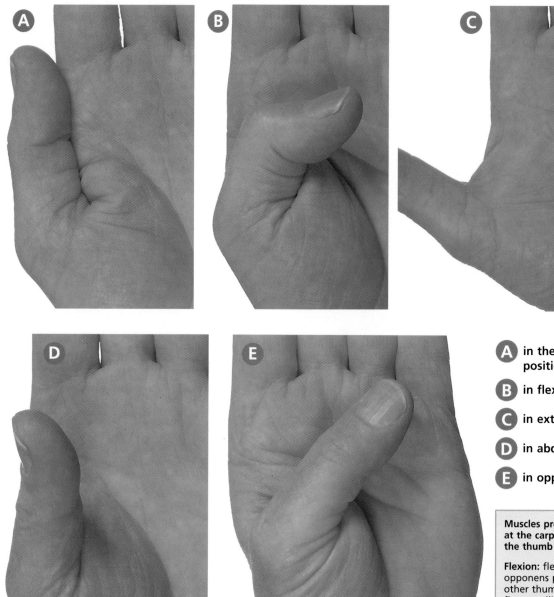

A in the anatomical position

B in flexion

C in extension

D in abduction

E in opposition

Muscles producing movements at the carpometacarpal joint of the thumb

Flexion: flexor pollicis brevis, opponens pollicis, and (when the other thumb joints are flexed) flexor pollicis longus.

Extension: abductor pollicis longus, extensor pollicis longus, extensor pollicis brevis.

Abduction: abductor pollicis brevis, abductor pollicis longus.

Adduction: adductor pollicis.

Opposition: opponens pollicis, flexor pollicis brevis, reinforced by adductor pollicis and flexor pollicis longus.

With the thumb in the anatomical position (A), the thumb nail is at right angles to the fingers because the first metacarpal is at right angles to the others (pages 123–124). This is a rather artificial position; in the normal position of rest, the thumb makes an angle of about 60° with the plane of the palm (i.e. it is partially abducted). Flexion (B) means bending the thumb across the palm, keeping the phalanges at right angles to the palm. Extension (C) is the opposite movement, away from the palm. In abduction (D) the thumb is lifted forwards from the plane of the palm, and continuation of this movement inevitably leads to opposition (E), with rotation of the first metacarpal, twisting the whole digit so that the pulp of the thumb can be brought towards the palm at the base of the little finger (or more commonly in everyday use, to contact or overlap any of the flexed fingers). Opposition is a combination of abduction with flexion and medial rotation at the carpometacarpal joint; it is not necessarily accompanied by flexion at the other thumb joints.

Palm of left hand

Ⓐ *palmar aponeurosis*

Removal of the palmar skin reveals the palmar aponeurosis.

Ⓑ *after removal of palmar aponeurosis*

Deeper dissection of the palm reveals the flexor retinaculum, the palmar branches of the median and ulnar nerves and the superficial palmar arch, flanked by the muscles of the thenar and hypothenar eminences.

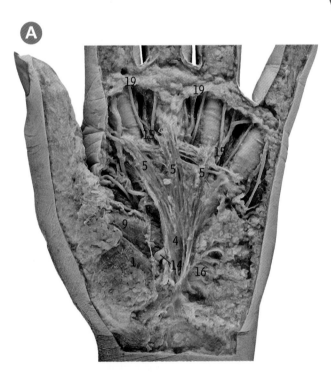

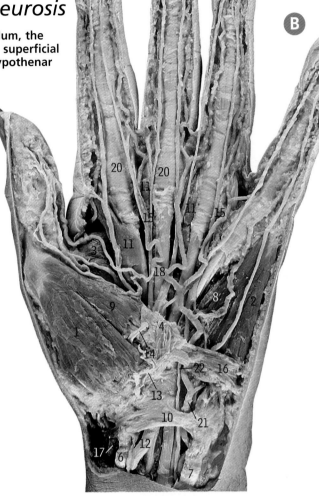

1	Abductor pollicis brevis	**12**	Median nerve
2	Abductor digiti minimi	**13**	Median nerve, palmar branch
3	Adductor pollicis	**14**	Median nerve, recurrent branch
4	Aponeurosis, central part	**15**	Palmar digital vessels and nerves
5	Aponeurosis, digital slips	**16**	Palmaris brevis
6	Flexor carpi radialis	**17**	Radial artery
7	Flexor carpi ulnaris	**18**	Superficial palmar arch
8	Flexor digiti minimi brevis	**19**	Superficial transverse metacarpal
9	Flexor pollicis brevis		ligaments
10	Flexor retinaculum	**20**	Synovial sheaths of flexor tendons
11	Lumbrical	**21**	Ulnar artery
		22	Ulnar nerve

CT 3D reconstruction to show flexor digitorum profundus tendons

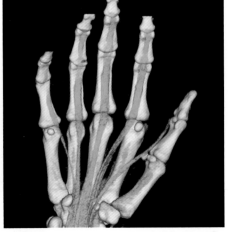

Arteriovenous fistula, Dupuytren's contracture, see pages 170–172.

A Palm of right hand *with synovial sheaths*

The synovial sheaths of the wrist and fingers have been emphasised by blue tissue. On the middle finger, the fibrous flexor sheath has been removed (but retained on the other fingers, as at 3) to show the whole length of the synovial sheath (22). On the index and ring fingers, the synovial sheath projects slightly proximal to the fibrous sheath. The synovial sheath of the little finger is continuous with the sheath surrounding the finger flexor tendons under the flexor retinaculum (the ulnar bursa, 24), and the sheath of flexor pollicis longus is the radial bursa (20), which also continues under the retinaculum (9).

1　Abductor digiti minimi
2　Abductor pollicis brevis
3　Fibrous flexor sheath
4　Flexor carpi radialis
5　Flexor carpi ulnaris
6　Flexor digiti minimi brevis
7　Flexor digitorum superficialis
8　Flexor pollicis brevis
9　Flexor retinaculum
10　Median nerve
11　Muscular (recurrent) branch of median nerve
12　Palmar branch of median nerve
13　Palmar branch of ulnar nerve
14　Palmar digital artery
15　Palmar digital nerve
16　Palmaris brevis
17　Palmaris longus
18　Pisiform bone
19　Radial artery
20　Radial bursa and flexor pollicis longus
21　Superficial palmar arch
22　Synovial sheath
23　Ulnar artery
24　Ulnar bursa
25　Ulnar nerve

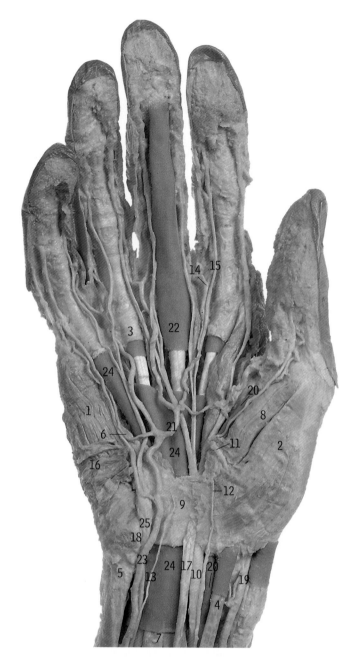

In the carpal tunnel (beneath the flexor retinaculum), one synovial sheath envelops the eight tendons of flexor digitorum superficialis and profundus (A24), another envelops the flexor pollicis longus tendon (A20), and flexor carpi radialis (in its own compartment of the flexor retinaculum) has its own sheath also (A4). The synovial sheaths for flexor carpi radialis and flexor pollicis longus extend as far as the tendon insertions.

The sheath of the long finger flexors is continuous with the digital synovial sheath of the little finger, but is *not* continuous with the digital synovial sheaths of the ring, middle or index fingers; these fingers have their own synovial sheaths whose proximal ends project slightly beyond the *fibrous* sheaths within which the digital *synovial* sheaths lie.

The muscular (recurrent) branch (A11) of the median nerve usually supplies abductor pollicis brevis, flexor pollicis brevis and opponens pollicis, but of all the muscles in the body flexor pollicis brevis (A8) is the one most likely to have an anomalous supply: in about one-third of hands by the median nerve, in another third by the ulnar nerve, and in the rest by both the median and ulnar nerves.

B Right index finger *long tendons, vincula and relations*

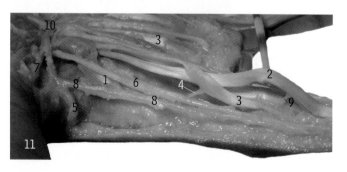

1　First lumbrical muscle
2　Flexor digitorum profundus
3　Flexor digitorum superficialis
4　Long vinculum of superficialis tendon
5　Metacarpal arterial branch
6　Palmar digital nerve
7　Princeps pollicis artery
8　Radialis indicis artery
9　Short vinculum of profundus tendon
10　Superficial palmar arterial arch
11　Thumb

Digital nerve block, hand infections, mallet finger, see pages 170–172.

Left wrist and hand
A *palmar surface* B *axial MR image*

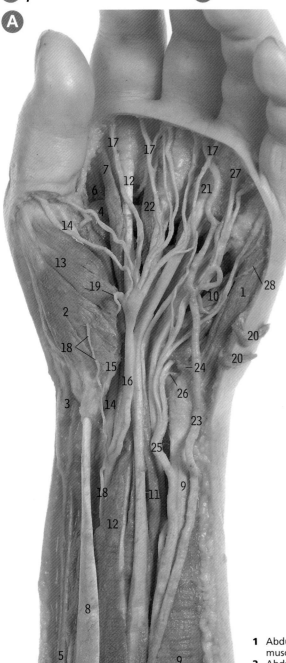

Parts of the fibrous flexor sheaths of the fingers (A21) have also been excised to show the contained tendons of flexor digitorum superficialis (A12) and flexor digitorum profundus (A11). In the palm, the lumbrical muscles (A7 and 22) arise from the profundus tendons. Compare features in the MR image with the dissection.

1 Abductor digiti minimi	**17** Median nerve, digital branch
2 Abductor pollicis brevis	**18** Median nerve, palmar
3 Abductor pollicis longus	cutaneous branch
4 Adductor pollicis	**19** Median nerve, recurrent
5 Brachioradialis	branch
6 First dorsal interosseous	**20** Palmaris brevis
7 First lumbrical	**21** Remaining parts of fibrous
8 Flexor carpi radialis	flexor sheath
9 Flexor carpi ulnaris	**22** Second lumbrical
10 Flexor digiti minimi brevis	**23** Ulnar artery
11 Flexor digitorum profundus	**24** Ulnar artery, deep branch
12 Flexor digitorum superficialis	**25** Ulnar nerve
13 Flexor pollicis brevis	**26** Ulnar nerve, deep branch
14 Flexor pollicis longus	**27** Ulnar nerve, digital branch
15 Flexor retinaculum cut edge	**28** Ulnar nerve, muscular branch
16 Median nerve	

The lumbrical muscles have no bony attachments. They arise from the tendons of flexor digitorum profundus (A11) – the first and second (A7 and A22) from the tendons of the index and middle fingers respectively, and the third and fourth from adjacent sides of the middle and ring, and ring and little fingers respectively. Each is attached distally to the radial side of the dorsal digital expansion of each finger (page 166).

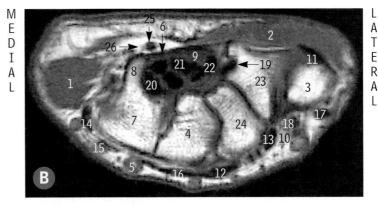

1 Abductor digiti minimi muscle	**13** Tendon of extensor carpi radialis longus muscle	**20** Tendon of flexor digitorum profundus muscle
2 Abductor pollicis brevis muscle	**14** Tendon of extensor carpi ulnaris muscle	**21** Tendon of flexor digitorum superficialis muscle
3 Base of first metacarpal	**15** Tendon of extensor digiti minimi muscle	**22** Tendon of flexor pollicis longus muscle
4 Capitate	**16** Tendon of extensor digitorum muscle	**23** Trapezium
5 Dorsal venous arch	**17** Tendon of extensor pollicis brevis muscle	**24** Trapezoid
6 Flexor retinaculum	**18** Tendon of extensor pollicis longus muscle	**25** Ulnar artery
7 Hamate	**19** Tendon of flexor carpi radialis muscle	**26** Ulnar nerve
8 Hook of hamate		
9 Median nerve		
10 Radial artery		
11 Tendon of abductor pollicis longus muscle		
12 Tendon of extensor carpi radialis brevis muscle		

Carpal tunnel syndrome, median nerve palsy, see pages 170–172.

Superficial palmar arch

A *incomplete in the left hand*

B *complete in the right hand*

In two-thirds of hands, the superficial palmar arch is not complete (as in A29). In the other third, it is usually completed by the superficial palmar branch of the radial artery (B30).

In the palm the superficial arterial arch (29) and its branches (as at 1) lie superficial to the common palmar digital nerves (22 and 7), but on the fingers the palmar digital nerves (as at 3) lie superficial (anterior) to the palmar digital arteries (as at 2).

1   A common palmar digital artery
2   A palmar digital artery
3   A palmar digital nerve
4   Abductor digiti minimi
5   Abductor pollicis brevis
6   Abductor pollicis longus
7   Common palmar digital branch of ulnar nerve
8   Common origin of 28 and 26
9   Deep branch of ulnar artery
10 Deep branch of ulnar nerve
11 Deep palmar arch
12 First lumbrical
13 Flexor carpi radialis
14 Flexor carpi ulnaris and pisiform
15 Flexor digitorum profundus
16 Flexor digitorum superficialis
17 Flexor pollicis brevis
18 Flexor pollicis longus
19 Flexor retinaculum
20 Fourth lumbrical
21 Median nerve
22 Median nerve dividing into common palmar digital branches
23 Muscular (recurrent) branch of median nerve
24 Opponens digiti minimi
25 Palmaris brevis
26 Princeps pollicis artery
27 Radial artery
28 Radialis indicis artery
29 Superficial palmar arch
30 Superficial palmar branch of radial artery
31 Ulnar artery
32 Ulnar nerve

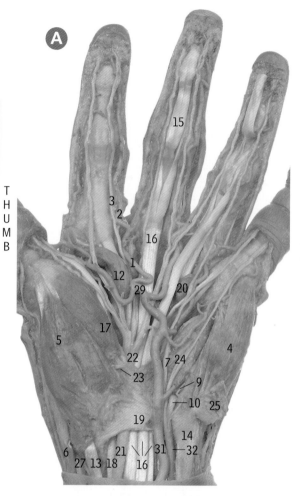

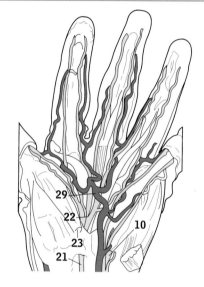

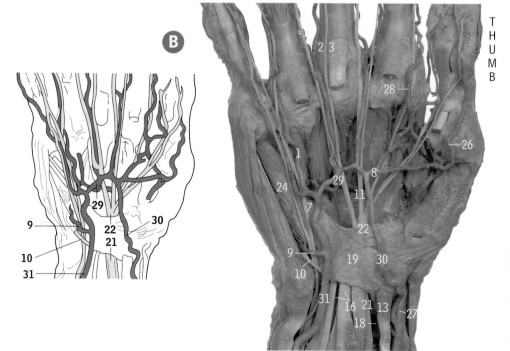

Arterial puncture at the wrist, Guyon's canal syndrome, see pages 170–172.

Palm of right hand

C *deep palmar arch* **D** *arteriogram of palmar arteries*

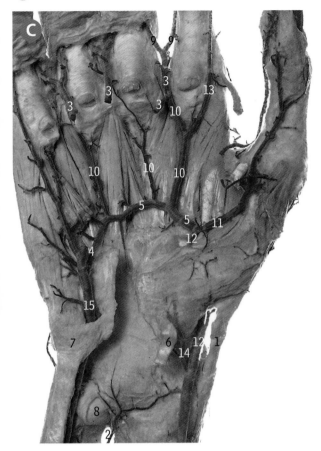

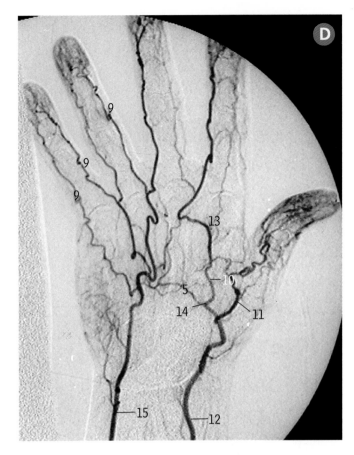

Most muscles and tendons have been removed and the arteries have been distended by injection. The deep palmar arch (5) is seen giving off the palmar metacarpal arteries (10) which join the common palmar digital arteries (3) from the superficial arch. Compare C with the vessels in the arteriogram.

1 Abductor pollicis longus
2 Branch of anterior interosseous artery to anterior carpal arch
3 Common palmar digital arteries (from superficial arch)
4 Deep branch of ulnar artery
5 Deep palmar arch
6 Flexor carpi radialis
7 Flexor carpi ulnaris and pisiform

8 Head of ulna
9 Palmar digital arteries
10 Palmar metacarpal arteries
11 Princeps pollicis artery
12 Radial artery
13 Radialis indicis artery (anomalous origin)
14 Superficial palmar branch of radial artery
15 Ulnar artery

Trigger finger, see pages 170–172.

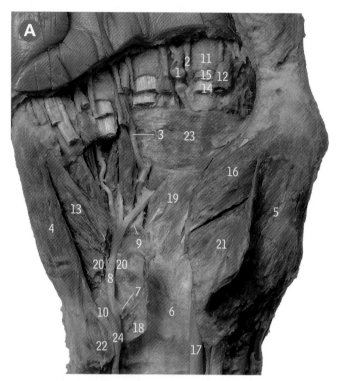

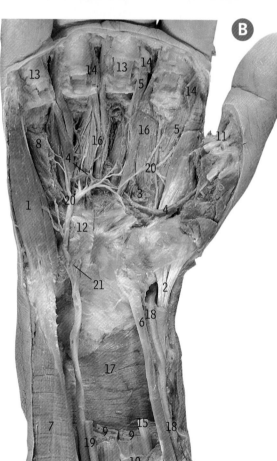

A Palm of right hand
deep branch of the ulnar nerve

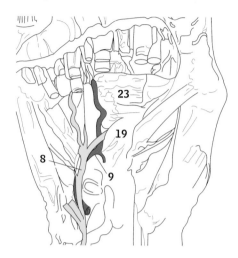

The long flexor tendons (15 and 14) and lumbricals (12) have been cut off near the heads of the metacarpals, and parts of the hypothenar muscles removed to show the deep branches of the ulnar nerve and artery (8 and 7) running into the palm and curling laterally to pass between the transverse and oblique heads of adductor pollicis (23 and 19).

1 A common palmar digital artery	**13** Flexor digiti minimi brevis
2 A palmar digital nerve	**14** Flexor digitorum profundus
3 A palmar metacarpal artery	**15** Flexor digitorum superficialis
4 Abductor digiti minimi	**16** Flexor pollicis brevis
5 Abductor pollicis brevis	**17** Flexor pollicis longus
6 Carpal tunnel	**18** Flexor retinaculum (cut edge)
7 Deep branch of ulnar artery	**19** Oblique head of adductor pollicis
8 Deep branch of ulnar nerve	**20** Opponens digiti minimi
9 Deep palmar arch	**21** Opponens pollicis
10 Digital branches of ulnar nerve	**22** Pisiform
11 Fibrous flexor sheath	**23** Transverse head of adductor pollicis
12 First lumbrical	**24** Ulnar nerve

B Palm of right hand
deep dissection

Deep to the adductor pollicis and the flexor tendons lie the pronator quadratus proximally and the extensive deep palmar branches of the ulnar nerve and deep palmar arch distally.

1 Abductor digiti minimi	**12** Flexor retinaculum – cut
2 Abductor pollicis longus	**13** Flexor tendon sheaths
3 Adductor pollicis – cut	**14** Lumbrical – cut
4 Deep palmar arch	**15** Median nerve – cut
5 Dorsal interossei	**16** Palmar interossei
6 Flexor carpi radialis	**17** Pronator quadratus
7 Flexor carpi ulnaris	**18** Radial artery
8 Flexor digiti minimi – cut	**19** Ulnar artery – cut
9 Flexor digitorum profundus – cut	**20** Ulnar nerve, deep branches to intrinsic hand muscles
10 Flexor digitorum superficialis – cut	**21** Ulnar nerve, superficial branch (cut at wrist)
11 Flexor pollicis longus	

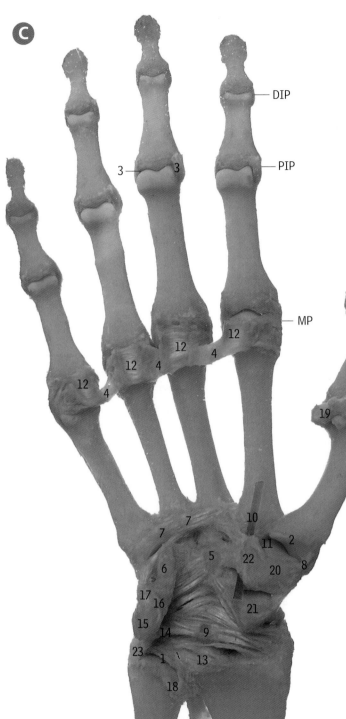

- DIP
- PIP
- MP

C Palm of right hand
ligaments and joints

The capsule of the carpometacarpal joint of the thumb (between the base of the first metacarpal and the trapezium) has been removed, to show the saddle-shaped joint surfaces, which allow the unique movement of opposition of the thumb to occur. The palmar and lateral ligaments (11 and 8) of the joint remain intact. The capsule of the distal radio-ulnar joint has also been removed to show the articular disc, but the wrist joint, the ulnar part of which lies distal to the disc, has not been opened.

1 Articular disc of distal radio-ulnar joint
2 Base of first metacarpal
3 Collateral ligament of interphalangeal joint
4 Deep transverse metacarpal ligament
5 Head of capitate
6 Hook of hamate
7 Interosseous metacarpal ligament
8 Lateral ligament of carpometacarpal joint of thumb
9 Lunate
10 Marker in groove on trapezium for flexor carpi radialis tendon
11 Palmar ligament of carpometacarpal joint of thumb
12 Palmar ligament of metacarpophalangeal joint with groove for flexor tendon
13 Palmar radiocarpal ligament
14 Palmar ulnocarpal ligament
15 Pisiform
16 Pisohamate ligament
17 Pisometacarpal ligament
18 Sacciform recess of capsule of distal radio-ulnar joint
19 Sesamoid bones of flexor pollicis brevis tendons (with adductor pollicis on ulnar side)
20 Trapezium
21 Tubercle of scaphoid
22 Tubercle of trapezium
23 Ulnar collateral ligament of wrist joint

The collateral ligaments of the metacarpophalangeal and interphalangeal joints (D2, C3) pass obliquely forwards from the posterior part of the side of the head of the proximal bone to the anterior part of the side of the base of the distal bone.

Opposition of the thumb is a combination of flexion and abduction with medial rotation of the first metacarpal (page 156). The saddle-shape of the joint between the base of the first metacarpal and the trapezium, together with the way that the capsule and its reinforcing ligaments are attached to the bones, ensures that when flexor pollicis brevis and opponens pollicis contract they produce the necessary metacarpal rotation.

The articular disc (1) holds the lower ends of the radius and ulna together, and separates the distal radio-ulnar joint from the wrist joint, so that the cavities of these joints are not continuous (unlike those of the elbow and proximal radio-ulnar joints, which have one continuous cavity – page 146).

DIP distal interphalangeal joint
PIP proximal interphalangeal joint
MP metacarpophalangeal joint

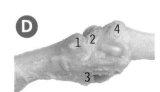

D Right index finger
metacarpophalangeal (MP) joint, from the radial side

Part of the capsule has been removed to define the collateral ligament (2).

1 Base of proximal phalanx
2 Collateral ligament
3 Fibrous flexor sheath
4 Head of second metacarpal

Gamekeeper's thumb, see pages 170–172.

Dorsum of left hand
A Radial side view of 'Anatomical snuff box'

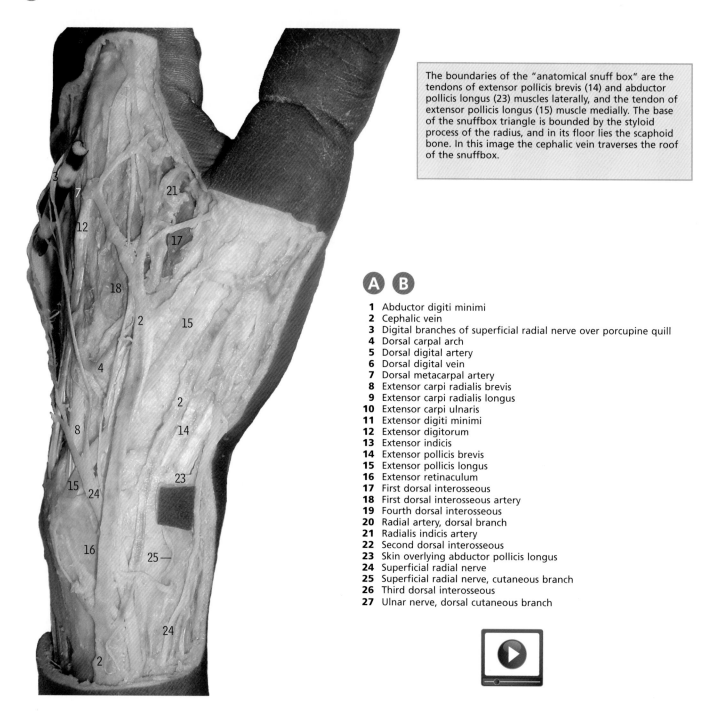

The boundaries of the "anatomical snuff box" are the tendons of extensor pollicis brevis (14) and abductor pollicis longus (23) muscles laterally, and the tendon of extensor pollicis longus (15) muscle medially. The base of the snuffbox triangle is bounded by the styloid process of the radius, and in its floor lies the scaphoid bone. In this image the cephalic vein traverses the roof of the snuffbox.

A B

1 Abductor digiti minimi
2 Cephalic vein
3 Digital branches of superficial radial nerve over porcupine quill
4 Dorsal carpal arch
5 Dorsal digital artery
6 Dorsal digital vein
7 Dorsal metacarpal artery
8 Extensor carpi radialis brevis
9 Extensor carpi radialis longus
10 Extensor carpi ulnaris
11 Extensor digiti minimi
12 Extensor digitorum
13 Extensor indicis
14 Extensor pollicis brevis
15 Extensor pollicis longus
16 Extensor retinaculum
17 First dorsal interosseous
18 First dorsal interosseous artery
19 Fourth dorsal interosseous
20 Radial artery, dorsal branch
21 Radialis indicis artery
22 Second dorsal interosseous
23 Skin overlying abductor pollicis longus
24 Superficial radial nerve
25 Superficial radial nerve, cutaneous branch
26 Third dorsal interosseous
27 Ulnar nerve, dorsal cutaneous branch

B Dorsum of left hand

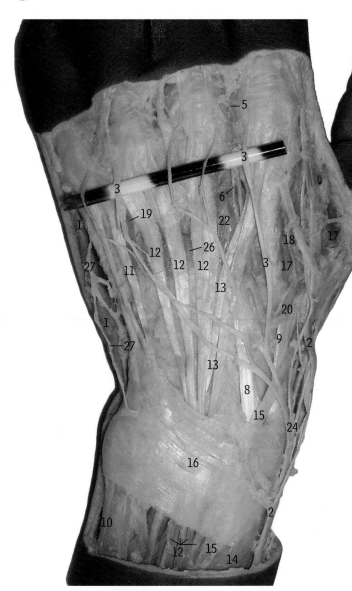

C Dorsum of right wrist and hand
synovial sheaths

Fascia and cutaneous branches of the ulnar nerve have been removed; the extensor reticulum (13) and the radial nerve (2) have been preserved and the synovial sheaths have been emphasised by blue tissue. From the radial to the ulnar side, the six compartments of the extensor retinaculum contain the tendons of: (a) abductor pollicis longus and extensor pollicis brevis (1 and 11); (b) extensor carpi radialis longus and brevis (6 and 5); (c) extensor pollicis longus (12); (d) extensor digitorum and extensor indicis (9 and 10); (e) extensor digiti minimi (8); (f) extensor carpi ulnaris (7).

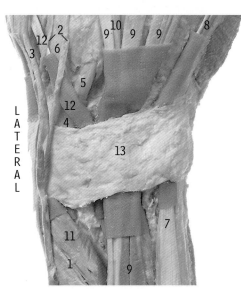

C

1. Abductor pollicis longus
2. Branches of radial nerve
3. Cephalic vein
4. Common sheath for 5 and 6
5. Extensor carpi radialis brevis
6. Extensor carpi radialis longus
7. Extensor carpi ulnaris
8. Extensor digiti minimi
9. Extensor digitorum
10. Extensor indicis
11. Extensor pollicis brevis
12. Extensor pollicis longus
13. Extensor retinaculum

Nail abnormalities, wrist ganglion, see pages 170–172.

Ⓐ Dorsum of right hand *arteries*

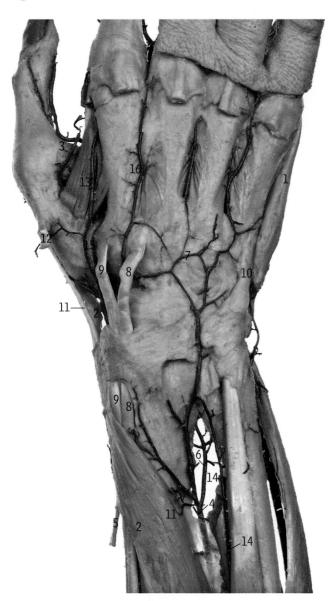

The arteries have been injected and the long finger tendons removed to display the dorsal carpal arch (7) and dorsal metacarpal arteries (as at 13 and 16). Above the wrist pronator quadratus has been removed to show the branch (6) of the anterior interosseous artery (4), which continues towards the palm; the anterior interosseous itself passes to the dorsal surface to join the posterior interosseous artery (14).

Ⓑ Left ring finger *extensor expansion (dorsal digital expansion)*

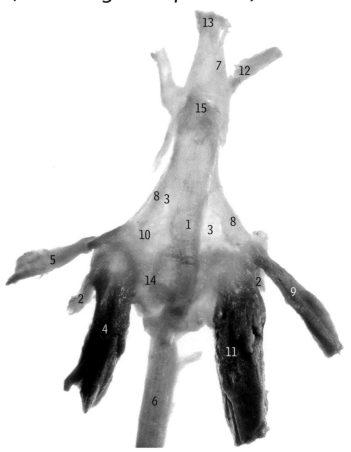

1	Abductor digiti minimi	**9**	Extensor carpi radialis longus
2	Abductor pollicis longus	**10**	Extensor carpi ulnaris
3	Adductor pollicis and branch of princeps pollicis artery	**11**	Extensor pollicis brevis
		12	Extensor pollicis longus
4	Anterior interosseous artery	**13**	First dorsal interosseous and first dorsal metacarpal artery
5	Brachioradialis		
6	Branch of anterior interosseous artery to anterior carpal arch	**14**	Posterior interosseous artery
		15	Radial artery
7	Dorsal carpal arch	**16**	Second dorsal interosseous and second dorsal metacarpal artery
8	Extensor carpi radialis brevis		

1	Common extensor tendon	**8**	Lateral tendon "wing tendon"
2	Deep transverse metacarpal ligament	**9**	Lumbrical muscle
		10	Oblique interosseous fibres
3	Dorsal digital expansion	**11**	Palmar interosseous muscle
4	Dorsal interosseous muscle	**12**	Retinacular ligament, transverse band
5	Dorsal interosseous muscle, phalangeal attachment		
		13	Terminal conjoint extensor tendon
6	Extensor digitorum tendon		
7	Lateral conjoined extensor tendon	**14**	Transverse ligament
		15	Triangular ligament

Three tendons pass to different levels of the thumb: abductor pollicis longus (A2) to the base of the first metacarpal, extensor pollicis brevis (A11) to the base of the proximal phalanx, and extensor pollicis longus (A12) to the base of the distal phalanx.

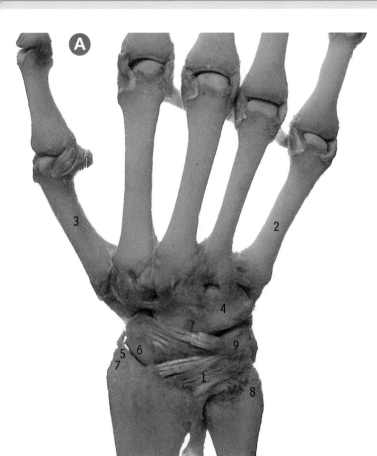

A Dorsum of right hand
ligaments and joints

Most joint capsules have been removed, including the radial parts of the wrist joint capsule, thus showing the articulation between the scaphoid (6) and the lower end of the radius (7).

1 Dorsal radiocarpal ligament
2 Fifth metacarpal
3 First metacarpal
4 Hamate
5 Radial collateral ligament of wrist joint
6 Scaphoid
7 Styloid process of radius
8 Styloid process of ulna
9 Triquetral

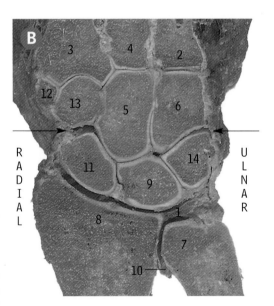

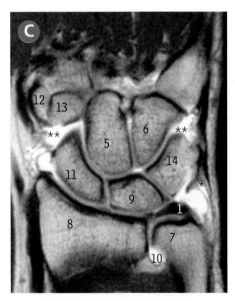

Right wrist
coronal section

B dissection

C coronal MR arthrogram

1 Articular disc (triangular fibrocartilage)
2 Base of fourth metacarpal
3 Base of second metacarpal
4 Base of third metacarpal
5 Capitate
6 Hamate
7 Head of ulna
8 Lower end of radius
9 Lunate
10 Sacciform recess of distal radio-ulnar joint
11 Scaphoid
12 Trapezium
13 Trapezoid
14 Triquetral
* Normal vascular penetration of triangular fibrocartilage peripherally
** Contrast in midcarpal joint indicates abnormal communication between radiocarpal and midcarpal joints

Viewed from the dorsal surface, the section has passed through the wrist near this surface, and the first and fifth metacarpals have not been included in the cut. The arrows between the two rows of carpal bones indicate the line of the midcarpal joint. Compare the MR image with the section.

Avascular necrosis of the scaphoid, dislocation of the lunate, see pages 170–172.

Right midcarpal and wrist joints

A *midcarpal joint, opened up in forced flexion*

B *wrist joint, opened up in forced extension*

BACK OF RIGHT THUMB EDGE

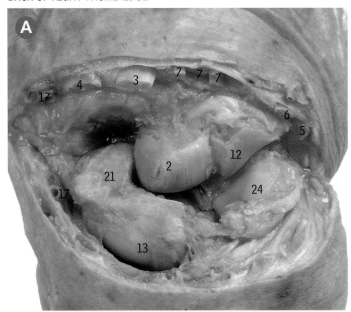

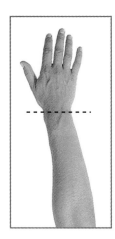

1 Articular disc
2 Capitate
3 Extensor carpi radialis brevis
4 Extensor carpi radialis longus
5 Extensor carpi ulnaris
6 Extensor digiti minimi
7 Extensor digitorum
8 Flexor carpi radialis tendon
9 Flexor carpi ulnaris tendon
10 Flexor digitorum profundus tendon
11 Flexor digitorum superficialis tendon
12 Hamate
13 Lunate
14 Median nerve
15 Palmar arch vein
16 Palmaris longus tendon
17 Radial artery
18 Radial artery, palmar arch branch
19 Radial surface for lunate
20 Radial surface for scaphoid
21 Scaphoid
22 Styloid process of radius
23 Styloid process of ulna
24 Triquetral
25 Ulnar artery

FRONT OF RIGHT THUMB EDGE

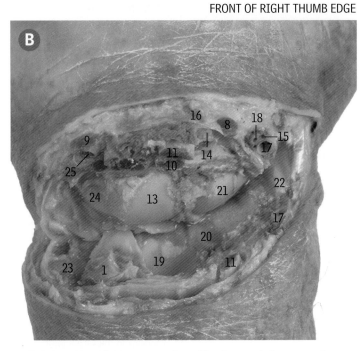

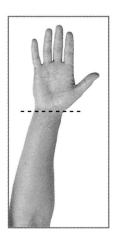

Both joints have been opened up (far beyond the normal range of movement) in order to demonstrate the bones of the joint surfaces. The wrist joint in B has been forced open in extension. A has been forced open in flexion. The proximal (wrist joint) surfaces of the scaphoid (21), lunate (13) and triquetral (24) are seen in B, and their distal (midcarpal joint) surfaces in A.

Wrist and hand *radiographs*

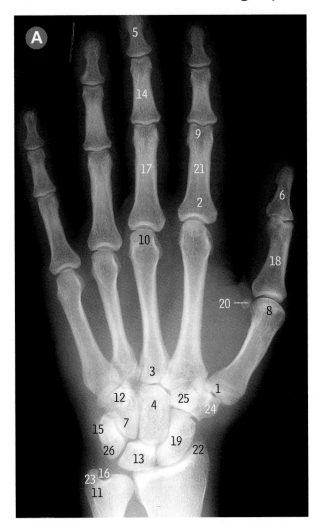

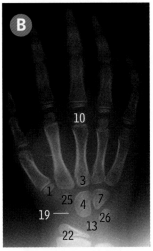

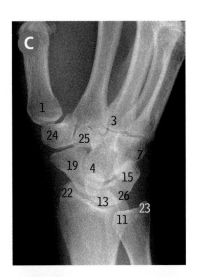

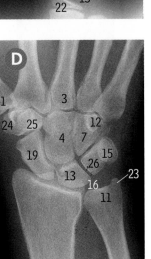

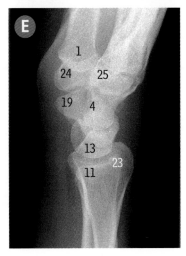

A dorsopalmar projection

B of a 4-year-old child

C oblique projection

D posteroanterior projection

E lateral projection

The epiphysis at the lower end of the radius appears on a radiograph at 2 years and in the ulna at 6 years. The first carpal bone to appear is the capitate at 1 year.

Compare the epiphyses of the metacarpals and phalanges seen in B with the bony specimens in J and K on page 125.

1 Base of first metacarpal	**16** Position of articular disc (triangular fibrocartilage)
2 Base of phalanx	
3 Base of third metacarpal	**17** Proximal phalanx of middle finger
4 Capitate	
5 Distal phalanx of middle finger	**18** Proximal phalanx of thumb
6 Distal phalanx of thumb	**19** Scaphoid
7 Hamate	**20** Sesamoid bone in flexor pollicis brevis
8 Head of first metacarpal	
9 Head of phalanx	**21** Shaft of phalanx
10 Head of third metacarpal	**22** Styloid process at lower end of radius
11 Head of ulna	
12 Hook of hamate	**23** Styloid process of ulna
13 Lunate	**24** Trapezium
14 Middle phalanx of middle finger	**25** Trapezoid
15 Pisiform	**26** Triquetral

Upper limb

Clinical thumbnails, see website for details and further clinical images to download into your own notes.

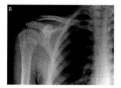

Accessory ossicles

Acromioclavicular separation

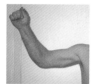

Anterior interosseous nerve entrapment

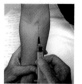

Arterial puncture at the elbow

Arterial puncture at the wrist

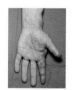

Arteriovenous fistula

Auscultation of the brachial pulse

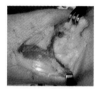

Avascular necrosis of the scaphoid

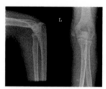

Avulsion medial epicondyle

Axillary artery aneurysm

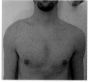

Axillary-subclavian vein thrombosis

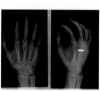

Bar room fracture

Biceps tendon reflex

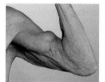

Bicipital tendinitis and rupture

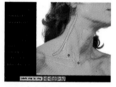

Brachial plexus block

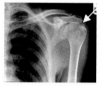

Calcific tendinitis

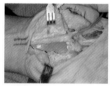

Carpal tunnel syndrome

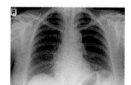

Cervical rib

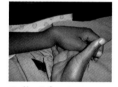

Colles' fracture

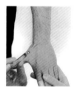

de Quervain's disease

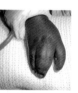

Digital development abnormality

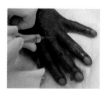

Digital nerve block

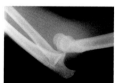

Dislocation of the elbow

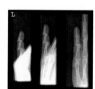

Dislocation of the finger

Dislocation of humerus

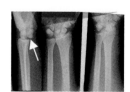

Dislocation of the lunate

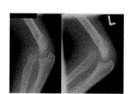

Dislocation of the radial head

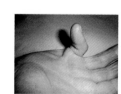

Dupuytren's contracture

Elbow arthroscopy

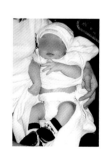

Erb's palsy

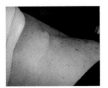

Fractured clavicle

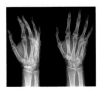

Fractured hamate

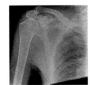

Fractured scapula

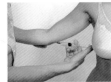

Gamekeeper's thumb

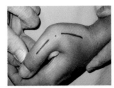

Golfer's elbow – injection

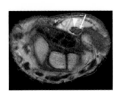

Guyon's canal syndrome

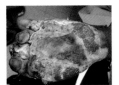

Hand infections

Intramuscular injection – deltoid

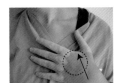

Klumpke's paralysis

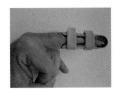

Mallet finger

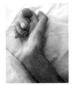

Median nerve palsy

Nail abnormalities

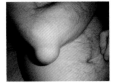

Olecranon bursitis

Painful arc syndrome/ rotator cuff tear

Posterior dislocation of the shoulder

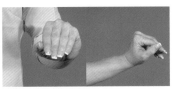

Posterior interosseous nerve entrapment

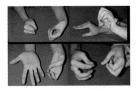

Radial nerve palsy

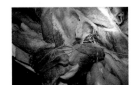

Scapular arterial anastomoses

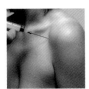

Shoulder joint injection

Smith's fracture

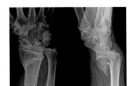

Sternoclavicular dislocation

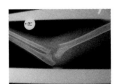

Supracondylar fracture of the humerus

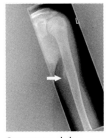

Supracondylar spur

Tennis elbow

Traction of forearm fractures

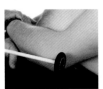

Triceps tendon reflex

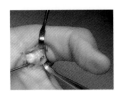

Trigger finger

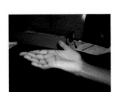

Ulnar nerve palsy

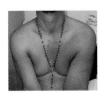

Vascular abnormalities

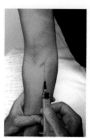
Venepuncture of the upper limb

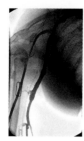
Venous cutdown

Volkmann's ischaemic contracture

Winging of the scapula

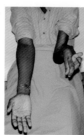
Wrist arthroscopy

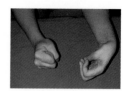
Wrist drop

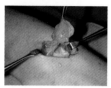
Wrist ganglion

Thorax

  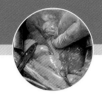 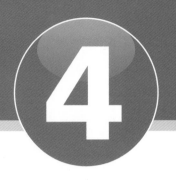

Thorax Ⓐ *surface anatomy, from the front*
Ⓑ *axial skeleton, from behind*
Ⓒ *3D CT reconstruction of thorax*

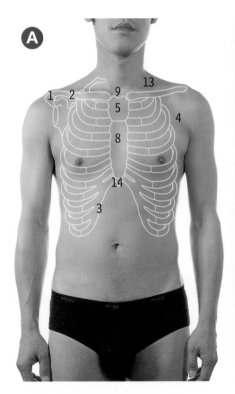 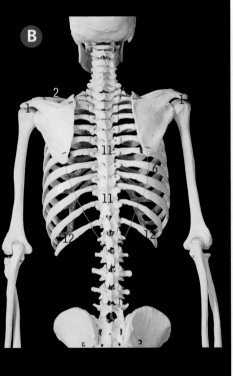 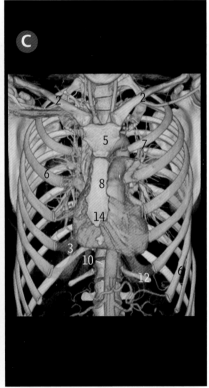

1	Acromion	**8**	Sternal body
2	Clavicle	**9**	Suprasternal notch
3	Costal margin	**10**	Thoracic vertebra, body
4	Deltopectoral groove	**11**	Thoracic vertebra, spine
5	Manubrium	**12**	Twelfth rib
6	Rib	**13**	Trapezius
7	Second rib	**14**	Xiphisternum

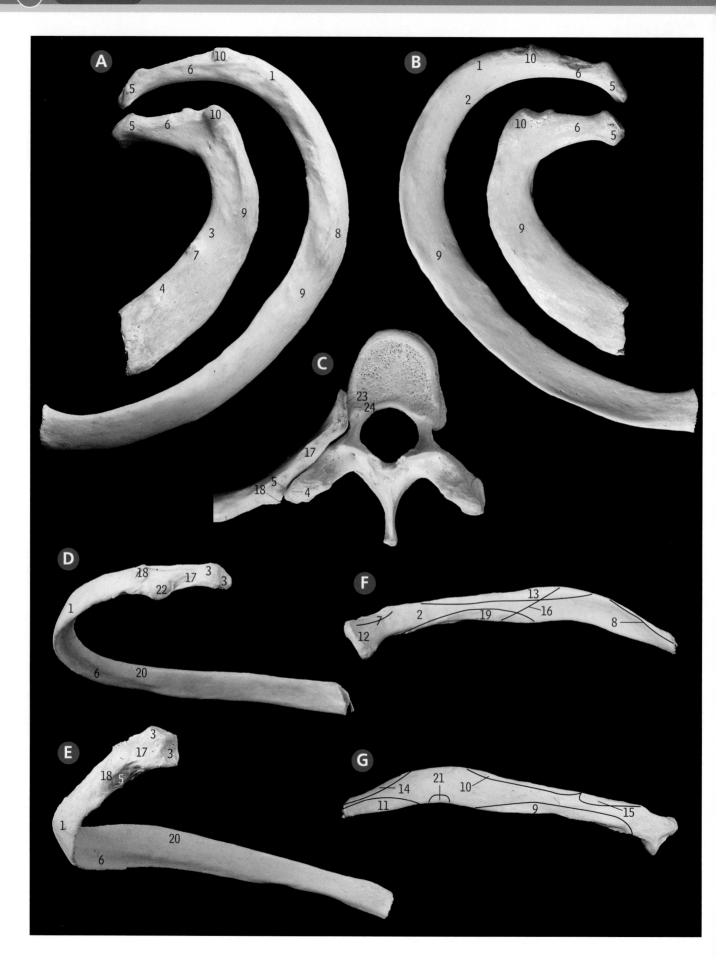

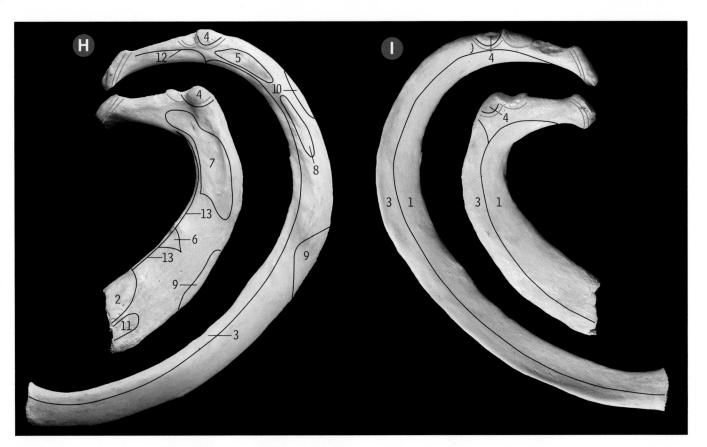

Left first rib (inner) and second rib (outer)

A from above

B from below

1 Angle
2 Costal groove
3 Groove for subclavian artery and first thoracic nerve
4 Groove for subclavian vein
5 Head
6 Neck
7 Scalene tubercle
8 Serratus anterior tuberosity
9 Shaft
10 Tubercle

The atypical ribs are the first, second, tenth, eleventh and twelfth.

The **first rib** has a head with one facet (A5), a prominent tubercle (A10), no angle and no costal groove. The shaft has superior and inferior surfaces.

The **second rib** has a head with two facets (B5), an angle (B1) near the tubercle (B10), a broad costal groove (B2) posteriorly, and an external surface facing upwards and outwards with the inner surface facing correspondingly downwards and inwards.

The **twelfth rib** has a head with one facet (F12) but there is no tubercle, no angle and no costal groove. The shaft tapers at its end (the ends of all other ribs widen slightly).

Ribs and relationships

C a typical rib and vertebra articulated, from above

D the left fifth rib from behind (a typical upper rib)

E the left seventh rib from behind (a typical lower rib)

F the left twelfth rib from the front, with attachments

G the left twelfth rib from behind, with attachments

1 Angle of rib
2 Area covered by pleura
3 Articular facet of head
4 Articular facet of transverse process
5 Articular part of tubercle
6 Costal groove
7 Costotransverse ligament
8 Diaphragm
9 Erector spinae
10 External intercostal
11 External oblique
12 Head
13 Internal intercostal
14 Latissimus dorsi
15 Levator costae
16 Line of pleural reflexion
17 Neck of rib
18 Non-articular part of tubercle
19 Quadratus lumborum
20 Shaft of rib
21 Serratus posterior inferior
22 Tubercle
23 Upper costal facet of head of rib
24 Upper costal facet of vertebral body

Left first rib (inner) and second rib (outer), attachments

H from above

I from below

Blue lines, epiphysial lines; green lines, capsule attachments of costovertebral joints

1 Area covered by pleura
2 Costoclavicular ligament
3 Intercostal muscles and membranes
4 Lateral costotransverse ligament
5 Levator costae
6 Scalenus anterior
7 Scalenus medius
8 Scalenus posterior
9 Serratus anterior
10 Serratus posterior superior
11 Subclavius
12 Superior costotransverse ligament
13 Suprapleural membrane

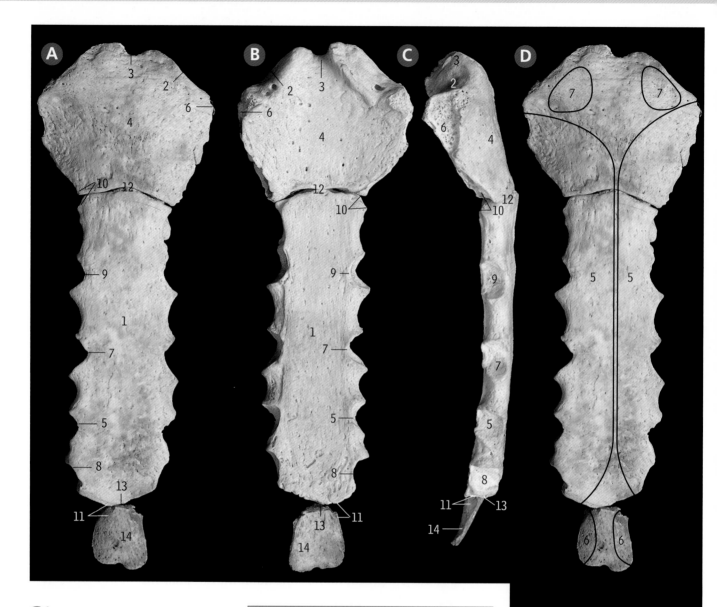

Sternum

A from the front

B from behind

C from the right

1 Body
2 Clavicular notch
3 Jugular notch
4 Manubrium
5 Notch for fifth costal cartilage
6 Notch for first costal cartilage
7 Notch for fourth costal cartilage
8 Notch for sixth costal cartilage
9 Notch for third costal cartilage
10 Notches for second costal cartilage
11 Notches for seventh costal cartilage
12 Sternal angle and manubriosternal joint
13 Xiphisternal joint
14 Xiphoid process

The sternum consists of the manubrium (4), body (1) and xiphoid process (14).

The body of the sternum (1) is formed by the fusion of four sternebrae, the sites of the fusion sometimes being indicated by three slight transverse ridges.

The manubrium (4) and body (1) are bony but the xiphoid process (14), which varies considerably in size and shape, is cartilaginous although it frequently shows some degree of ossification.

The manubriosternal and xiphisternal joints (12 and 13) are both symphyses, the surfaces being covered by hyaline cartilage and united by a fibrocartilaginous disc.

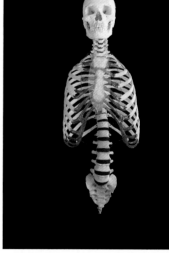

Median sternotomy, sternal variants, see pages 215–216.

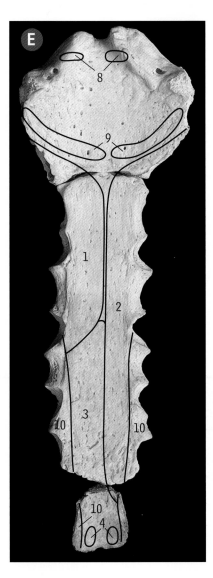

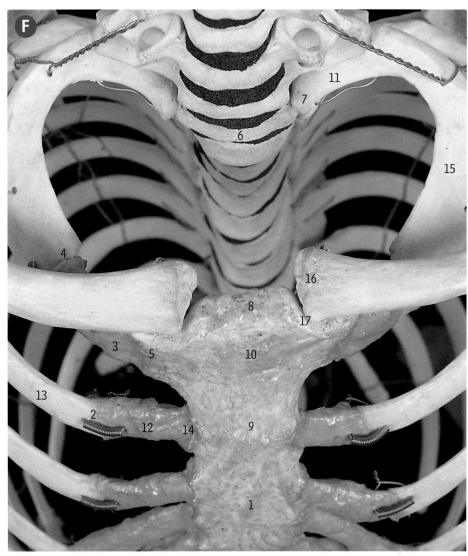

Sternum attachments

D from the front

E from behind

1 Area covered by left pleura
2 Area covered by right pleura
3 Area in contact with pericardium
4 Diaphragm
5 Pectoralis major
6 Rectus abdominis
7 Sternocleidomastoid
8 Sternohyoid
9 Sternothyroid
10 Transversus thoracis

The two pleural sacs are in contact from the levels of the second to fourth costal cartilages (E2 and 1).

F Thoracic inlet *in an articulated skeleton, from above and in front*

The thoracic inlet or outlet (upper aperture of the thorax) is approximately the same size and shape as the outline of the kidney, and is bounded by the first thoracic vertebra (6), first ribs (15), and costal cartilages (3) and the upper border of the manubrium of the sternum (jugular notch, 8). It does not lie in a horizontal plane but slopes downwards and forwards.

The second costal cartilage (12) joins the manubrium and body of the sternum (10 and 1) at the level of the manubriosternal joint (9). This is an important landmark, since the joint line is palpable as a ridge at the slight angle between the manubrium and body, and the second costal cartilage and rib can be identified lateral to it. Other ribs can be identified by counting down from the second.

1 Body of sternum
2 Costochondral joint
3 First costal cartilage
4 First costochondral joint
5 First sternocostal joint
6 First thoracic vertebra
7 Head of first rib
8 Jugular notch
9 Manubriosternal joint
   (angle of Louis)
10 Manubrium of sternum
11 Neck of first rib
12 Second costal cartilage
13 Second rib
14 Second sternocostal joint
15 Shaft of first rib
16 Sternal end of clavicle
17 Sternoclavicular joint

Costochondral pathology, flail chest, see pages 215–216.

Heart, left pleura and lung *surface markings, in the female*

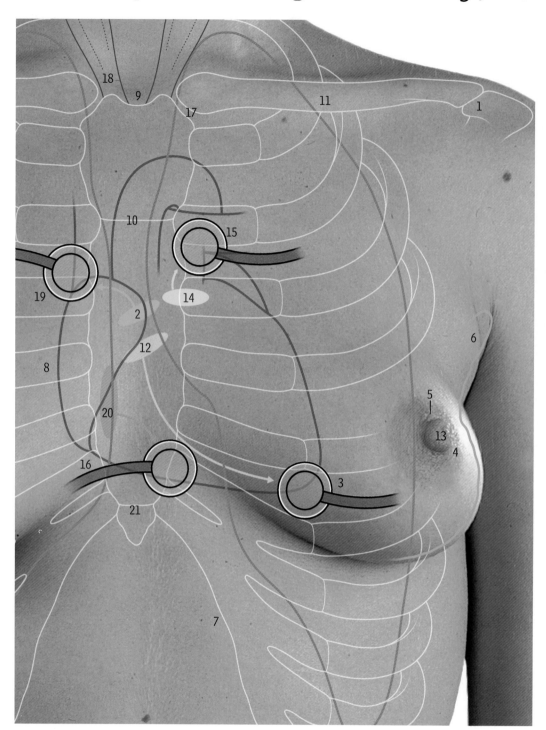

Brown line, heart; purple line, pleura; green line, axillary tail of breast

The positions of the four heart valves are indicated by coloured ellipses, and the sites where the sounds of the corresponding valves are best heard with the stethoscope are shown.

The manubriosternal joint (10) is palpable and a guide to identifying the second costal cartilage (15) which joins the sternum at this level (see page 177, F9, 14 and 12).

The pleura and lung extend into the neck for 2.5 cm above the medial third of the clavicle.

In the midclavicular line the lower limit of the *pleura* reaches the eighth costal cartilage, in the midaxillary line it reaches the tenth rib, and at the lateral border of the erector spinae muscle it crosses the twelfth rib. The lower border of the *lung* is about two ribs higher than the pleural reflection.

Behind the sternum, the pleural sacs are adjacent to one another in the midline from the level of the second to fourth costal cartilages, but then diverge owing to the mass of the heart on the left.

1 Acromioclavicular joint	**7** Costal margin (at eighth costal cartilage)	**12** Mitral valve	**18** Sternocleidomastoid
2 Aortic valve	**8** Fourth costal cartilage	**13** Nipple of breast	**19** Third costal cartilage
3 Apex of heart	**9** Jugular notch	**14** Pulmonary valve	**20** Tricuspid valve
4 Areola of breast	**10** Manubriosternal joint	**15** Second costal cartilage	**21** Xiphisternal joint
5 Areolar glands of breast	**11** Midpoint of clavicle	**16** Sixth costal cartilage	
6 Axillary tail of breast (of Spence)		**17** Sternoclavicular joint	

Auscultation of heart sounds, see pages 215–216.

Female breast *mammary gland*

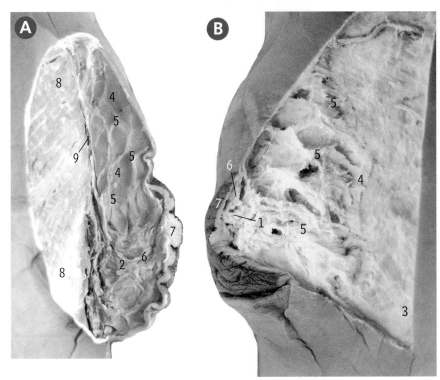

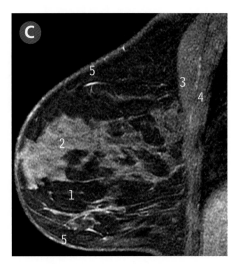

A median parasagittal section

B dissection of areola, nipple and breast tissue

C MR sagittal breast

1 Ampulla of lactiferous duct
2 Condensed glandular tissue
3 Fascia over pectoralis major muscle
4 Fat
5 Fibrous septum

6 Lactiferous duct
7 Nipple
8 Pectoralis major muscle
9 Retromammary space

1 Adipose tissue
2 Fibroglandular tissue
3 Pectoralis major muscle
4 Pectoralis minor muscle
5 Skin

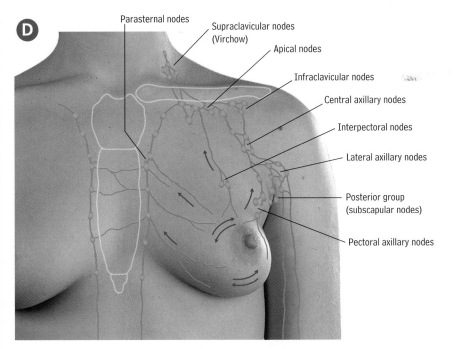

Parasternal nodes
Supraclavicular nodes (Virchow)
Apical nodes
Infraclavicular nodes
Central axillary nodes
Interpectoral nodes
Lateral axillary nodes
Posterior group (subscapular nodes)
Pectoral axillary nodes

D Breast *lymph drainage*

There is a diffuse network of anastomosing lymphatic channels within the breast, including the overlying skin, and *lymph in any part may travel to any other part.* Larger channels drain most of the lymph to axillary nodes, but some from the medial part pass through the thoracic wall near the sternum to parasternal nodes adjacent to the internal thoracic vessels. These are the commonest and initial sites for cancerous spread, but other nodes may be involved (especially in the later spread of disease); these include infraclavicular and supraclavicular (deep cervical) nodes, nodes in the mediastinum, and nodes in the abdomen (via the diaphragm and rectus sheath). Spread to the opposite breast may also occur.

Breast examination, breast abnormalities, carcinoma of the breast, mastectomy, orange-peel skin, see pages 215–216.

Ⓐ Right side of the thorax *from behind with the arm abducted*

With the arm fully abducted, the medial (vertebral) border of the scapula (5) comes to lie at an angle of about 60° to the vertical, and indicates approximately the line of the oblique fissure of the lung (interrupted line).

1 Deltoid
2 Fifth intercostal space
3 Inferior angle of scapula
4 Latissimus dorsi
5 Medial border of scapula
6 Spine of scapula
7 Spinous process of third thoracic vertebra
8 Teres major
9 Trapezius

The line of the oblique fissure of the lung runs from the level of the spine of the third thoracic vertebra (7) to the sixth costal cartilage at the lateral border of the sternum (see B). With the arm fully abducted, the vertebral border of the scapula (5) is a good guide to the direction of this fissure.

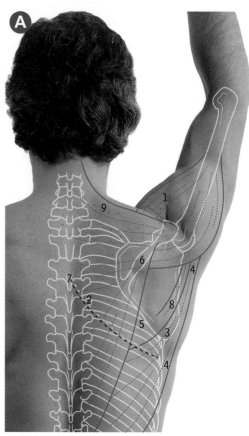

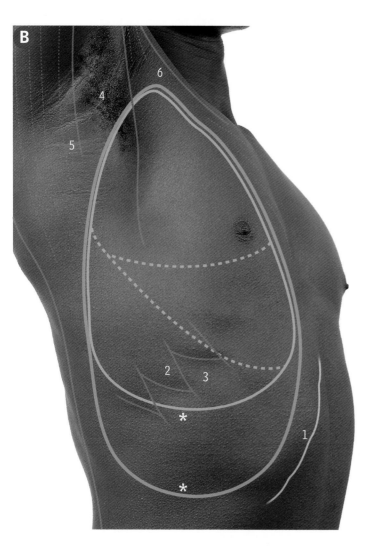

Ⓑ Right side of the thorax *surface markings, from the right, with the arm abducted*

The purple line indicates the extent of the pleura, and the solid orange line the lower limit of the lung; note the gap between the two at the lower part of the thorax, indicating the costodiaphragmatic recess of pleura, which does not contain any lung. The transverse and oblique fissures of the lung are represented by the interrupted orange lines.

1 Costal margin
2 Digitations of serratus anterior
3 External oblique
4 Floor of axilla
5 Latissimus dorsi
6 Pectoralis major

The transverse fissure of the right lung is represented by a line drawn horizontally backwards from the fourth costal cartilage until it meets the line of the oblique fissure (described in A) running forwards to the sixth costal cartilage. The triangle so outlined indicates the middle lobe of the lung, with the superior lobe above it and the inferior lobe below and behind it. It is the area covered by the right breast.

On the left side, where the lung has only two lobes, superior and inferior, there is no transverse fissure; the surface marking for the oblique fissure is similar to that on the right.

* The asterisks represent the places where the lower edges of the lung and pleura cross the eighth and tenth ribs, respectively in the mid-axillary line.

Anterior chest wall muscles of the thorax
from the front

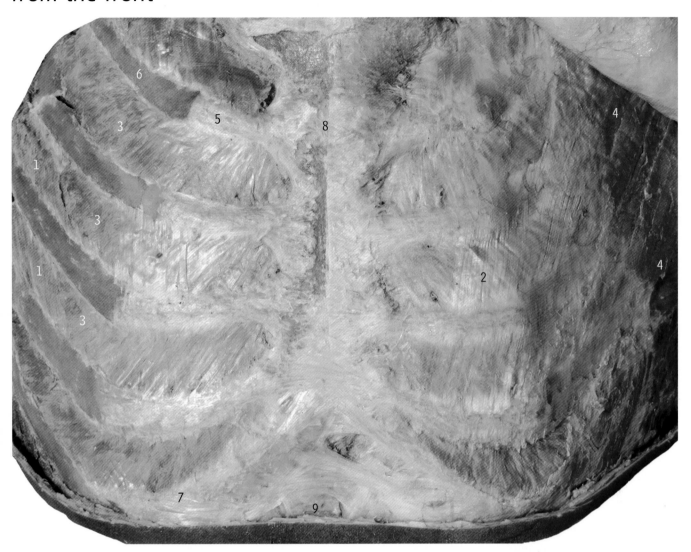

1 External intercostal muscle	**5** Second costal cartilage
2 External intercostal membrane	**6** Second rib
3 Internal intercostal muscle	**7** Sixth costal cartilage
4 Pectoralis minor muscle	**8** Sternal angle (Louis)
	9 Xiphoid process

The fibres of the **external intercostal muscles** (1) run downwards and medially, and near the costochondral junctions (as between 5 and 6) give place to the anterior intercostal membrane (here removed); these are thin sheets of connective tissue through which the underlying internal intercostal muscles (3) can be seen.

The fibres of the **internal intercostal muscles** (3) run downwards and laterally. At the front, they are covered by the anterior intercostal membranes, and at the back of the thorax they give place to the posterior intercostal membranes. The different directions of the muscle fibres enable the two muscle groups to be distinguished – down and medially for the externals (1), down and laterally for the internals (3).

The seventh costal cartilage is the lowest to join the sternum and together with the eighth, ninth and tenth cartilages forms the costal margin.

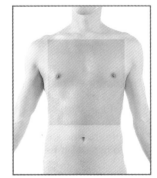

Coronal CT of chest

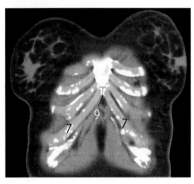

Flail chest, see pages 215–216.

Muscles of the thorax *right intercostal muscles*

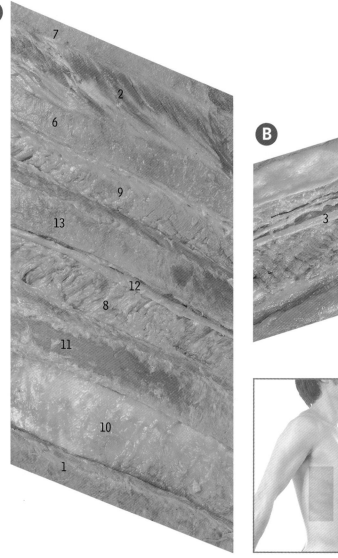

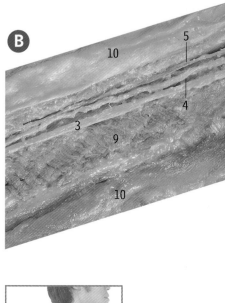

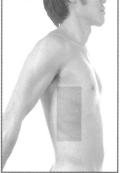

A from the outside

B from the inside

1 Eighth rib
2 External intercostal
3 Fifth intercostal nerve
4 Fifth posterior intercostal artery
5 Fifth posterior intercostal vein
6 Fifth rib
7 Fourth rib
8 Innermost intercostal
9 Internal intercostal
10 Pleura
11 Seventh rib
12 Sixth intercostal nerve
13 Sixth rib

> The **internal intercostal muscles** are continuous posteriorly with the posterior intercostal membranes which are covered up by the medial ends of the external intercostals (as at 2).

In A, each intercostal space has been dissected to a different depth, showing from above downwards an external intercostal muscle (2), internal intercostal (9), innermost intercostal (8) and pleura (10). The main intercostal vessels and nerve lie between the internal and innermost muscles; the nerve (12) is seen in the sixth interspace immediately below the sixth rib (13) and lying on the outer surface of the innermost intercostal (8), but the artery and vein are under cover of the costal groove. The vessels as well as the nerve are seen in the fifth intercostal space when this is dissected from the inside of the thorax, as in B; here the pleura and innermost intercostal muscle have been removed, and the vessels (5 and 4) and fifth intercostal nerve (3) lie against the inner surface of the internal intercostal (9).

Intercostal nerve block, see pages 215–216.

Muscles of the thorax

A *internal view thorax, from behind (inside view)*

B *left lower intercostal muscles*

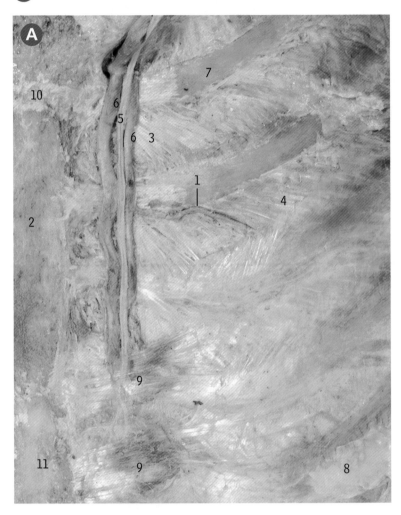

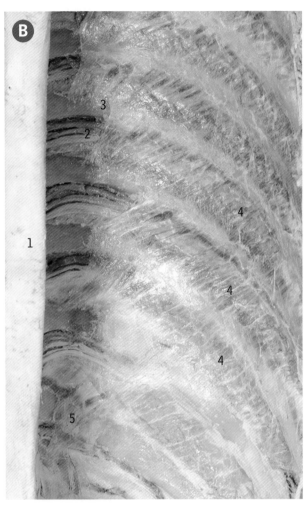

This view of the internal surface of the thoracic wall shows the posterior surface of the right half of the sternum and adjacent wall, with the pleura removed. The internal thoracic artery (4) is seen passing deep to the slips of transversus thoracis (9, previously called sternocostalis).

1	Anterior intercostal vein	**7**	Second rib
2	Body of sternum	**8**	Sixth rib
3	Innermost intercostal membrane	**9**	Slips of transversus thoracis muscle
4	Internal intercostal muscle	**10**	Sternal angle (Louis)
5	Internal thoracic artery	**11**	Xiphoid process
6	Internal thoracic veins		

This view of the lower left hemithorax is seen from the right and in front, with the pleura, vessels and nerves removed, and shows part of the innermost layer of thoracic wall muscles (4).

1	Descending thoracic aorta
2	Eighth intercostal neurovascular bundle
3	Eighth rib
4	Innermost intercostal muscle
5	Twelfth rib

Costochondral pathology, see pages 215–216.

Lungs, pericardium and pleura *from the front*

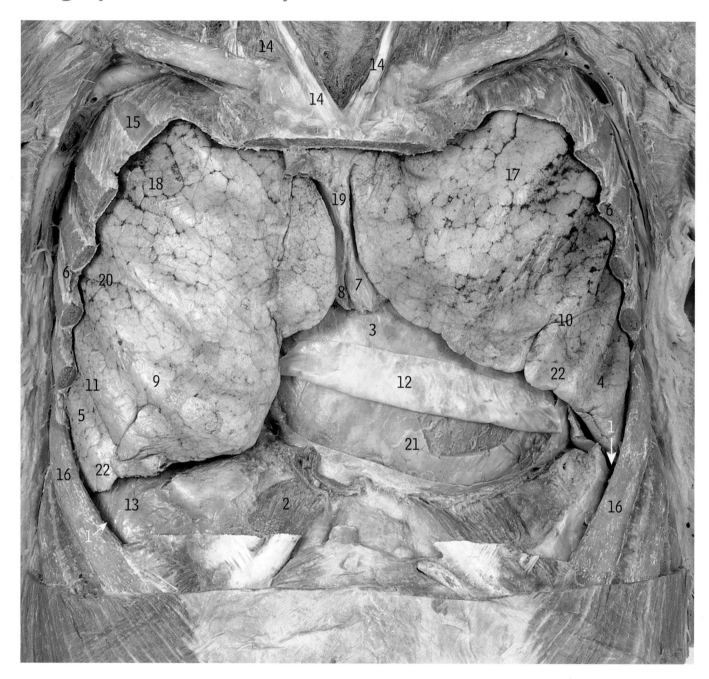

1 Costodiaphragmatic recess
2 Diaphragm
3 Fibrous pericardium
4 Inferior lobe of left lung
5 Inferior lobe of right lung
6 Intercostal muscles
7 Line of anterior reflection of left pleura
8 Line of anterior reflection of right pleura

9 Middle lobe of right lung
10 Oblique fissure of left lung
11 Oblique fissure of right lung
12 Parietal pericardium
13 Parietal diaphragmatic pleura
14 Sternocleidomastoid
15 Second rib
16 Seventh rib

17 Superior lobe of left lung
18 Superior lobe of right lung
19 Thymic remnants, see page 360
20 Transverse fissure of right lung
21 Visceral pericardium overlying myocardium
22 Visceral pleura

Cardiopulmonary resuscitation (CPR), thymus, see pages 215–216.

Heart and pericardium

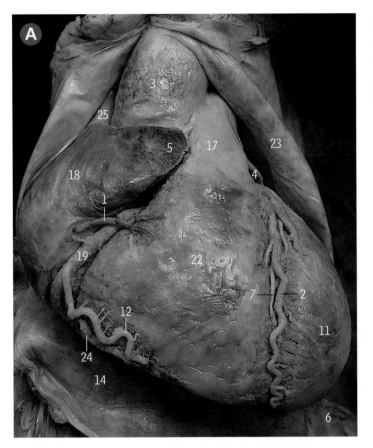

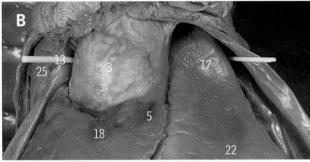

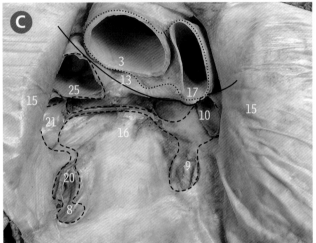

A from the front

B with marker in the transverse sinus

C oblique sinus after removal of the heart

1 Anterior cardiac vein
2 Anterior interventricular branch of left coronary artery
3 Ascending aorta
4 Auricle of left atrium
5 Auricle of right atrium
6 Diaphragm
7 Great cardiac vein
8 Inferior vena cava
9 Left inferior pulmonary vein
10 Left superior pulmonary vein
11 Left ventricle
12 Marginal branch of right coronary artery
13 Marker in transverse sinus
14 Pericardium fused with central tendon of diaphragm
15 Pericardium turned laterally over lung
16 Posterior wall of pericardial cavity and oblique sinus
17 Pulmonary trunk
18 Right atrium
19 Right coronary artery
20 Right inferior pulmonary vein
21 Right superior pulmonary vein
22 Right ventricle
23 Serous pericardium overlying fibrous pericardium (turned laterally)
24 Small cardiac vein
25 Superior vena cava

The **right border of the heart** is formed by the right atrium (A18).

The **left border** is formed mostly by the left ventricle (A11) with at the top the uppermost part (infundibulum) of the right ventricle (A22) and the tip of the left auricle (A4).

The **inferior border** is formed by the right ventricle (A22) with a small part of the left ventricle at the apex.

Anterior interventricular branch of left coronary artery = **left anterior descending (LAD)** as often used by clinicians.

In A, the pericardium has been incised and turned back (23) to display the anterior surface of the heart. The pulmonary trunk (17) leaves the right ventricle (22) in front and to the left of the ascending aorta (3), which is overlapped by the auricle (5) of the right atrium (18). The superior vena cava (25) is to the right of the aorta and still largely covered by pericardium. The anterior interventricular branch (2) of the left coronary artery and the great cardiac vein (7) lie in the interventricular groove between the right and left ventricles (22 and 11), and the right coronary artery (19) is in the atrioventricular groove between the right ventricle (22) and right atrium (18). In B, only the upper part of another heart is shown, with a marker in the transverse sinus, the space behind the aorta (3) and pulmonary trunk (17). In C, the heart has been removed from the pericardium, leaving the orifices of the great vessels. The dotted line indicates the attachment of the single sleeve of serous pericardium surrounding the aorta (3) and pulmonary trunk (17). The interrupted line indicates the attachment of another more complicated but still single sleeve of serous pericardium surrounding all the other six great vessels (the four pulmonary veins, 10, 9, 20 and 21, and the superior and inferior venae cavae, 25 and 8). The narrow interval between the two sleeves is the transverse sinus; the solid line in C indicates the path of the marker in B. The area of the pericardium (16) between the pulmonary veins and limited above by the reflection of the serious pericardium on to the back of the heart is the oblique sinus.

Cardiac tamponade, pericardial effusion, see pages 215–216.

Heart *with blood vessels injected* Ⓐ *from the front* Ⓑ *from behind*

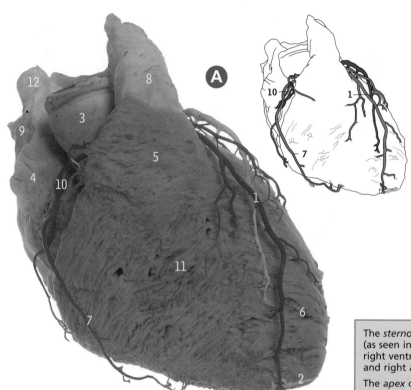

The coronary arteries have been injected with red latex and the cardiac veins with grey latex. The pulmonary trunk (8) passes upwards from the infundibulum (5) of the right ventricle (11), and at its commencement it is just in front and to the left of the ascending aorta (3).

1 Anterior interventricular branch of left coronary artery and great cardiac vein in interventricular groove
2 Apex
3 Ascending aorta
4 Auricle of right atrium (displaced laterally)
5 Infundibulum of right ventricle (conus arteriosus)
6 Left ventricle
7 Marginal branch of right coronary artery
8 Pulmonary trunk
9 Right atrium
10 Right coronary artery in anterior atrioventricular groove
11 Right ventricle
12 Superior vena cava

The *sternocostal* surface of the heart is the *anterior* surface (as seen in A on page 185 and A here) formed mainly by the right ventricle (A11, D7), with parts of the left ventricle (A6) and right atrium (A9 and D10).

The *apex* of the heart (A2) is formed by the left ventricle.

The *base* of the heart is the *posterior* surface, formed mainly by the left atrium (B8) with a small part of the right atrium (B13).

The *inferior* surface is the *diaphragmatic* surface, formed by the two ventricles (mainly the left) (B10 and B15).

Anterior interventricular branch of left coronary artery = *left anterior descending (LAD)* as often used by clinicians.

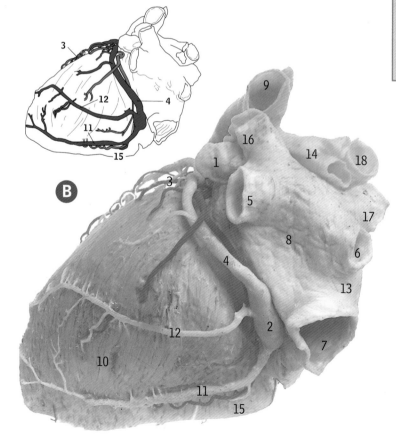

1 Auricle of left atrium
2 Coronary sinus in posterior atrioventricular groove
3 Great cardiac vein and anterior interventricular branch of left coronary artery
4 Great cardiac vein and circumflex branch of left coronary artery
5 Inferior left pulmonary vein
6 Inferior right pulmonary vein
7 Inferior vena cava
8 Left atrium
9 Left pulmonary artery
10 Left ventricle
11 Middle cardiac vein and posterior interventricular branch of right coronary artery in posterior interventricular groove
12 Posterior vein of left ventricle
13 Right atrium
14 Right pulmonary artery
15 Right ventricle
16 Superior left pulmonary vein
17 Superior right pulmonary vein
18 Superior vena cava

Coronary artery bypass grafting (CABG), myocardial infarction, see pages 215–216.

C Right atrium *from the front and right*

The anterior wall has been incised near its left margin and reflected to the right, showing on its internal surface the vertical crista terminalis (2) and horizontal pectinate muscles (7). The fossa ovalis (3) is on the interatrial septum, and the opening of the coronary sinus (6) is to the left of the inferior vena caval opening (4).

1 Auricle
2 Crista terminalis
3 Fossa ovalis
4 Inferior vena cava
5 Limbus
6 Opening of coronary sinus
7 Pectinate muscles
8 Position of atrioventricular node

9 Position of intervenous tubercle (lower)
10 Superior vena cava
11 Tricuspid valve
12 Valve of coronary sinus (Thebesian valve)
13 Valve of inferior vena cava (Eustachian valve)

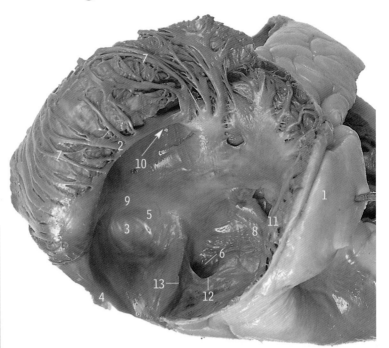

The fossa ovalis (3) forms part of the interatrial septum, and is part of the embryonic primary septum.

The limbus (5), which forms the margin of the fossa ovalis (3), represents the lower margin of the embryonic secondary septum. Before the primary and secondary septa fuse (at birth), the gap between them forms the foramen ovale.

The sinuatrial node (SA node, not illustrated) is embedded in the anterior wall of the atrium at the upper end of the crista terminalis, just below the opening of the superior vena cava.

The atrioventricular node (AV node, 8) is embedded in the interatrial septum, just above and to the left of the opening of the coronary sinus (6).

D Right ventricle *from the front*

1 Anterior cusp of tricuspid valve
2 Anterior papillary muscle
3 Ascending aorta
4 Auricle of right atrium
5 Chordae tendineae
6 Inferior vena cava
7 Infundibulum of right ventricle (conus arteriosus)
8 Posterior papillary muscle
9 Pulmonary trunk
10 Right atrium
11 Septomarginal trabeculation (moderator band)
12 Septal papillary muscle (of conus)
13 Superior vena cava

The septomarginal trabeculum (11), which conducts part of the right limb of the atrioventricular bundle from the interventricular septum (13) to the anterior papillary muscle (2), was formerly known as the moderator band.

The chordae tendineae (5) connect the cusps of the tricuspid valve to the papillary muscles.

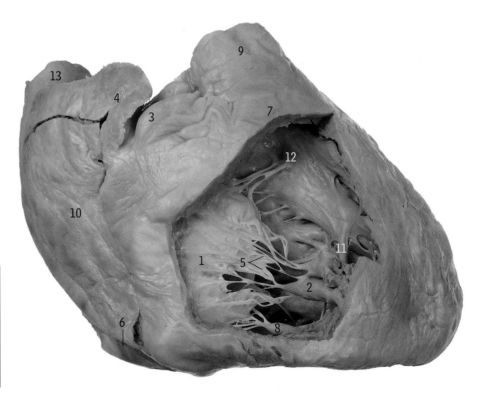

Artificial cardiac pacemaker, cardiac pacemaker, left ventricular enlargement, see pages 215–216.

Ⓐ Left ventricle
from the left and below

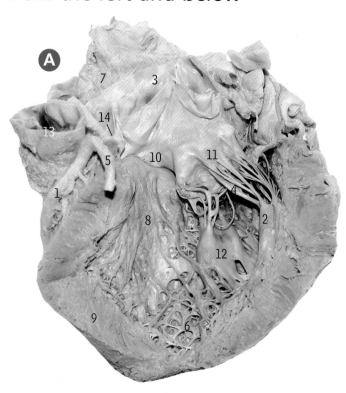

Ⓑ Heart
coronal section of the ventricles

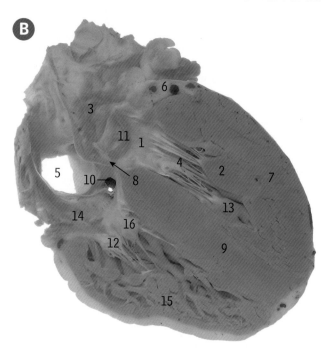

The heart has been cut in two in the coronal plane, and this is the posterior section seen from the front, looking towards the back of both ventricles. The section has passed immediately in front of the anterior cusp of the mitral valve (1) and the posterior cusp of the aortic valve (11).

1 Anterior interventricular artery
2 Anterolateral papillary muscle
3 Aorta
4 Chordae tendineae
5 Circumflex coronary artery
6 Coarse trabeculations
7 Left atrium
8 Left bundle branch
9 Left ventricle open
10 Membranous septum
11 Mitral valve
12 Posteromedial papillary muscle
13 Pulmonary valve
14 Right coronary orifice

The cusps of the aortic and pulmonary valves are here given their official names but some English texts use slightly different alternatives, as follows:

	Official	**English**
Aortic	Right	Anterior
	Left	Left posterior
	Posterior	Right posterior
Pulmonary	Left	Posterior
	Anterior	Left anterior
	Right	Right anterior

1 Anterior cusp of mitral valve
2 Anterolateral papillary muscle
3 Ascending aorta
4 Chordae tendineae
5 Inferior vena cava
6 Left coronary artery branches and great cardiac vein
7 Left ventricular wall
8 Membranous part of interventricular septum
9 Muscular part of interventricular septum
10 Opening of coronary sinus
11 Posterior cusp of aortic valve
12 Posterior cusp of tricuspid valve
13 Posterior papillary muscle
14 Right atrium
15 Right ventricular wall
16 Septal cusp of tricuspid valve

Mitral valve disease, see pages 215–216.

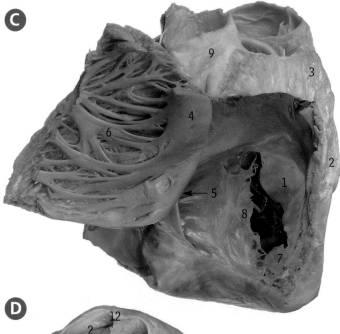

C Tricuspid valve *from the right atrium*

The atrium has been opened by incising the anterior wall (2) and turning the flap outwards so that the atrial surface of the atrioventricular orifice is seen, guarded by the three cusps of the tricuspid valve – anterior (1), posterior (7) and septal (8).

1 Anterior cusp of tricuspid valve	**6** Pectinate muscles
2 Anterior wall of right atrium	**7** Posterior cusp of tricuspid valve
3 Auricle of right atrium	
4 Crista terminalis	**8** Septal cusp of tricuspid valve
5 Interatrial septum	**9** Superior vena cava

The posterior cusp (7) of the tricuspid valve is the smallest.

D Pulmonary, aortic and mitral valves *from above*

The pulmonary trunk (12) and ascending aorta (3) have been cut off immediately above the three cusps of the pulmonary and aortic valves (7, 2 and 15, and 14, 10 and 6). The upper part of the left atrium (5) has been removed to show the upper surface of the mitral valve cusps (11 and 1).

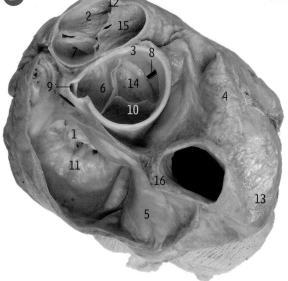

1 Anterior cusp of mitral valve	**9** Ostium of left coronary artery
2 Anterior cusp of pulmonary valve	**10** Posterior cusp of aortic valve
3 Ascending aorta	**11** Posterior cusp of mitral valve
4 Auricle of right atrium	**12** Pulmonary trunk
5 Left atrium	**13** Right atrium
6 Left cusp of aortic valve	**14** Right cusp of aortic valve
7 Left cusp of pulmonary valve	**15** Right cusp of pulmonary valve
8 Marker in ostium of right coronary artery	**16** Superior vena cava

E Heart *fibrous framework*

The heart is seen from the right and behind after removing both atria, looking down on to the fibrous rings (4) that surround the mitral and tricuspid orifices and form the attachments for the bases of the valve cusps. The cusps of the pulmonary valve (7, 2 and 13) are seen at the top of the infundibulum of the right ventricle (5), and the aortic valve cusps (12, 9 and 6) have been dissected out from the beginning of the ascending aorta.

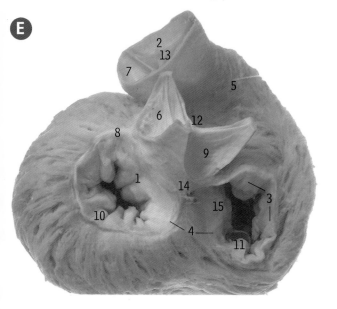

1 Anterior cusp of mitral valve	**8** Left fibrous trigone
2 Anterior cusp of pulmonary valve	**9** Posterior cusp of aortic valve
3 Anterior cusp of tricuspid valve	**10** Posterior cusp of mitral valve
4 Fibrous ring	**11** Posterior cusp of tricuspid valve
5 Infundibulum of right ventricle	**12** Right cusp of aortic valve
6 Left cusp of aortic valve	**13** Right cusp of pulmonary valve
7 Left cusp of pulmonary valve	**14** Right fibrous trigone
	15 Septal cusp of tricuspid valve

Coronary arteries

A left coronary arteriogram, lateral projection

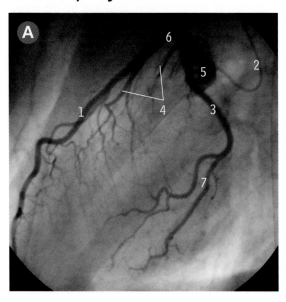

B right coronary arteriogram, left anterior oblique projection

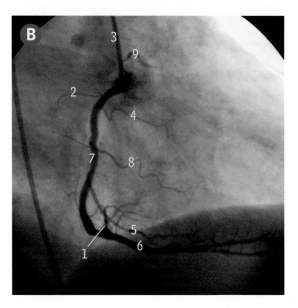

1 Anterior interventricular artery
2 Catheter in ascending aorta
3 Circumflex artery
4 Diagonal branches
5 Left coronary sinus (Valsalva)
6 Left main stem
7 Marginal artery

1 Atrio-ventricular nodal branch
2 Atrial branch
3 Catheter at aortic root
4 Conus artery
5 Marginal branch right coronary artery
6 Posterior interventricular artery
7 Right coronary artery
8 Right ventricular branch
9 Sinu-atrial nodal branch

C cast of the coronary arteries, from the front

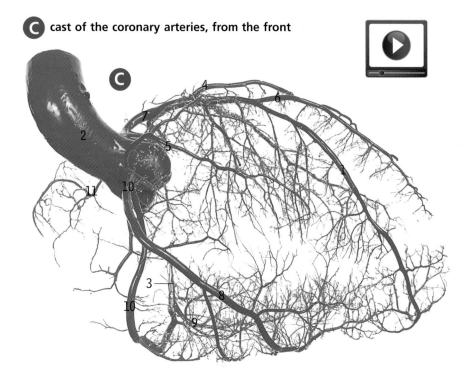

1 Anterior interventricular artery
2 Ascending aorta
3 Atrioventricular nodal artery
4 Circumflex artery
5 Conal artery
6 Diagonal artery
7 Left main stem
8 Marginal branch of right coronary artery
9 Posterior interventricular branch of right coronary artery
10 Right coronary artery
11 Sinu-atrial nodal branch

The interventricular branches are often called by clinicians the descending branches (anterior interventricular, left anterior descending; posterior interventricular, posterior descending).

Angina pectoris, coronary angiography, see pages 215–216.

D Coronary arteries *3D CT reconstruction*

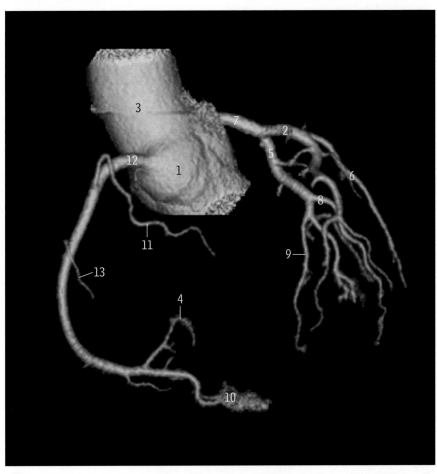

1 Anterior aortic sinus
2 Anterior interventricular, left anterior descending branch, left coronary artery (LAD)
3 Aorta, ascending
4 Atrioventricular nodal artery
5 Circumflex branch, left coronary artery
6 Diagonal artery
7 Left coronary main stem
8 Marginal artery, left coronary artery
9 Obtuse marginal branch, left coronary artery
10 Posterior interventricular branch, right coronary artery
11 Right conal artery
12 Right coronary artery
13 Right ventricular branch, right coronary artery

E Cast of the heart and great vessels *from below and behind*

This cast shows the coronary sinus (4) in the atrioventricular groove, and various tributaries (see notes).

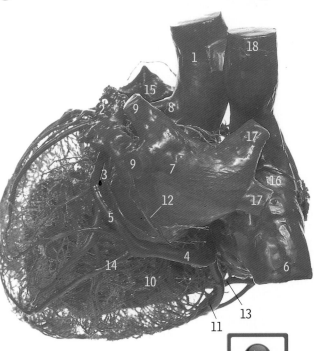

1 Ascending aorta
2 Auricle of left atrium
3 Circumflex branch of left coronary artery
4 Coronary sinus
5 Great cardiac vein
6 Inferior vena cava
7 Left atrium
8 Left coronary artery
9 Left pulmonary veins
10 Left ventricle
11 Middle cardiac vein
12 Oblique vein of left atrium
13 Posterior interventricular branch of right coronary artery
14 Posterior vein of left ventricle
15 Pulmonary trunk
16 Right atrium
17 Right pulmonary veins
18 Superior vena cava

The base of the heart is its posterior surface, formed largely by the left atrium (E7). Note that the base is not the part of the heart which joins the superior vena cava, aorta and pulmonary trunk; this part has no special name.

The very small oblique vein of the left atrium (E12) marks the point where the great cardiac vein (E5) becomes the coronary sinus (E4), but in E, the junction is unusually far to the right so that the posterior vein of the left ventricle (E14) joins the great cardiac vein (E5) instead of the coronary sinus itself.

The coronary sinus (E4), which receives most of the venous blood from the heart, lies in the posterior part of the atrioventricular groove between the left atrium and left ventricle and opens into the right atrium.

The coronary sinus normally receives as tributaries the great cardiac vein (E5), middle cardiac vein (E11), and the small cardiac vein, the posterior vein of the left ventricle (E14) and the oblique vein of the left atrium (E12).

Coronary abnormalities, dextrocardia, see pages 215–216.

Ⓐ Right lung root and mediastinal pleura

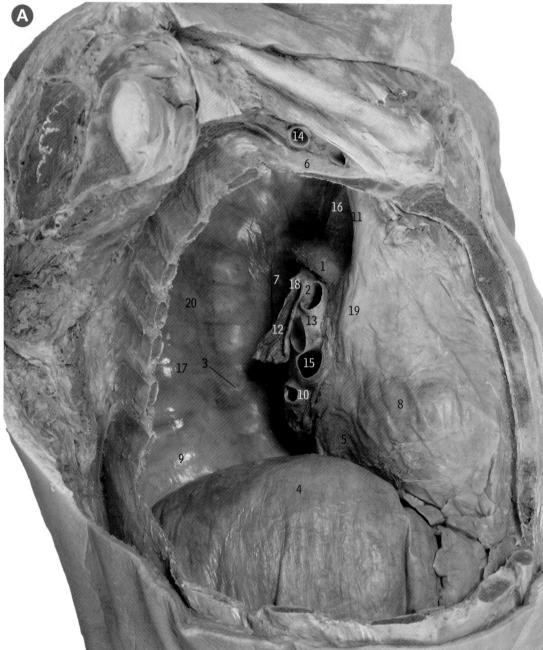

Ⓐ

This is the view of the right side of the mediastinum after removing the lung but with the parietal pleura still intact.

1 Azygos vein
2 Branch of right pulmonary artery to superior lobe
3 Branches of sympathetic trunk to greater splanchnic nerve
4 Diaphragm
5 Inferior vena cava
6 Neck of first rib
7 Oesophagus
8 Pericardium over right atrium
9 Pleura, costal
10 Right inferior pulmonary vein
11 Right phrenic nerve
12 Right principal bronchus
13 Right pulmonary artery
14 Right subclavian artery
15 Right superior pulmonary vein
16 Right vagus nerve
17 Sixth right posterior intercostal vessels under parietal pleura
18 Superior lobe bronchus
19 Superior vena cava
20 Sympathetic trunk and ganglion

Ⓑ Right lung root and mediastinum

In a similar specimen to A, most of the pleura has been removed to display the underlying structures. The azygos vein (1) arches over the structures forming the lung root to enter the superior vena cava (24). The highest structures in the lung root are the artery (2) and bronchus (14) to the superior lobe of the lung. The right superior pulmonary vein (18) is in front of the right pulmonary artery, with the right inferior pulmonary vein (12) the lowest structure in the root. Above the arch of the azygos vein the trachea (28), with the right vagus nerve (19) in contact with it, lies in front of the oesophagus (8). Part of the first rib has been cut away to show the structures lying in front of its neck (5), the sympathetic trunk (27), supreme intercostal vein (22), superior intercostal artery (20) and the ventral ramus of the first thoracic nerve. The right recurrent laryngeal nerve hooks underneath the right subclavian artery (16). The right phrenic nerve (13) runs down over the superior vena cava (24) and the pericardium overlying the right atrium (9), and pierces the diaphragm (4) beside the inferior vena cava. Contributions from the sympathetic trunk (3) pass over the sides of vertebral bodies superficial to posterior intercostal arteries and veins (as at 20 and 21) to form the greater splanchnic nerve. The lower part of the oesophagus (8) behind the lung root and heart has the azygos vein (1) on its right side.

Surgical emphysema, see pages 215–216.

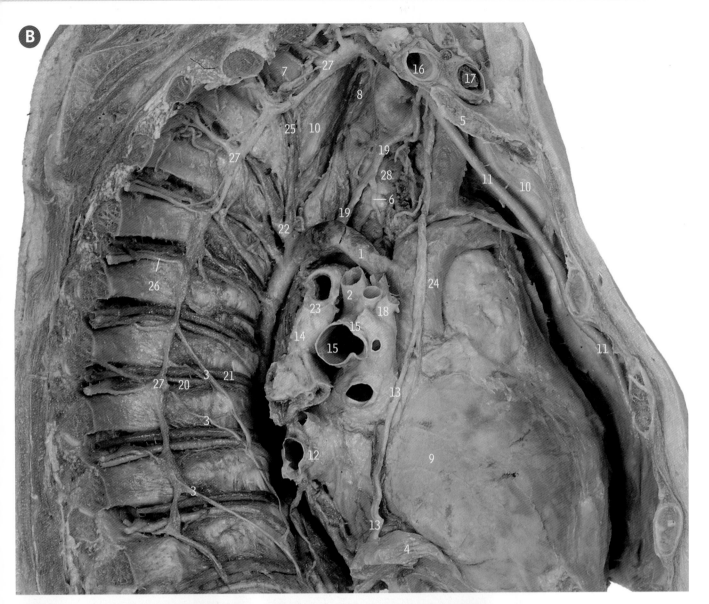

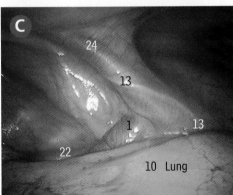

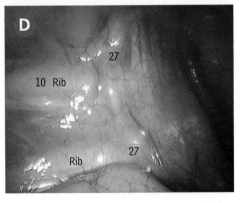

C D Thoracoscopies

1 Azygos vein (arch)
2 Branch of right pulmonary artery to superior lobe
3 Branches of sympathetic trunk to greater splanchnic nerve
4 Diaphragm
5 First rib (sectioned)
6 Inferior cardiac branches of vagus nerve
7 Neck of first rib
8 Oesophagus
9 Pericardium over right atrium
10 Pleura
11 Right internal thoracic artery
12 Right inferior pulmonary vein
13 Right phrenic nerve
14 Right principal bronchus
15 Right pulmonary artery
16 Right subclavian artery
17 Right subclavian vein (NB thrombus)
18 Right superior pulmonary vein
19 Right vagus nerve
20 Sixth right posterior intercostal artery
21 Sixth right posterior intercostal vein
22 Superior intercostal vein
23 Superior lobe bronchus
24 Superior vena cava
25 Supreme intercostal vein
26 Sympathetic rami communicantes
27 Sympathetic trunk and ganglion
28 Trachea

Pleural effusion, thoracoscopy, transthoracic sympathectomy, see pages 215–216.

Left lung root and mediastinal pleura

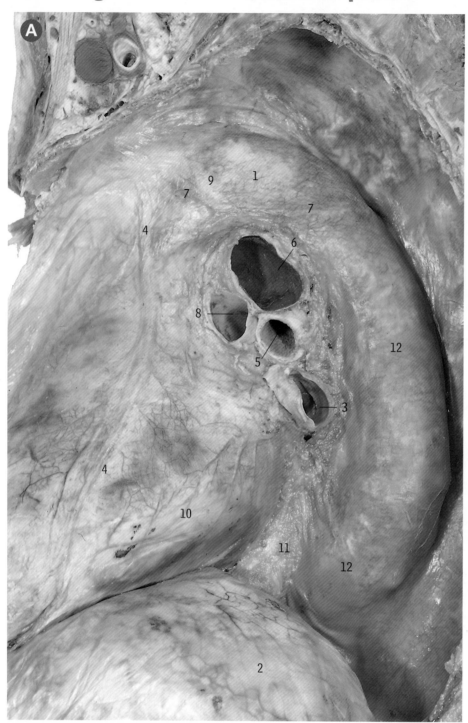

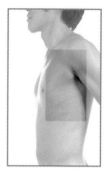

1 Arch of aorta
2 Diaphragm
3 Left inferior pulmonary vein
4 Left phrenic nerve and
  pericardiophrenic vessels
5 Left principal bronchus
6 Left pulmonary artery
7 Left superior intercostal vein
8 Left superior pulmonary vein
9 Left vagus nerve
10 Mediastinal pleura and pericardium
   overlying left ventricle
11 Oesophagus
12 Thoracic aorta, descending

Left parasagittal CT

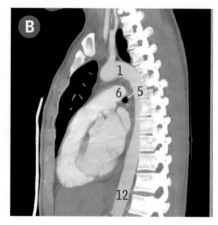

On the left side above the diaphragm,
the lower end of the oesophagus lies in
a triangle bounded by the diaphragm
below (2), the heart in front (10) and
the descending aorta behind (12).

This is the view of the left side of the mediastinum after removing the lung
but with the parietal pleura still intact. Compare the features seen here with
those in the dissection opposite (a different specimen), from which the
pleura has been removed.

Pneumothorax, thoracic aortic aneurysm, see pages 215–216.

Left lung root and mediastinum

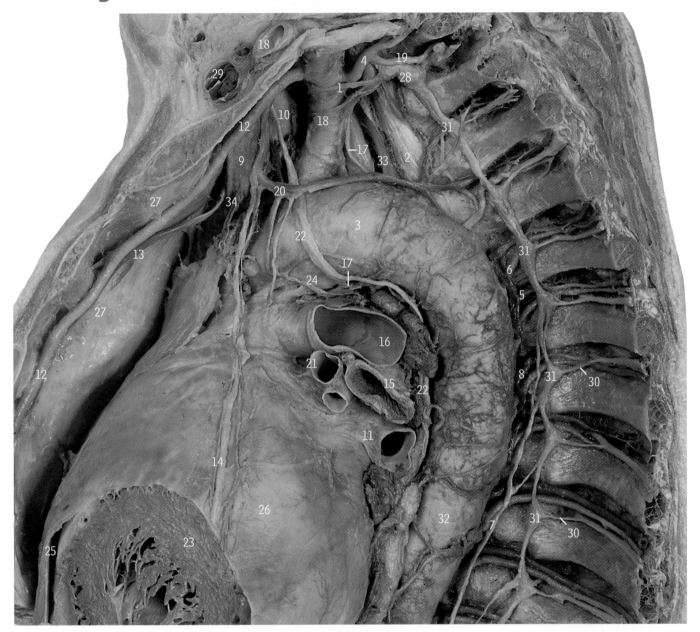

1 Ansa subclavia	**9** Left brachiocephalic vein	**19** Left superior intercostal artery
2 Anterior longitudinal ligament	**10** Left common carotid artery	**20** Left superior intercostal vein
3 Arch of aorta	**11** Left inferior pulmonary vein	**21** Left superior pulmonary vein
4 Costocervical trunk	**12** Left internal thoracic artery	**22** Left vagus nerve
5 Fifth left posterior intercostal vein	**13** Left internal thoracic vein	**23** Left ventricle (NB thick-walled cavity)
6 Fourth left posterior intercostal artery	**14** Left phrenic nerve and pericardiophrenic vessels	**24** Ligamentum arteriosum
7 Greater splanchnic nerve	**15** Left principal bronchus	**25** Pericardial cavity (space)
8 Hemi-azygos vein	**16** Left pulmonary artery	**26** Pericardium overlying left ventricle
	17 Left recurrent laryngeal nerve	
	18 Left subclavian artery	

27 Pleura (cut edge)	
28 Stellate ganglion	
29 Subclavian vein	
30 Sympathetic rami communicantes	
31 Sympathetic trunk and ganglion	
32 Thoracic aorta	
33 Thoracic duct (page 209)	
34 Thymic veins (page 360)	

Coarctation of the aorta, subclavian arterial stent, see pages 215–216.

Axial CT images *with contrast*

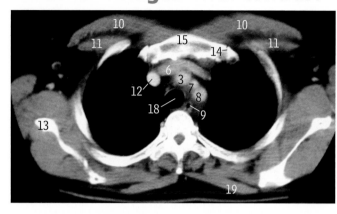

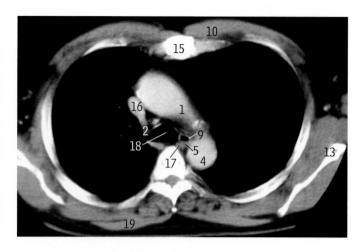

A Level of T2

1 Arch aorta
2 Azygos vein
3 Brachiocephalic trunk (artery)
4 Descending aorta
5 Hemi-azygos vein

6 Left brachiocephalic vein
7 Left common carotid artery
8 Left subclavian artery
9 Oesophagus
10 Pectoralis major

B Level of T4

11 Pectoralis minor
12 Right brachiocephalic vein
13 Scapula
14 Sternoclavicular joint
15 Sternum

16 Superior vena cava
17 Thoracic duct
18 Trachea
19 Trapezius

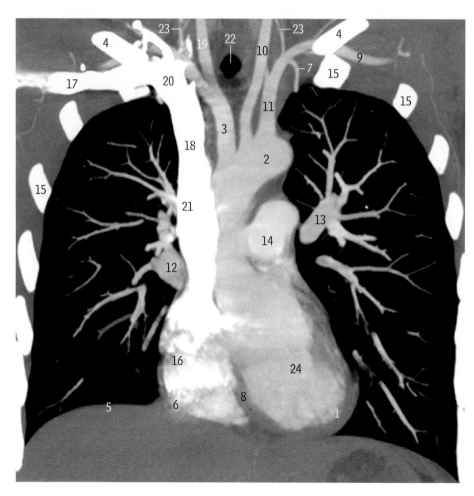

C Thorax
coronal 64 slice CT reconstruction – venous phase

1 Apex of heart
2 Arch of aorta
3 Brachiocephalic trunk
4 Clavicle
5 Dome of diaphragm, right
6 Inferior vena cava
7 Internal thoracic artery
8 Interventricular septum
9 Left axillary artery
10 Left common carotid artery
11 Left subclavian artery
12 Pulmonary artery, right
13 Pulmonary artery, upper lobe branch
14 Pulmonary trunk
15 Ribs
16 Right atrium
17 Right axillary vein
18 Right brachiocephalic vein
19 Right common carotid artery
20 Right subclavian vein
21 Superior vena cava
22 Trachea
23 Vertebral artery
24 Ventricle, left

Phrenic nerve palsy, see pages 215–216.

Cast of the lower trachea and bronchi

A *vertical from the front* **B** *oblique from the left*

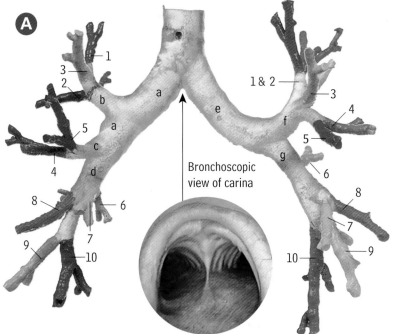

The principal and lobar bronchi are labelled with letters; the segmental bronchi are labelled with their conventional numbers. In the side view in B, the cast has been tilted to avoid overlap, and the right side is more anterior than the left.

Bronchoscopic view of carina

Right lung
Lobar bronchi
a Principal
b Superior lobe
c Middle lobe
d Inferior lobe

Left lung

e Principal
f Superior lobe
g Inferior lobe

Segmental bronchi
Superior lobe
1 Apical
2 Posterior
3 Anterior

Superior lobe
1 & 2 Apicoposterior
3 Anterior
4 Superior lingular
5 Inferior lingular

Middle lobe
4 Lateral
5 Medial

Inferior lobe
6 Apical (superior)
7 Medial basal
8 Anterior basal
9 Lateral basal
10 Posterior basal

Inferior lobe
6 Apical (superior)
7 Medial basal
8 Anterior basal
9 Lateral basal
10 Posterior basal

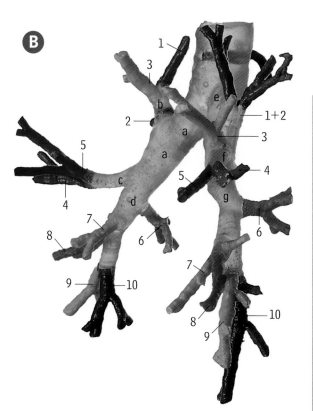

The trachea divides into right and left principal bronchi (a and e).

The right principal bronchus (a) is shorter, wider and more vertical than the left (e).

The left principal bronchus (e) is longer and narrower and lies more transversely than the right. Foreign bodies are therefore more likely to enter the right principal bronchus than the left.

The right principal bronchus (a) gives off a superior lobe bronchus (b) and then enters the hilum of the right lung before dividing into middle and inferior lobe bronchi (c and d).

The left principal bronchus (e) enters the hilum of the lung before dividing into superior and inferior lobe bronchi (f and g).

The branches of the lobar bronchi are called segmental bronchi and each supplies a segment of lung tissue – bronchopulmonary segment. The segmental bronchi and the bronchopulmonary segments have similar names, and the ten segments of each lung are officially numbered (as here and page 198) as well as being named.

The segmental bronchi of the left and right lungs are essentially similar except that the apical and posterior bronchi of the superior lobe of the left lung arise from a common stem, thus called the apicoposterior bronchus and labelled here as 1 and 2; also there is no middle lobe of the left lung, and so the corresponding segments bear similar numbers; and the medial basal bronchus (7) of the left lung usually arises in common with the anterior basal (8).

The apical (superior) bronchus of the inferior lobe (6) of both lungs is the first or highest bronchus to arise from the posterior surface of the bronchial tree, as illustrated in B. When lying on the back fluid may therefore gravitate into this bronchus.

Cast of the bronchial tree

The bronchi and bronchopulmonary segments have been coloured and labelled with their conventional numbers.

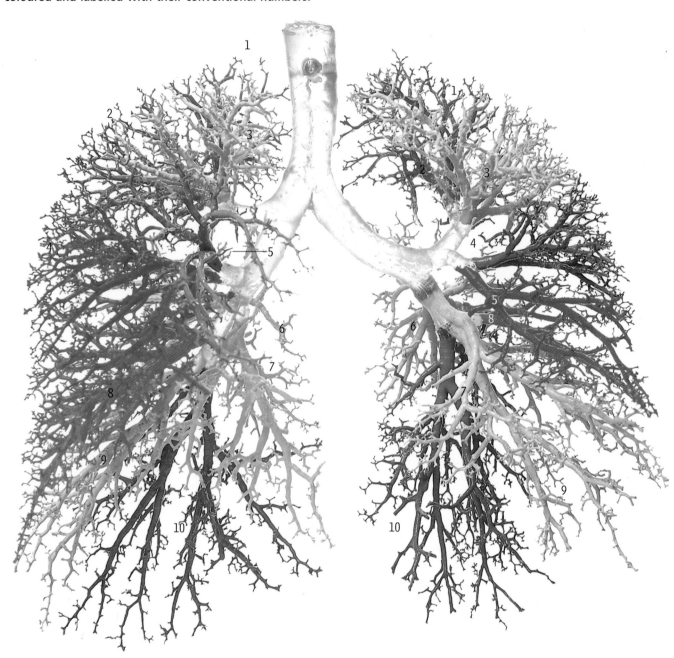

Right lung

Superior lobe
1 Apical
2 Posterior
3 Anterior

Middle lobe
4 Lateral
5 Medial

Inferior lobe
6 Apical (superior)
7 Medial basal
8 Anterior basal
9 Lateral basal
10 Posterior basal

Left lung

Superior lobe
1 Apical
2 Posterior
3 Anterior
4 Superior lingular
5 Inferior lingular

Inferior lobe
6 Apical (superior)
7 Medial basal (cardiac)
8 Anterior basal
9 Lateral basal
10 Posterior basal

Bronchoscopy, empyema, see pages 215–216.

Bronchopulmonary segments of the right lung

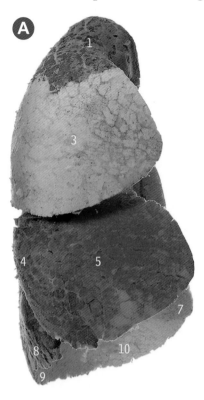

Ⓐ

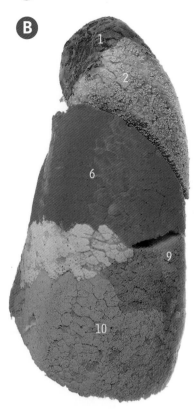

Ⓑ

Ⓐ *from the front*
Ⓑ *from behind*

Superior lobe
1 Apical
2 Posterior
3 Anterior

Middle lobe
4 Lateral
5 Medial

Inferior lobe
6 Apical (superior)
7 Medial basal
8 Anterior basal
9 Lateral basal
10 Posterior basal

A subapical (subsuperior) segmental bronchus and bronchopulmonary segment are present in over 50% of lungs; in this specimen, this additional segment is shown in white.

The posterior basal segment (10) is coloured with two different shades of yellow ochre.

Bronchopulmonary segments of the left lung

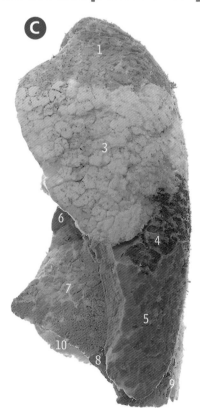

Ⓒ

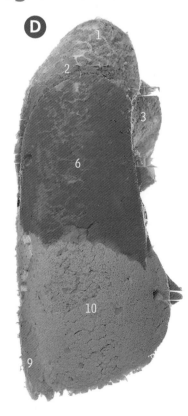

Ⓓ

Ⓒ *from the front*
Ⓓ *from behind*

Superior lobe
1 Apical
2 Posterior
3 Anterior
4 Superior lingular
5 Inferior lingular

Inferior lobe
6 Apical (superior)
7 Medial basal (cardiac)
8 Anterior basal
9 Lateral basal
10 Posterior basal

The apical and posterior segments (1 and 2) are both coloured green, having been filled from the common apicoposterior bronchus (see page 197).

A Bronchopulmonary segments of the right lung
from the lateral sides

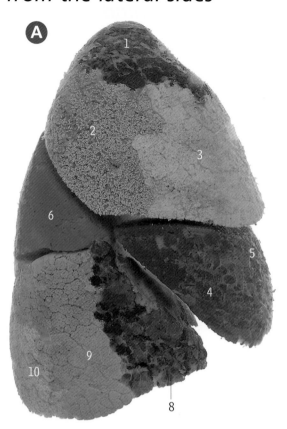

B Right bronchogram

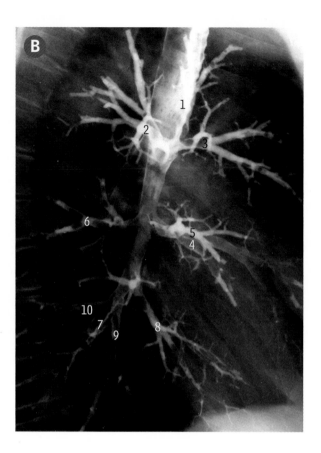

Coronal CT, lung windows*

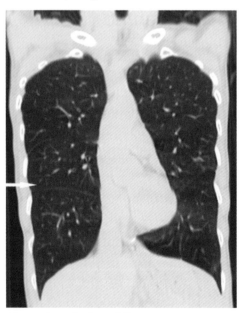

*Arrow shows horizontal fissure.

Superior lobe
1 Apical
2 Posterior
3 Anterior

Middle lobe
4 Lateral
5 Medial

Inferior lobe
6 Apical (superior)
7 Medial basal
8 Anterior basal
9 Lateral basal
10 Posterior basal

The medial basal segment (7) is not seen in the view in A.

The posterior basal segment in A (10) is coloured with two different shades of green.

Empyema, see pages 215–216.

C Bronchopulmonary segments of the left lung *from the lateral side*

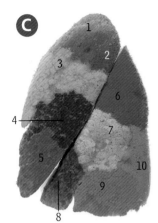

Superior lobe
1 Apical
2 Posterior
3 Anterior
4 Superior lingular
5 Inferior lingular

Inferior lobe
6 Apical (superior)
7 Medial basal (cardiac)
8 Anterior basal
9 Lateral basal
10 Posterior basal

The apical and posterior segments (1 and 2) are both coloured green, having been filled from the common apicoposterior bronchus (see page 199, D).

D Left bronchogram

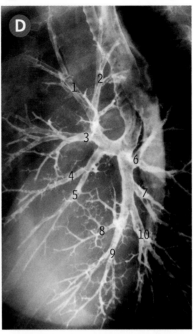

1 Anterior segmental bronchi
2 Anterior segmental vein
3 Apicoposterior segmental bronchi
4 Apicoposterior segmental vein
5 Inferior lingular segmental bronchus
6 Inferior lingular segmental vein
7 Inferior lobar bronchus
8 Inferior lobe
9 Left inferior pulmonary vein
10 Left main bronchus
11 Left pulmonary artery
12 Left superior pulmonary vein
13 Lingular bronchus
14 Oblique fissure
15 Superior division bronchus
16 Superior lingular segmental bronchus
17 Superior lingular segmental vein
18 Superior lobar bronchus
19 Superior lobe

E Lungs, detailed dissections to show bronchopulmonary segments of left lung

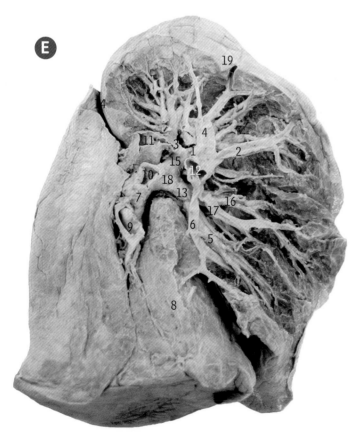

Sagittal CT, lung windows*

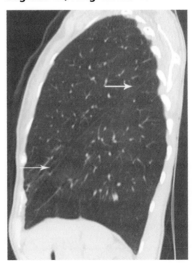

*Arrows show oblique fissure.

Haemothorax, see pages 215–216.

A Cast of the bronchial tree and pulmonary vessels *from the front*

B Lung roots and bronchial arteries *right side from above*

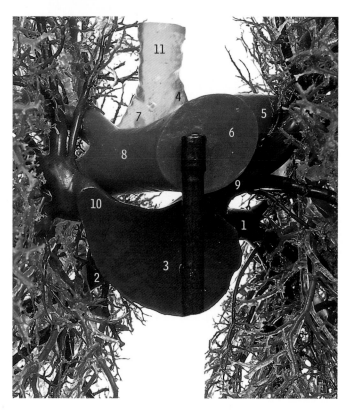

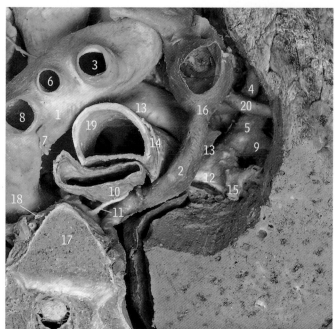

The thorax has been sectioned transversely at the level of the third thoracic vertebra (17), just above the arch of the aorta (1) whose three larger branches have been removed (8, 6 and 3), and lung tissue at the hilum has been dissected away from above. The oesophagus (10) and trachea (19) have been tilted forwards to show one of the bronchial arteries (11).

The pulmonary trunk (6) divides into the left and right pulmonary arteries (5 and 8), and these vessels have been injected with red resin. The four pulmonary veins (9, 1, 2 and 10) which drain into the left atrium (3) have been filled with blue resin. Note that in the living body the pulmonary veins are filled with oxygenated blood from the lungs and would normally be represented by a red colour; similarly the pulmonary arteries contain deoxygenated blood and should be represented by a blue colour.

1 Arch of aorta	**12** Right principal bronchus
2 Azygos vein	**13** Right pulmonary artery
3 Brachiocephalic trunk	**14** Right vagus nerve
4 Inferior lobe artery	**15** Superior lobe bronchus
5 Inferior lobe bronchus	**16** Superior vena cava
6 Left common carotid artery	**17** Third thoracic vertebra
7 Left recurrent laryngeal nerve	**18** Thoracic duct
8 Left subclavian artery	**19** Trachea
9 Middle lobe bronchus	**20** Tributary of inferior
10 Oesophagus	pulmonary vein
11 Right bronchial artery	

1 Inferior left pulmonary vein	**7** Right principal bronchus
2 Inferior right pulmonary vein	**8** Right pulmonary artery
3 Left atrium	**9** Superior left pulmonary vein
4 Left principal bronchus	**10** Superior right pulmonary vein
5 Left pulmonary artery	
6 Pulmonary trunk	**11** Trachea

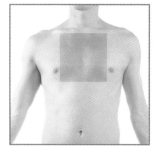

Carcinoma of the oesophagus, pulmonary embolism, see pages 215–216.

C Cast of the pulmonary arteries and bronchi *from the front*

D Pulmonary arteriogram

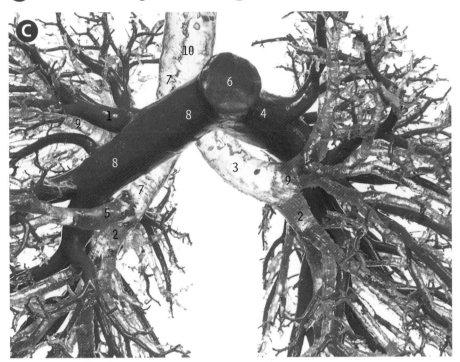

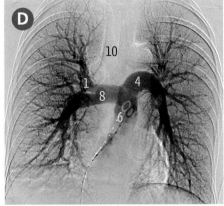

The upper part of the pulmonary trunk (6) is seen end-on after cutting off the lower part, and the bifurcation of the trunk into the left (4) and right (8) pulmonary arteries is in front of the beginning of the left main bronchus (3). In the living body, these pulmonary vessels contain deoxygenated blood and would normally be represented by a blue colour, but here they have been filled with red resin. Compare the vessels in the cast with those in the arteriogram D.

1 Branch of right pulmonary artery to superior lobe
2 Inferior lobe bronchus
3 Left principal bronchus
4 Left pulmonary artery
5 Middle lobe bronchus
6 Pulmonary trunk
7 Right principal bronchus
8 Right pulmonary artery
9 Superior lobe bronchus
10 Trachea

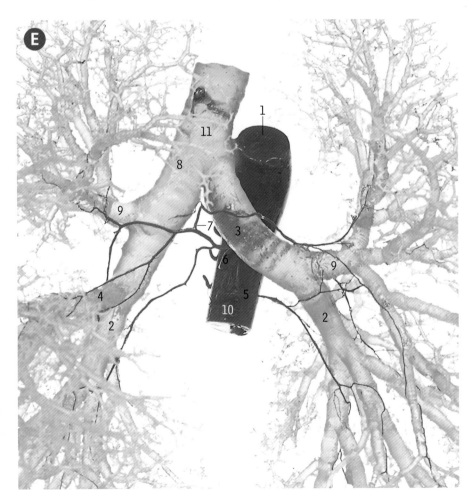

E Cast of the bronchi and bronchial arteries *from the front*

Part of the aorta (1 and 10) has been injected with red resin to fill the bronchial arteries. These vessels normally run behind the bronchi and their branches but in this specimen, they are in front.

1 Arch of aorta
2 Inferior lobe bronchus
3 Left principal bronchus
4 Middle lobe bronchus
5 Origin of lower left bronchial artery
6 Origin of right bronchial artery
7 Origin of upper left bronchial artery
8 Right principal bronchus
9 Superior lobe bronchus
10 Thoracic aorta
11 Trachea

A Right lung *medial surface*

B Left lung *medial surface*

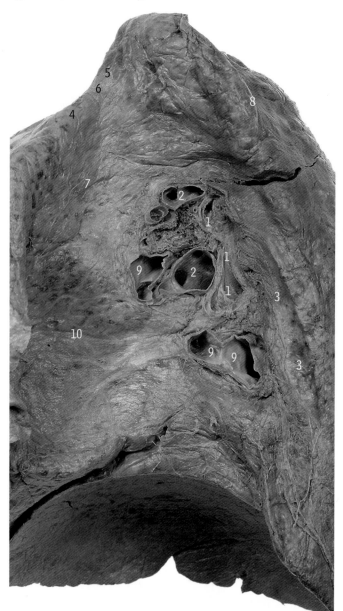

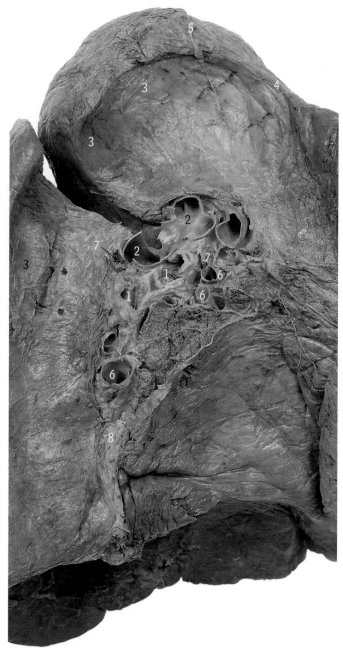

In the hardened dissecting room specimen, adjacent structures make impressions on the medial surface of the lung. The most prominent feature on the right side is the groove for the azygos vein (3), above and behind the structures of the lung root (9, 2 and 1).

1 Branches of right principal bronchus
2 Branches of right pulmonary artery
3 Groove for azygos vein
4 Groove for first rib
5 Groove for subclavian artery
6 Groove for subclavian vein
7 Groove for superior vena cava
8 Oesophageal and tracheal area
9 Right pulmonary veins
10 Transverse fissure

The upper end of the medial surface of the right lung lies against the oesophagus and trachea (A8) with only the pleura intervening, but on the left, the subclavian artery (B5) (and the left common carotid in front of it) keep the lung further away from these structures.

Compare with the right lung in A, and note the large size of the impression made by the aorta on the left lung (B3), in contrast to the smaller azygos groove on the right (A3).

1 Branches of left principal bronchus
2 Branches of left pulmonary artery
3 Groove for aorta
4 Groove for first rib
5 Groove for left subclavian artery
6 Left pulmonary veins
7 Lymph node, containing carbon
8 Pulmonary ligament

Carcinoma of the lung, mesothelioma, tuberculosis, see pages 215–216.

Lower neck and upper thorax *surface markings*

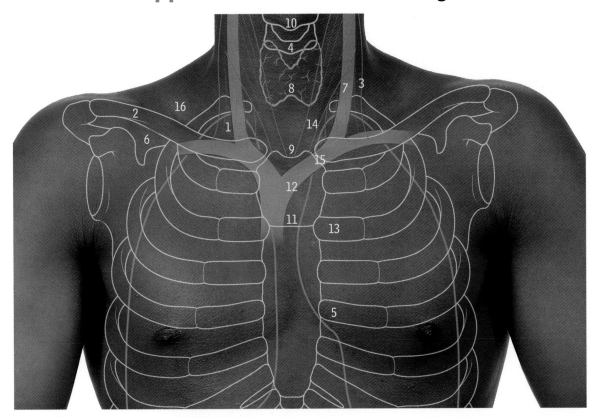

The purple line indicates the extent of the pleura and lung on each side; the apices of the pleura and lung (1) rise into the neck for about 3 cm above the medial third of the clavicle. The lower end of the internal jugular vein (7) lies behind the interval between the sternal (14) and clavicular (3) heads of sternocleidomastoid. Behind the sternoclavicular joint (15) the internal jugular and subclavian veins unite to form the brachiocephalic vein. The trachea (8) is felt in the midline above the jugular notch (9), and the arch of the cricoid cartilage (4) is 4–5 cm above the notch. The manubriosternal joint is at the level of the second costal cartilage (13) and opposite the lower border of the body of the fourth thoracic vertebra, and the horizontal plane through these points indicates the junction between the superior and inferior parts of the mediastinum. The left brachiocephalic vein passes behind the upper half of the manubrium to unite with the right brachiocephalic at the lower border of the right first costal cartilage (to form the superior vena cava). The midpoint of the manubrium (12) marks the highest level of the arch of the aorta and the origin of the brachiocephalic trunk. Compare many of the features mentioned here with the structures in the dissection on page 206.

1 Apex of pleura and lung
2 Clavicle
3 Clavicular head of sternocleidomastoid
4 Cricoid cartilage
5 Fourth costal cartilage
6 Infraclavicular fossa
7 Internal jugular vein
8 Isthmus of thyroid gland overlying trachea
9 Jugular notch (suprasternal)
10 Laryngeal prominence of the thyroid cartilage
11 Manubriosternal joint
12 Midpoint of manubrium of sternum
13 Second costal cartilage
14 Sternal head of sternocleidomastoid
15 Sternoclavicular joint
16 Supraclavicular fossa

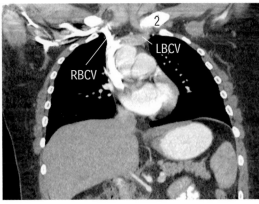

Coronal CT, venous phase of chest showing right (RBCV) and left (LBCV) brachiocephalic veins

Superior vena cava obstruction, variations in great veins, see pages 215–216.

Thoracic inlet and mediastinum *from the front*

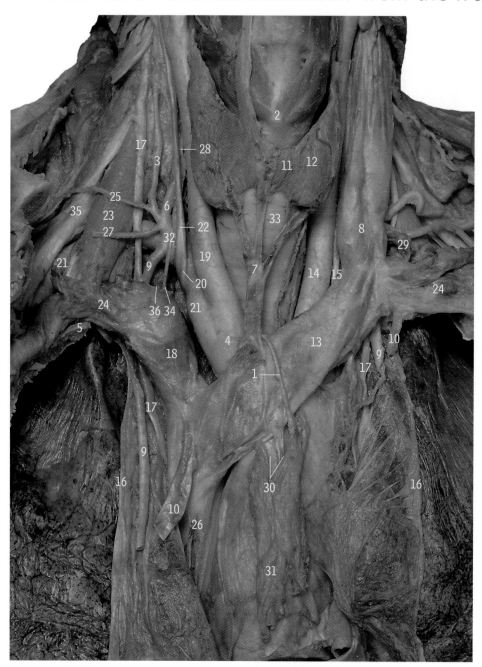

The anterior thoracic wall and the medial ends of the clavicles have been removed, but part of the parietal pleura (16) remains over the medial part of each lung. The right internal jugular vein has also been removed, displaying the thyrocervical trunk (32) and the origin of the internal thoracic artery (9). Inferior thyroid veins (7) run down over the trachea (33) to enter the left brachiocephalic vein (13). The thymus (31) has been dissected out from mediastinal fat; thymic veins (30) enter the left brachiocephalic vein, and an unusual thymic artery (1) arises from the brachiocephalic trunk (4).

The remains of the thymus (31) are in front of the pericardium, but in the child, where the thymus is much larger (see page 184), it may extend upwards in front of the great vessels as high as the lower part of the thyroid gland (12).

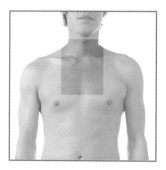

1 A thymic artery	**13** Left brachiocephalic vein	**25** Superficial cervical artery
2 Arch of cricoid cartilage	**14** Left common carotid artery	**26** Superior vena cava
3 Ascending cervical artery	**15** Left vagus nerve	**27** Suprascapular artery
4 Brachiocephalic trunk	**16** Parietal pleura (cut edge) over lung	**28** Sympathetic trunk
5 First rib cut edge	**17** Phrenic nerve	**29** Thoracic duct
6 Inferior thyroid artery	**18** Right brachiocephalic vein	**30** Thymic veins
7 Inferior thyroid veins	**19** Right common carotid artery	**31** Thymus
8 Internal jugular vein	**20** Right recurrent laryngeal nerve	**32** Thyrocervical trunk
9 Internal thoracic artery	**21** Right subclavian artery	**33** Trachea
10 Internal thoracic vein	**22** Right vagus nerve	**34** Unusual cervical tributary of 18
11 Isthmus of thyroid gland	**23** Scalenus anterior	**35** Upper trunk of brachial plexus
12 Lateral lobe of thyroid gland	**24** Subclavian vein	**36** Vertebral vein

Pancoast tumour, thoracic outlet syndromes, see pages 215–216.

Thoracic inlet and superior mediastinum
axilla and root of neck

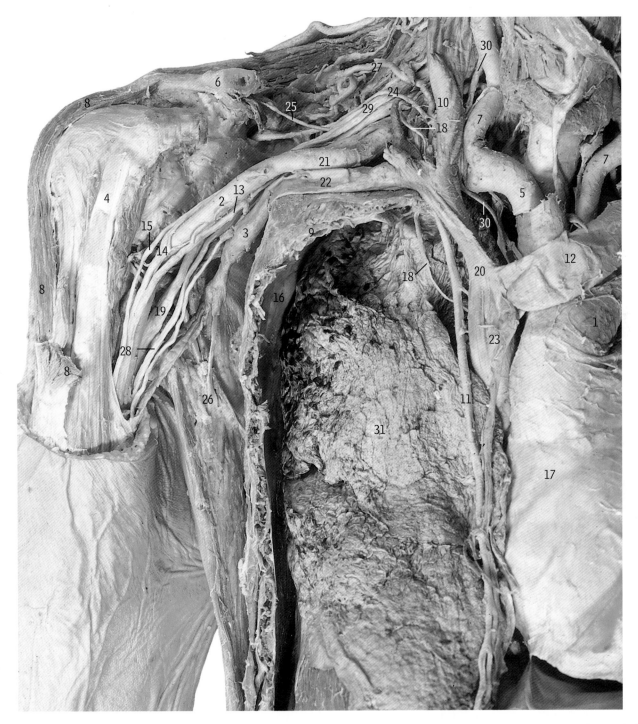

1 Aortic arch	**10** Internal jugular vein	**18** Phrenic nerve	**27** Transverse cervical artery
2 Axillary artery	**11** Internal thoracic artery	**19** Radial nerve	**28** Ulnar nerve
3 Axillary vein	**12** Left brachiocephalic vein	**20** Right brachiocephalic vein	**29** Upper trunk, brachial plexus
4 Biceps, short head	**13** Medial cord, brachial plexus	**21** Subclavian artery	**30** Vagus nerve
5 Brachiocephalic trunk	**14** Median nerve	**22** Subclavian vein	**31** Visceral pleura covering lung
6 Clavicle (cut and removed)	**15** Musculocutaneous nerve	**23** Superior vena cava	
7 Common carotid artery	**16** Parietal pleural covering of	**24** Suprascapular artery	
8 Deltoid	chest wall	**25** Suprascapular nerve	
9 First rib	**17** Pericardium, fibrous layer	**26** Thoracodorsal vein	

Bronchiectasis, sarcoidosis, see pages 215–216.

Thoracic inlet *right upper ribs, from below*

ANTERIOR

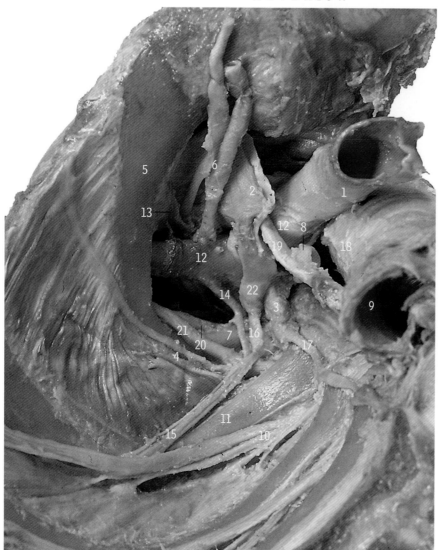

MEDIAL

1 Brachiocephalic trunk
2 Brachiocephalic vein
3 Cervicothoracic (stellate) ganglion
4 First intercostal nerve
5 First rib
6 Internal thoracic vessels
7 Neck of first rib
8 Recurrent laryngeal nerve
9 Right principal bronchus
10 Second intercostal nerve
11 Second rib
12 Subclavian artery
13 Subclavian vein
14 Superior intercostal artery
15 Superior intercostal vein
16 Supreme intercostal vein (unusually large)
17 Sympathetic trunk
18 Trachea
19 Vagus nerve
20 Ventral ramus of eighth cervical nerve
21 Ventral ramus of first thoracic nerve
22 Vertebral vein

The neck of the first rib (7) is crossed in order from medial to lateral by the sympathetic trunk (17), supreme intercostal vein (16), superior intercostal artery (14) and the ventral ramus of the first thoracic nerve (21).

This is the view looking upwards into the right side of the thoracic inlet – the region occupied by the cervical pleura, here removed. The under-surface of most of the first rib (5) is seen from below, with the subclavian artery (12) passing over the top of it after giving off the internal thoracic branch (6) which runs towards the top of the picture (to the anterior thoracic wall), and the costocervical trunk whose superior intercostal branch (14) runs down over the neck of the first rib (7). The vertebral vein (22) has come down from the neck and is labelled on its posterior surface before entering the brachiocephalic vein (2, labelled at its opened cut edge). The vertebral vein receives an unusually large supreme intercostal vein (16). On its medial side is the sympathetic trunk (17) with the cervicothoracic ganglion (3). The neck of the first rib (7) has the ventral ramus of the first thoracic nerve (21) below it.

Catheterisation of subclavian vein, thoracic outlet syndromes, see pages 215–216.

Posterior mediastinum *from the right hand side of the chest*

1 Azygos arch
2 Azygos vein
3 Gray and white communicating rami
4 Greater splanchnic nerve
5 Intercostal artery
6 Intercostal nerve
7 Intercostal vein
8 Oesophageal plexus
9 Oesophagus
10 Phrenic nerve
11 Sympathetic chain
12 Sympathetic ganglion
13 Thoracic duct

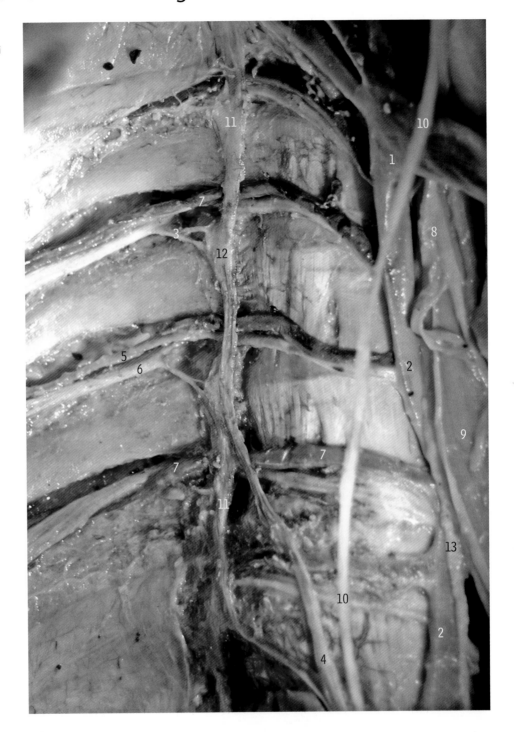

Azygos lobe, see pages 215–216.

A Oesophagus *lower thoracic part, from the front*

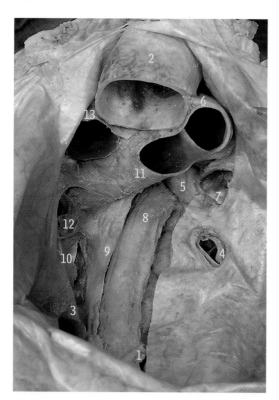

The heart has been removed from the pericardial cavity by transecting the great vessels, the pulmonary trunk being cut at the point where it divides into the two pulmonary arteries (11 and 6). Part of the pericardium (9) at the back has been removed to reveal the oesophagus (8). It is seen below the left principal bronchus (5) and is being crossed by the beginning of the right pulmonary artery (11).

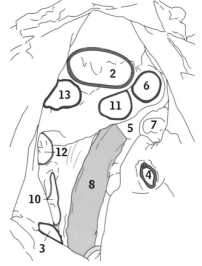

1 Anterior oesophageal trunk
2 Ascending aorta
3 Inferior vena cava
4 Left inferior pulmonary vein
5 Left principal bronchus
6 Left pulmonary artery
7 Left superior pulmonary vein
8 Oesophagus
9 Pericardium (cut edge)
10 Right inferior pulmonary vein
11 Right pulmonary artery
12 Right superior pulmonary vein
13 Superior vena cava

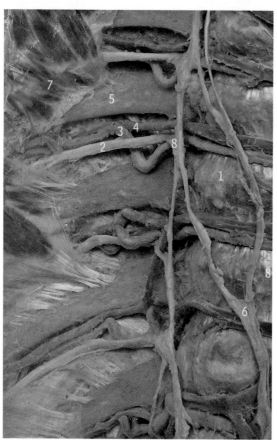

B Intercostal spaces
posterior internal view

This dissection shows the medial ends of some intercostal spaces of the right side, viewed from the front and slightly from the right. The pleura has been removed, revealing subcostal muscles (7) laterally, the nerves and vessels (4, 3 and 2) in the intercostal spaces, and the sympathetic trunk (8) and greater splanchnic nerve (6) on the sides of the vertebral bodies (as at 1).

1 Body of ninth thoracic vertebra
2 Eighth intercostal nerve
3 Eighth posterior intercostal artery
4 Eighth posterior intercostal vein

5 Eighth rib
6 Greater splanchnic nerve
7 Subcostal muscle
8 Sympathetic trunk and ganglia

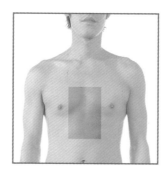

Intercostal drainage, see pages 215–216.

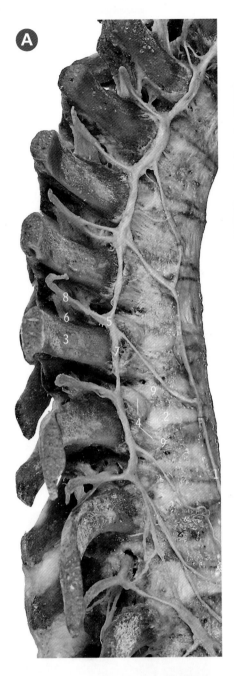
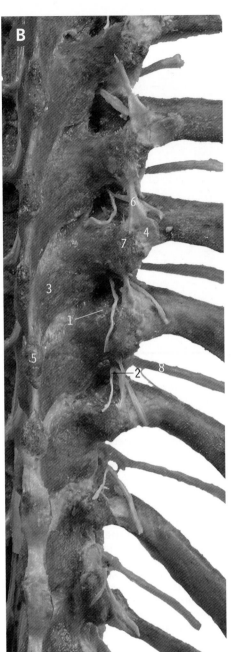

A Joints of the heads of the ribs *from the right*

In this part of the right mid-thoracic region, the ribs have been cut short beyond their tubercles, and the joints that the two facets of the head of a rib make with the facets on the sides of adjacent vertebral bodies and the intervening disc are shown, as at 4, 9 and 2, where the radiate ligament (4) covers the capsule of these small synovial joints.

1 Greater splanchnic nerve
2 Intervertebral disc
3 Neck of rib
4 Radiate ligament of head of rib
5 Rami communicantes
6 Superior costotransverse ligament
7 Sympathetic trunk
8 Ventral ramus of spinal nerve
9 Vertebral body

B Costotransverse joints *from behind*

In this view of the right half of the thoracic vertebral column from behind, costotransverse joints between the transverse processes of vertebrae and the tubercles of ribs are covered by the lateral costotransverse ligaments (as at 4). The dorsal rami of spinal nerves (2) pass medial to the superior costotransverse ligaments (6); ventral rami (8) run in front of these ligaments.

1 Costotransverse ligament
2 Dorsal ramus of spinal nerve
3 Lamina
4 Lateral costotransverse ligament
5 Spinous process
6 Superior costotransverse ligament
7 Transverse process
8 Ventral ramus of spinal nerve

C Costovertebral joints *disarticulated, from the right*

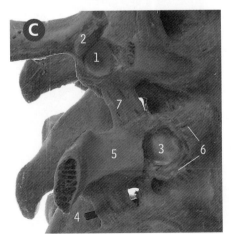

In the upper part of the figure, the upper rib has been severed through its neck (5) and the part with the tubercle attached has been turned upwards after cutting through the capsule of the costotransverse joint, to show the articular facet of the tubercle (2) and the transverse process (1). The head of the lower rib has been removed after transecting the radiate ligament (6) and underlying capsule of the joint of the head of the rib (3).

1 Articular facet of transverse process
2 Articular facet of tubercle of rib
3 Cavity of joint of head of rib
4 Marker between anterior and posterior parts of superior costotransverse ligament
5 Neck of rib
6 Radiate ligament
7 Superior costotransverse ligament

Varicella-zoster virus infection – chest wall, see pages 215–216.

Cast of the aorta and associated vessels

Ⓐ *from the right*   **Ⓑ** *from the left*

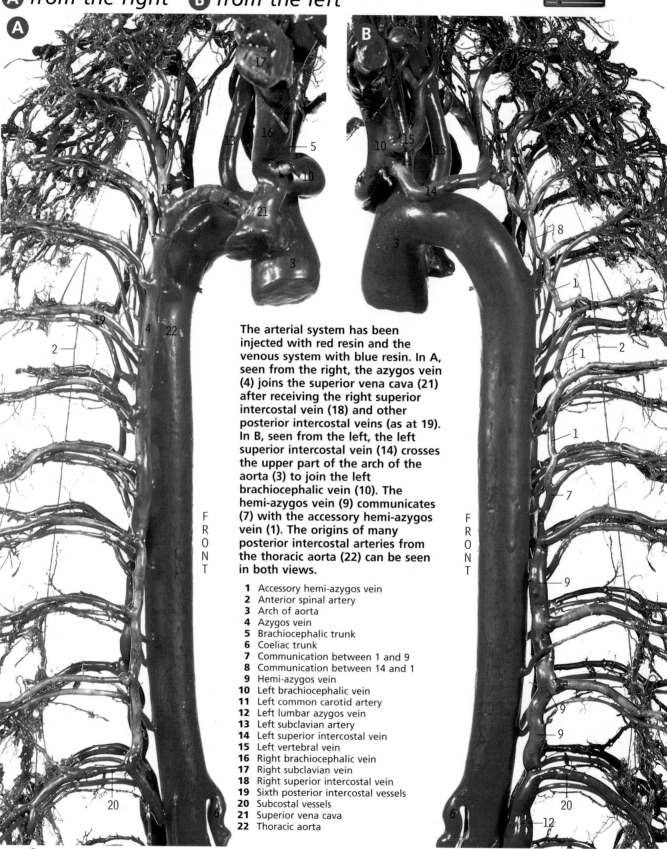

The arterial system has been injected with red resin and the venous system with blue resin. In A, seen from the right, the azygos vein (4) joins the superior vena cava (21) after receiving the right superior intercostal vein (18) and other posterior intercostal veins (as at 19). In B, seen from the left, the left superior intercostal vein (14) crosses the upper part of the arch of the aorta (3) to join the left brachiocephalic vein (10). The hemi-azygos vein (9) communicates (7) with the accessory hemi-azygos vein (1). The origins of many posterior intercostal arteries from the thoracic aorta (22) can be seen in both views.

1 Accessory hemi-azygos vein
2 Anterior spinal artery
3 Arch of aorta
4 Azygos vein
5 Brachiocephalic trunk
6 Coeliac trunk
7 Communication between 1 and 9
8 Communication between 14 and 1
9 Hemi-azygos vein
10 Left brachiocephalic vein
11 Left common carotid artery
12 Left lumbar azygos vein
13 Left subclavian artery
14 Left superior intercostal vein
15 Left vertebral vein
16 Right brachiocephalic vein
17 Right subclavian vein
18 Right superior intercostal vein
19 Sixth posterior intercostal vessels
20 Subcostal vessels
21 Superior vena cava
22 Thoracic aorta

Aortic dissection, variations in great arteries, see pages 215–216.

Diaphragm *from above*

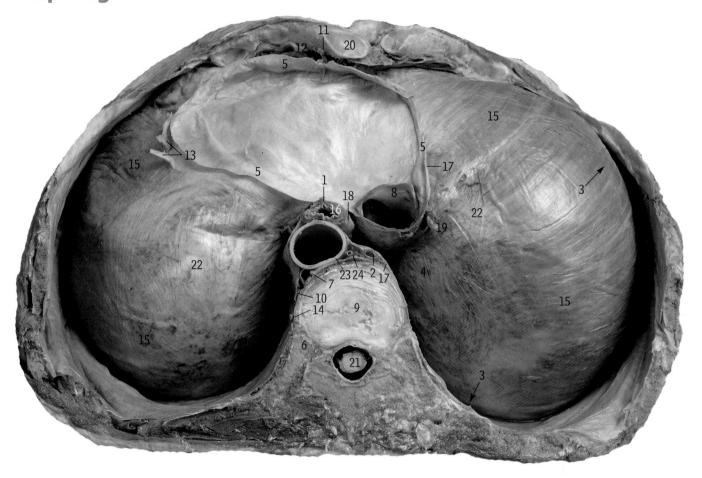

The thorax has been transected at the level of the disc between the ninth and tenth thoracic vertebrae.

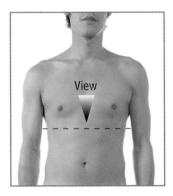

View

1	Anterior oesophageal plexus
2	Azygos vein
3	Costodiaphragmatic recess
4	Costomediastinal recess
5	Fibrous pericardium (cut edge)
6	Head of left ninth rib
7	Hemi-azygos vein
8	Inferior vena cava
9	Intervertebral disc
10	Left greater splanchnic nerve
11	Left internal thoracic artery
12	Left musculophrenic artery
13	Left phrenic nerve
14	Left sympathetic trunk
15	Muscle of diaphragm
16	Oesophagus
17	Pleura (cut edge)
18	Posterior oesophageal plexus
19	Right phrenic nerve
20	Seventh left costal cartilage
21	Spinal cord
22	Tendon of diaphragm
23	Thoracic aorta
24	Thoracic duct

According to the standard textbook description, the foramen for the vena cava is at the level of the disc between the eighth and ninth thoracic vertebrae, the oesophageal opening at the level of the tenth thoracic vertebra and the aortic opening opposite the twelfth thoracic vertebra. However, it is common for the oesophageal opening to be nearer the midline, as in this specimen (16), and the vena caval foramen (8) is lower than usual.

The vena caval foramen is in the tendinous part of the diaphragm and the oesophageal opening in the muscular part. The so-called aortic opening is not *in* the diaphragm but behind it (page 260).

The central tendon of the diaphragm has the shape of a trefoil leaf and has no bony attachment.

The right phrenic nerve (19) passes through the vena caval foramen in the tendinous part, but the left phrenic nerve (13) pierces the muscular part in front of the central tendon just lateral to the overlying pericardium.

The phrenic nerves are the *only motor* nerves to the diaphragm, including the crura. The supply from lower thoracic (intercostal and subcostal) nerves is purely sensory. Damage to one phrenic nerve completely paralyses its own half of the diaphragm.

Diaphragmatic hernia, gastro-oesophageal reflux, see pages 215–216.

Oesophageal radiographs *during a barium swallow*

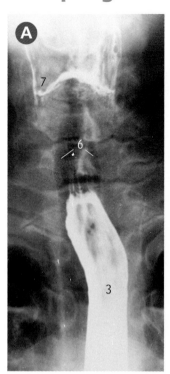

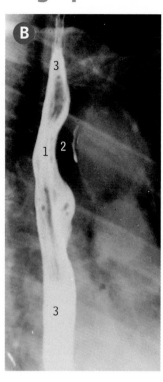

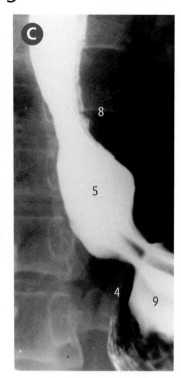

A lower pharynx and upper oesophagus

B middle part

C lower end

1 Aortic impression in oesophagus
2 Arch of aorta with plaque of calcification
3 Barium in oesophagus
4 Diaphragm
5 Lower thoracic oesophagus
6 Margins of trachea (translucent with contained air)
7 Piriform recess in laryngopharynx
8 Position of left atrium
9 Stomach

In A, viewed from the front, some of the barium paste adheres to the pharyngeal wall, outlining the piriform recesses (7), but most of it has passed into the oesophagus (3). In B, viewed obliquely from the left, the oesophagus is indented by the arch of the aorta (2) which shows some calcification in its wall – a useful aid to its identification. In C, there is some dilatation at the lower end of the thoracic oesophagus (5) and it is constricted where it passes through the diaphragm (4) to join the stomach (9). The left atrium of the heart (8) lies in front of the lower thoracic oesophagus (page 210, A8), but only when enlarged does the atrium cause an indentation in the oesophagus.

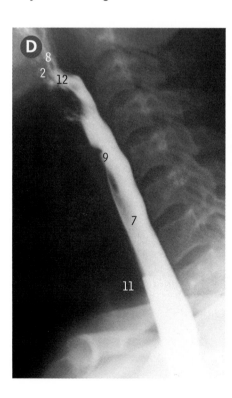

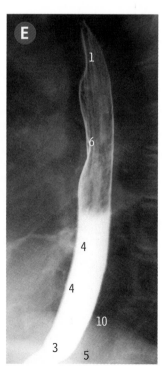

D cervical part

E thoracic part

1 Aortic arch impression
2 Base of tongue
3 Gastro-oesophageal junction
4 Left atrium position
5 Left hemidiaphragm
6 Left principal bronchus impression
7 Oesophagus
8 Oropharynx
9 Postcricoid venous plexus impression
10 Right hemidiaphragm
11 Trachea
12 Vallecula

Thorax

Clinical thumbnails, see website for details and further clinical images to download onto your own notes.

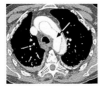

Angina pectoris

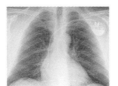

Aortic dissection

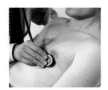

Artificial cardiac pacemaker

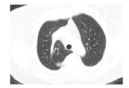

Auscultation of heart sounds

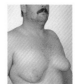

Azygos lobe

Breast abnormalities

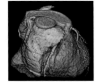

Breast examination

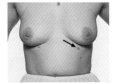

Bronchiectasis

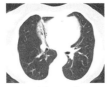

Bronchoscopy

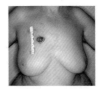

Carcinoma of the breast

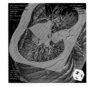

Carcinoma of the lung

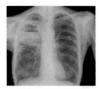

Carcinoma of the oesophagus

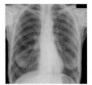

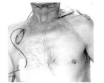

Cardiac pacemaker

Cardiac tamponade

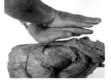

Cardiopulmonary resuscitation (CPR)

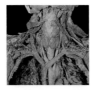

Catheterisation of subclavian vein

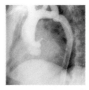

Coarctation of the aorta

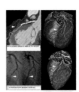

Coronary artery abnormalities

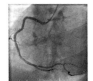

Coronary angiography

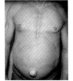

Coronary artery bypass grafting (CABG)

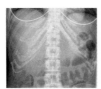

Costochondral pathology

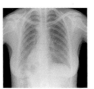

Dextrocardia

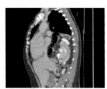

Diaphragmatic hernia

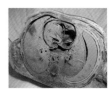

Empyema

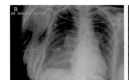

Flail chest

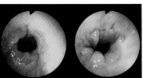

Gastro-oesophageal reflux

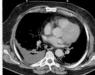

Haemothorax

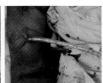

Intercostal drainage

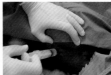

Intercostal nerve block

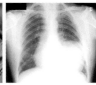

Left ventricular enlargement

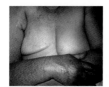

Mastectomy

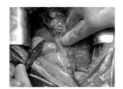

Median sternotomy

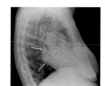

Mesothelioma

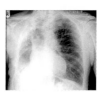

Mitral valve disease

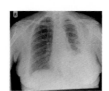

Myocardial infarction

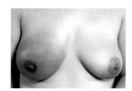

Orange peel texture of the skin and retraction of the nipple

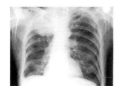

Pancoast tumour

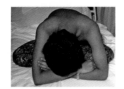

Pericardial effusion

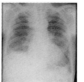

Phrenic nerve palsy

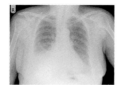

Pleural effusion

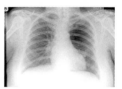

Pneumothorax

Pulmonary embolism

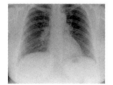

Sarcoidosis

Sternal variants

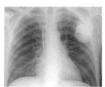

Subclavian arterial stent

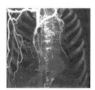

Superior vena cava obstruction

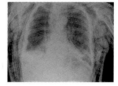

Surgical emphysema

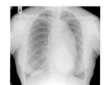

Thoracic aortic aneurysm

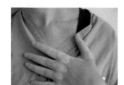

Thoracic outlet syndromes

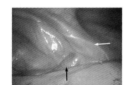

Thoracoscopy

Thymus

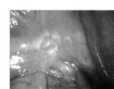

Transthoracic sympathectomy

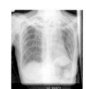

Tuberculosis

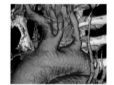

Variation in great arteries

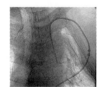

Variation in great veins

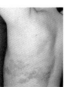

Varicella-zoster virus infection – chest wall

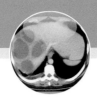
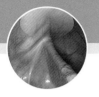
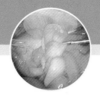

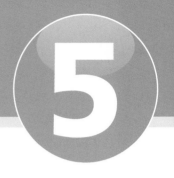

5

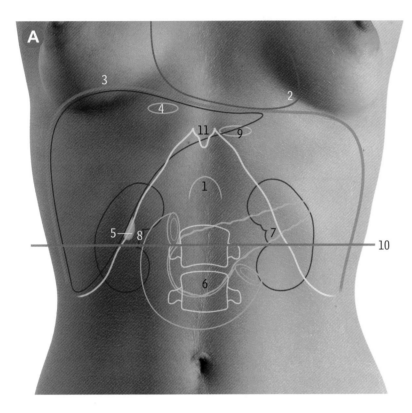

A Anterior abdominal wall *surface markings, above the umbilicus*

The solid white line indicates the costal margin. The blue line indicates the transpyloric plane. The C-shaped duodenum is outlined in pink, the kidneys and liver in brown and the pancreas in pale green.

1 Aortic opening in diaphragm
2 Apex of heart in fifth intercostal space
3 Dome of diaphragm and upper margin of liver
4 Foramen for inferior vena cava in diaphragm
5 Fundus of gall bladder, and junction of ninth costal cartilage and lateral border of rectus sheath
6 Head of pancreas and level of second lumbar vertebra
7 Hilum of left kidney
8 Hilum of right kidney
9 Oesophageal opening in diaphragm
10 Transpyloric plane
11 Xiphoid process

The transpyloric plane (10) lies midway between the jugular notch of the sternum and the upper border of the pubic symphysis, or approximately a hand's breadth below the xiphisternal joint (11), and level with the lower part of the body of the first lumbar vertebra.

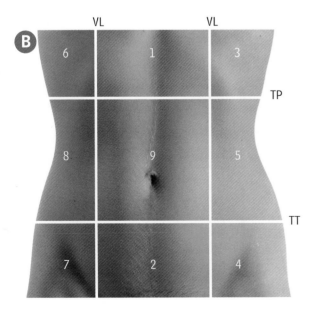

B Regions of the abdomen

The abdomen may be divided into regions by two vertical and two horizontal lines. The vertical lines (VL) pass through the midinguinal points: the upper horizontal line corresponds to the transpyloric plane (TP, A10), the lower line is drawn between the tubercles of the iliac crests (transtubercular [or supracristal] plane, TT).

1 Epigastric region
2 Hypogastrium or suprapubic region
3 Left hypochondrium
4 Left iliac region or iliac fossa
5 Left lumbar region
6 Right hypochondrium
7 Right iliac region or iliac fossa
8 Right lumbar region
9 Umbilical region

Varicella-zoster virus infection–abdominal wall, see pages 280–284.

A Anterior abdominal wall

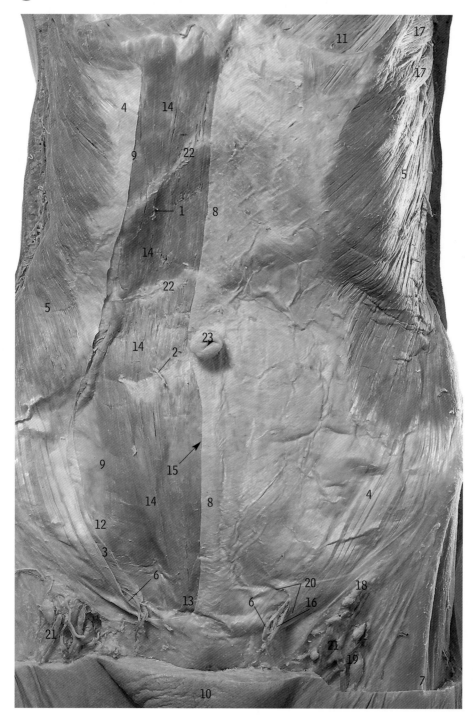

1 Anterior cutaneous nerve (eighth intercostal)
2 Anterior cutaneous nerve (tenth intercostal)
3 Anterior layer internal oblique aponeurosis
4 External oblique aponeurosis
5 External oblique muscle
6 Ilioinguinal nerve
7 Iliotibial tract
8 Linea alba
9 Linea semilunaris
10 Mons pubis
11 Pectoralis major, abdominal part
12 Posterior layer internal oblique aponeurosis
13 Pyramidalis muscle
14 Rectus abdominis
15 Rectus sheath, anterior
16 Round ligament of uterus
17 Serratus anterior muscle
18 Superficial inguinal lymph node (horizontal group)
19 Superficial inguinal lymph node (vertical group)
20 Superficial inguinal ring
21 Superficial inguinal veins
22 Tendinous intersection of rectus abdominis
23 Umbilicus

The rectus sheath (A15) is formed by the internal oblique aponeurosis (A3), which splits at the lateral border of the rectus muscle (A9) into two layers. The posterior layer (A12) passes behind the muscle to blend with the aponeurosis of transversus abdominis (B19) to form the posterior wall of the sheath (B13), and the anterior layer (A3) passes in front of the muscle to blend with the external oblique aponeurosis (A4) as the anterior wall (A15).

The anterior and posterior walls of the sheath unite at the medial border of the rectus muscle to form the midline linea alba (A8, B11).

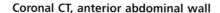

Coronal CT, anterior abdominal wall

Haematoma of the rectus sheath, Spigelian hernia, see pages 280–284.

B Rectus sheath

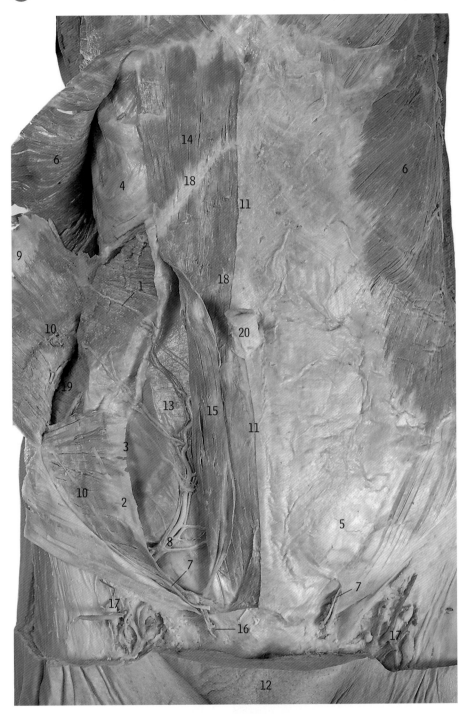

1 Anterior cutaneous nerve (tenth intercostal)
2 Anterior layer of internal oblique aponeurosis
3 Anterior wall of rectus sheath
4 Eighth rib
5 External oblique aponeurosis
6 External oblique muscle
7 Ilioinguinal nerve
8 Inferior epigastric vessels
9 Internal oblique aponeurosis
10 Internal oblique muscle
11 Linea alba
12 Mons pubis
13 Posterior wall of rectus sheath
14 Rectus abdominis
15 Rectus abdominis, reflected
16 Round ligament of uterus
17 Superficial inguinal lymph nodes
18 Tendinous intersection
19 Transversus abdominis
20 Umbilicus

Coronal CT

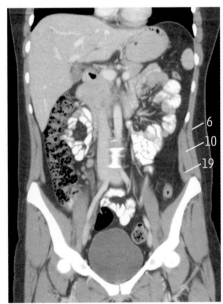

There is no posterior rectus sheath in the lower third of rectus abdominis, below the arcuate line (page 222, A1).

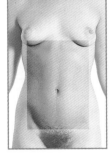

Cushing striations, see pages 280–284.

Groin in the male

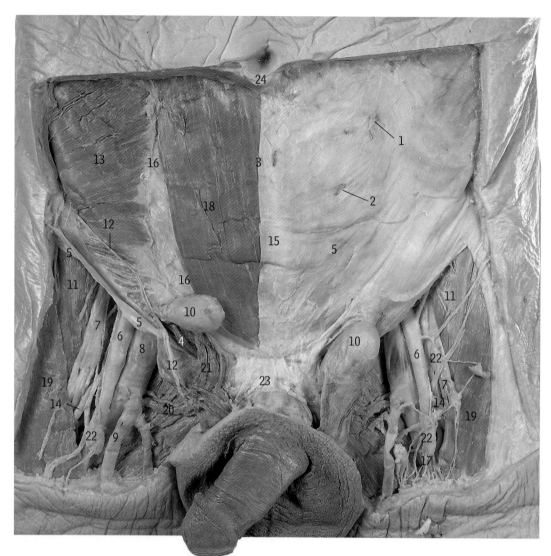

1 Anterior cutaneous nerve (eleventh intercostal)
2 Anterior cutaneous nerve (twelfth intercostal)
3 Anterior rectus sheath (cut edge)
4 Ductus (vas) deferens
5 External oblique aponeurosis
6 Femoral artery
7 Femoral nerve
8 Femoral vein
9 Great saphenous vein
10 Hernial sac (indirect)
11 Iliacus muscle
12 Ilioinguinal nerve
13 Internal oblique muscle
14 Lateral circumflex femoral artery
15 Linea alba
16 Linea semilunaris
17 Lymphatic vessels
18 Rectus abdominis muscle
19 Sartorius muscle
20 Scrotal venous connections
21 Spermatic cord
22 Superficial inguinal lymph node
23 Suspensory ligament of penis
24 Umbilicus

The hernial sacs (10), shown here, are not trueherniae but extraperitoneal fat herniating through the superficial inguinal ring; often seen in the dissection room.

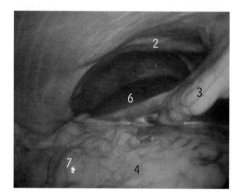

Laparoscopic view of upper abdominal cavity

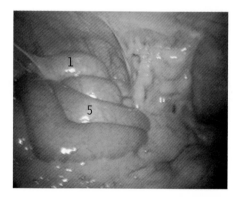

Laparoscopic view of lower abdominal cavity

1 Caecum
2 Diaphragm
3 Falciform ligament
4 Greater omentum
5 Ileum
6 Right lobe, liver
7 Transverse colon

Inguinal hernia repair, varicella-zoster virus infection–abdominal wall, see pages 280–284.

Adult anterior abdominal wall in the male *surface markings, right iliac fossa*

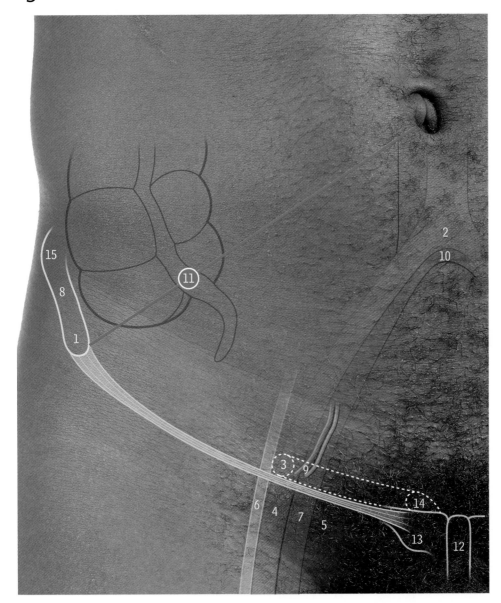

1 Anterior superior iliac spine
2 Bifurcation of aorta (fourth lumbar vertebra)
3 Deep inguinal ring
4 Femoral artery
5 Femoral canal
6 Femoral nerve
7 Femoral vein
8 Iliac crest
9 Inferior epigastric vessels
10 Lower end of inferior vena cava (fifth lumbar vertebra)
11 McBurney's point
12 Pubic symphysis
13 Pubic tubercle
14 Superficial inguinal ring
15 Tubercle of iliac crest

Cononal CT

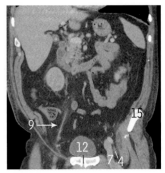

Sagittal CT

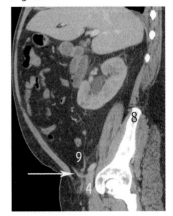

Arrows point to inferior epigastric artery

The caecum with the appendix opening into it from the left and the ascending colon continuing upwards from it are indicated by the brown line. The inguinal ligament, between the anterior superior iliac spine (1) and the pubic tubercle (13), is indicated by the light blue line. The femoral artery (4) has the femoral vein (7) on its medial side and the femoral nerve (6) on its lateral side. The femoral canal (5) is on the medial side of the vein. The deep inguinal ring (3) and inferior epigastric vessels (9) are above the femoral artery, while the superficial inguinal ring (14) is above and lateral to the pubic tubercle (13). McBurney's point (11) is a site on the surface of the anterior abdominal wall indicating the usual location of the base of the appendix internally. It lies one-third of the way along a line from the right anterior superior iliac spine to the umbilicus (red line).

The femoral artery (4, whose pulsation should normally be palpable) enters the thigh midway between the pubic symphysis (12) and the anterior superior iliac spine (1). This is often referred to as the midinguinal point.

Femoral hernia, McBurney's point, see pages 280–284.

(A) Adult anterior abdominal wall *umbilical folds, from behind*

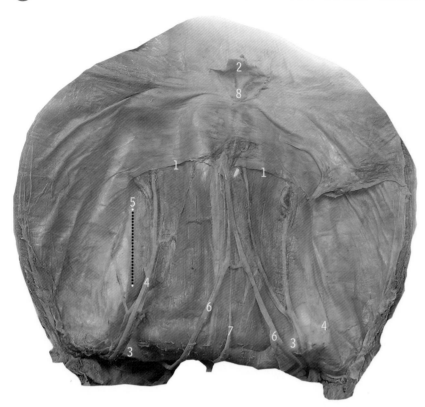

This view of the peritoneal surface of the central region of the anterior abdominal wall shows the peritoneal folds raised by underlying structures. There is one fold above the umbilicus – the falciform ligament – and there are five below it: the median umbilical fold (7) in the midline, and a pair of medial and lateral umbilical folds on each side (6 and 4).

1 Arcuate line
2 Falciform ligament
3 Inguinal triangle (Hesselbach)
4 Lateral umbilical fold which contains the inferior epigastric vessels
5 Linea semilunaris
6 Medial umbilical fold
7 Median umbilical fold
8 Umbilicus

The inguinal triangle of Hesselbach is a naturally weak region between rectus abdominis and the inferior epigastric vessels. Direct inguinal hernias appear through this region.

(B) Fetal anterior abdominal wall *from behind*

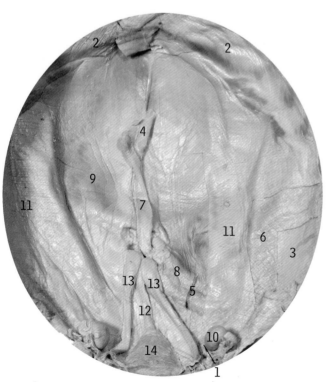

1 Deep inguinal ring
2 Diaphragm
3 External oblique muscle
4 Falciform ligament
5 Inferior epigastric vessels
6 Internal oblique muscle
7 Left umbilical vein
8 Rectus abdominis muscle
9 Rectus sheath (posterior layer)
10 Testis (undescended)
11 Transversus abdominis muscle
12 Urachus
13 Umbilical arteries
14 Urinary bladder

Caput medusae, postnatal umbilical vein catheter, omphalocele, umbilical and paraumbilical hernia, see pages 280–284.

A Right deep inguinal ring in adult male
laparoscopic view

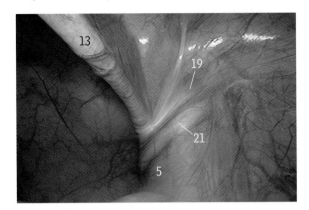

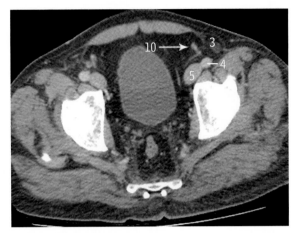

Axial CT, pelvis

B Anterior abdominal wall
abdominal view

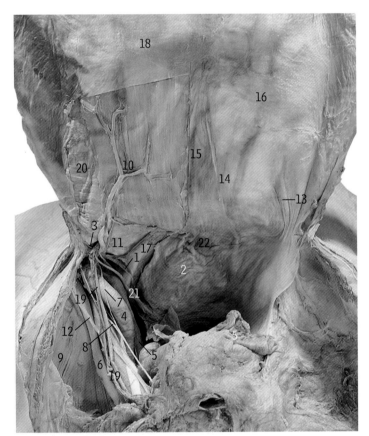

1. Accessory obturator artery
2. Bladder
3. Deep inguinal ring
4. External iliac artery
5. External iliac vein
6. Femoral nerve
7. Genitofemoral nerve, femoral branch
8. Genitofemoral nerve, genital branch
9. Iliacus
10. Inferior epigastric vessels
11. Inguinal triangle (Hesselbach)
12. Lateral cutaneous nerve of the thigh
13. Lateral umbilical fold (inferior epigastric vessels)
14. Medial umbilical fold (umbilical artery)
15. Median umbilical fold (urachus)
16. Parietal peritoneum
17. Pelvic brim
18. Posterior surface, rectus sheath
19. Testicular vessels
20. Transversus abdominis
21. Vas/ductus deferens
22. Visceral peritoneum, over bladder

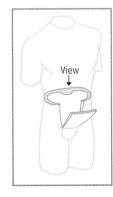

View

Abdominal viscera have been removed and the anterior abdominal wall detached laterally and reflected anteriorly and inferiorly to reveal the internal surface of the abdominal wall. The parietal peritoneum has been removed from the left side to show deeper structures in the pelvic and abdominal walls.

Inguinal hernia, indirect inguinal hernia, see pages 280–284.

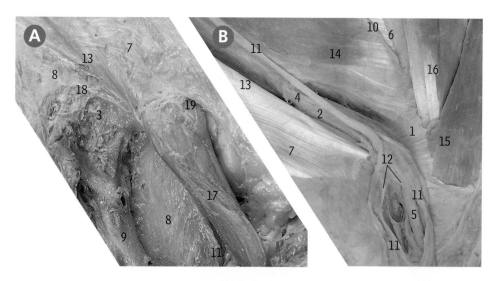

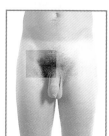

Right inguinal region *in the male*

A superficial dissection

B with the external oblique aponeurosis and spermatic cord incised

In A, the spermatic cord (17) is seen emerging from the superficial inguinal ring (19) and covered by the external spermatic fascia. In B, with the external oblique aponeurosis reflected and the anterior wall of the rectus sheath removed, the cord is emerging from the deep inguinal ring (4) with the cremasteric fascia (2) now the most superficial covering. All three coverings of the cord have been incised (12) to show the ductus/vas deferens (5).

1 Conjoint tendon	**11** Ilio-inguinal nerve
2 Cremasteric fascia and cremaster muscle over spermatic cord	**12** Incised margin of coverings of cord
3 Cribriform fascia	**13** Inguinal ligament
4 Deep inguinal ring	**14** Internal oblique
5 Ductus/vas deferens	**15** Pyramidalis
6 Edge of rectus sheath	**16** Rectus abdominis
7 External oblique aponeurosis	**17** Spermatic cord
8 Fascia lata	**18** Upper margin of saphenous opening
9 Great saphenous vein	**19** Upper margin of superficial inguinal ring
10 Iliohypogastric nerve	

Right inguinal region *in the female*

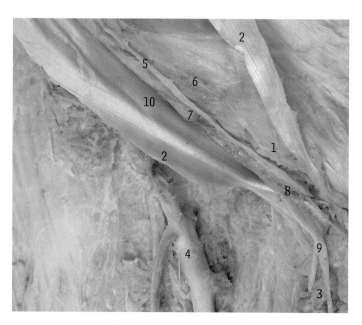

The external oblique aponeurosis (2) has been incised and reflected to show the position of the deep inguinal ring (7) which marks the lateral end of the inguinal canal. The round ligament of the uterus (9) emerges from the superficial inguinal ring (8), which marks the medial end of the canal, and becomes lost in the fat of the labium majus (3). The ilio-inguinal nerve (5) also passes through the canal and out of the superficial ring.

1 Conjoint tendon
2 External oblique aponeurosis
3 Fat of labium majus
4 Great saphenous vein
5 Ilio-inguinal nerve
6 Internal oblique
7 Position of deep inguinal ring
8 Position of superficial inguinal ring
9 Round ligament of uterus
10 Upper surface of inguinal ligament

In the female, the inguinal canal contains the round ligament of the uterus and the ilio-inguinal nerve.

The processus vaginalis is normally obliterated, but if it remains patent within the female inguinal canal, it is sometimes known as the canal of Nuck.

A Right deep inguinal ring and inguinal triangle *internal view*

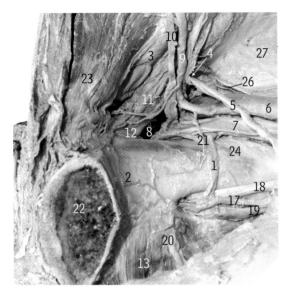

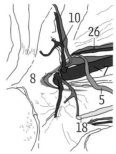

This is the view looking into the right half of the pelvis from the left, showing the posterior surface of the lower part of the anterior abdominal wall, above the pubic symphysis. The femoral ring (8), the entrance to the femoral canal, is below the medial end of the inguinal ligament (11). The inferior epigastric vessels (9, 10) lie medial to the deep inguinal ring (4).

The inguinal triangle (Hesselbach's triangle) is the area bounded laterally by the inferior epigastric vessels, medially by the lateral border of rectus abdominis and below by the inguinal ligament. A direct inguinal hernia passes forwards through this triangle, medial to the inferior epigastric vessels.

An indirect inguinal hernia passes through the deep inguinal ring lateral to the inferior epigastric vessels.

B Left deep inguinal ring in the male
internal peritoneal (view as seen at laparoscopy)

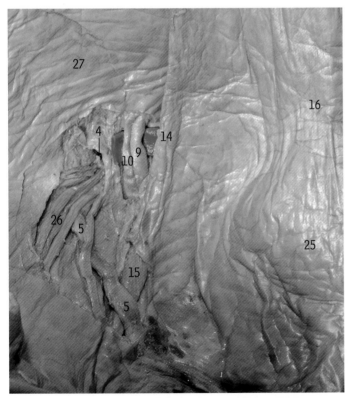

1 Abberant obturator vein
2 Body of pubis
3 Conjoint tendon
4 Deep inguinal ring
5 Ductus/vas deferens
6 External iliac artery
7 External iliac vein
8 Femoral ring
9 Inferior epigastric artery
10 Inferior epigastric vein
11 Inguinal ligament
12 Lacunar ligament
13 Levator ani muscle
14 Medial umbilical fold
15 Medial umbilical ligament
16 Median umbilical ligament
17 Obturator artery
18 Obturator nerve
19 Obturator vein
20 Origin of levator ani from fascia overlying obturator internus muscle
21 Pubic branches of the inferior epigastric vessels
22 Pubic ramus (transected)
23 Rectus abdominis muscle
24 Superior pubic ramus
25 Superior surface of bladder
26 Testicular vessels
27 Transversalis fascia overlying transversus abdominis muscle

Abdominal peritoneal folds *after removal of intra-abdominal organs, to show relations of ligaments and mesenteries*

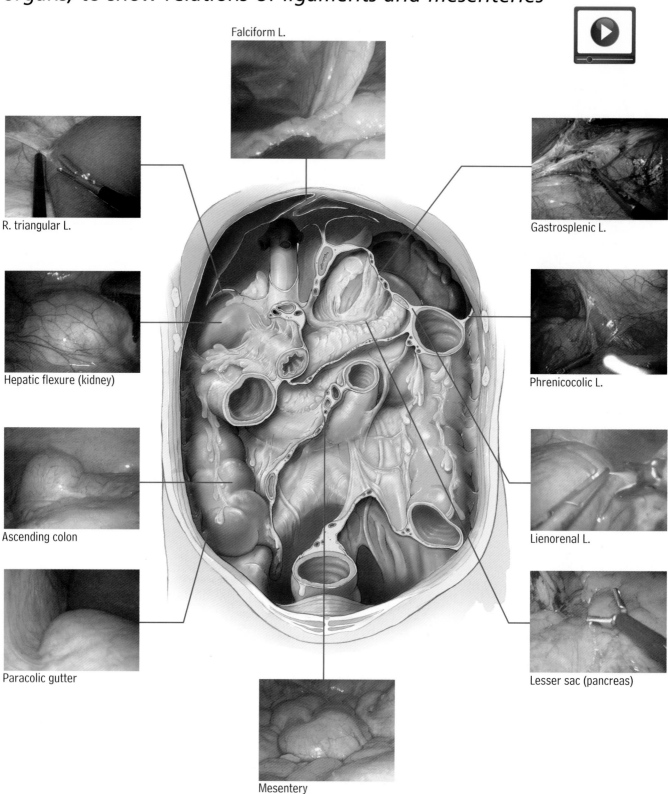

Falciform L.

R. triangular L.

Hepatic flexure (kidney)

Ascending colon

Paracolic gutter

Gastrosplenic L.

Phrenicocolic L.

Lienorenal L.

Lesser sac (pancreas)

Mesentery

 Drainage of subphrenic abscesses, peritoneal lavage, peritonitis, see pages 280–284.

Abdominal viscera *from the front*

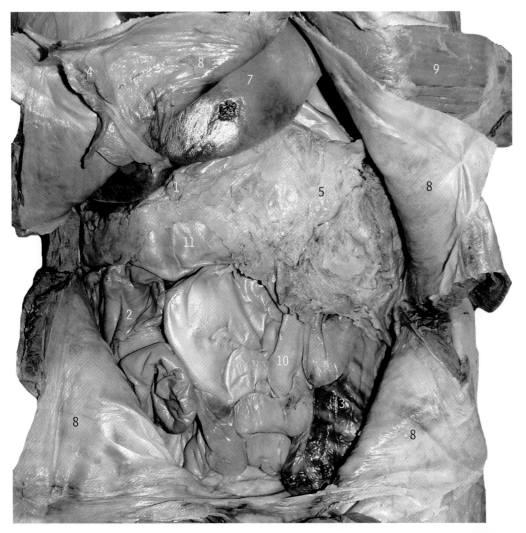

1 Appendices epiploicae
2 Ascending colon
3 Descending colon
4 Falciform ligament
5 Greater omentum
6 Ligamentum teres
   hepatis (round ligament)
7 Liver

8 Parietal peritoneum on
   anterior abdominal wall
9 Rectus abdominis
   muscle, reflected
   laterally
10 Small intestine
11 Transverse colon

For an explanation of peritoneal structures, see the
diagrams on pages 226, 233.

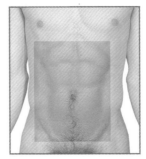

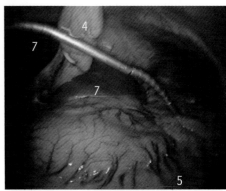

**Laparoscopic view of upper
abdominal viscera**

Liver biopsy, situs inversus totalis, see pages 280–284.

Abdominal viscera *from the front*

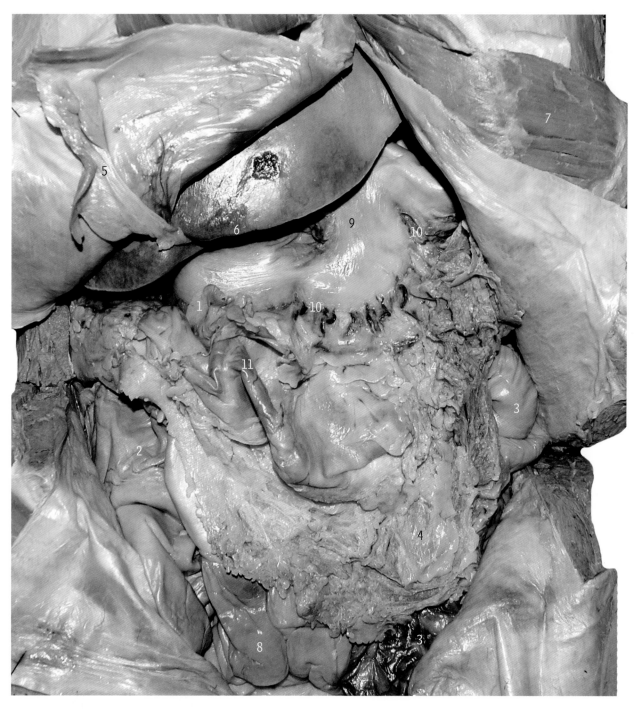

1 Appendices epiploicae	**7** Rectus abdominis muscle, reflected laterally
2 Ascending colon	**8** Small intestine
3 Descending colon	**9** Stomach
4 Greater omentum	**10** Stomach, greater curvature
5 Ligamentum teres hepatis in falciform ligament	**11** Transverse colon
6 Liver, left lobe	

Cholecystectomy, see pages 280–284.

Abdominal viscera *from the front*

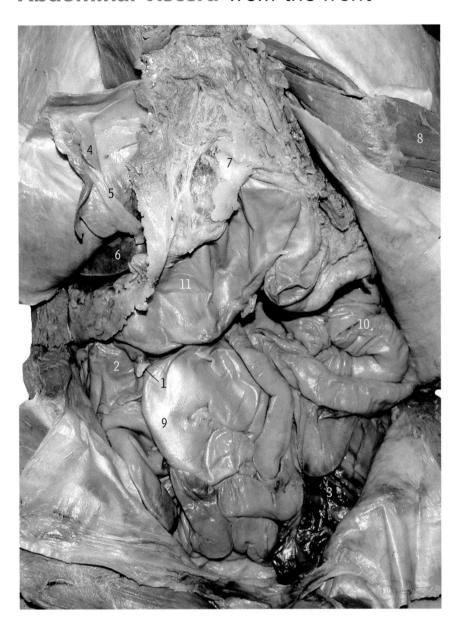

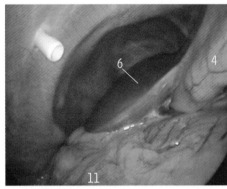

Laparoscopic view of abdominal viscera

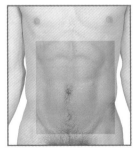

1 Appendices epiploicae
2 Ascending colon
3 Descending colon
4 Falciform ligament
5 Ligamentum teres hepatis
6 Liver, right lobe
7 Posterior surface of greater omentum
8 Rectus abdominis muscle, reflected laterally
9 Small intestine (ileum)
10 Small intestine (jejunum)
11 Transverse colon

The appendices epiploicae (1) are fat-filled appendages of peritoneum on the various parts of the colon (ascending, transverse, descending and sigmoid). They are not present on the small intestine or the rectum, and may be rudimentary on the caecum and appendix. In abdominal operations, they are one feature that helps to distinguish colon from other parts of the intestine.

Omental cake, see pages 280–284.

Lesser omentum and epiploic foramen

Ⓐ *from the front* Ⓑ *from the front and the right*

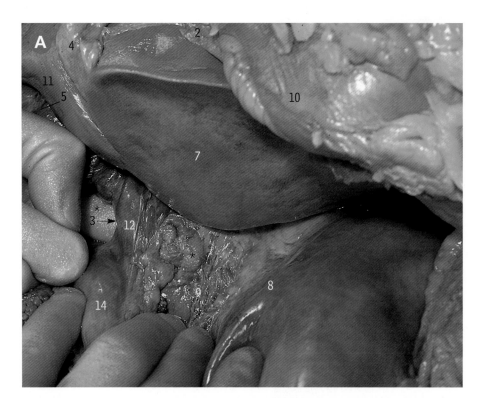

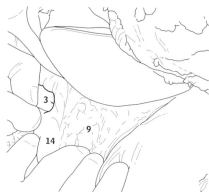

1 Descending (second) part of duodenum
2 Diaphragm
3 Epiploic foramen* (winslow)
4 Falciform ligament
5 Gall bladder
6 Inferior vena cava
7 Left lobe of liver
8 Lesser curvature of stomach
9 Lesser omentum
10 Pericardium
11 Quadrate lobe of liver
12 Right free margin of lesser omentum
13 Right lobe of liver
14 Superior (first) part of duodenum
15 Upper pole of right kidney

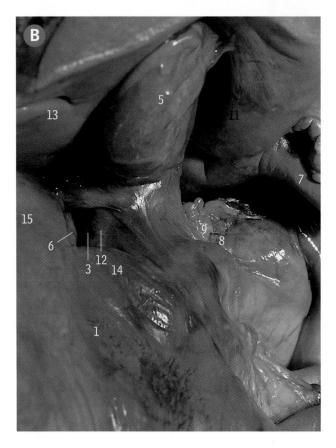

In A, a finger* has been placed in the epiploic foramen (3) behind the right free margin of the lesser omentum (12), and the tip can be seen in the lesser sac, through the transparent lesser omentum (9) which stretches between the liver (7) and the lesser curvature of the stomach (8). In the more lateral view in B, looking into the foramen from the right, the foramen (3) is identified between the right free margin of the lesser omentum (12) in front and the inferior vena cava (6) behind, above the first part of the duodenum (14).

The epiploic foramen (of Winslow, A3 and B3) is the communication between the general peritoneal cavity (sometimes called the greater sac) and the lesser sac (omental bursa), a space lined by peritoneum behind the stomach (A8 and B8) and lesser omentum (A9 and A12) and in front of parts of the pancreas and left kidney.

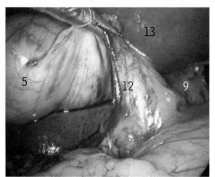

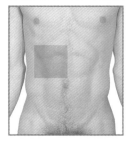

Laparoscopic view of lesser omentum (free margin)

Ⓐ Upper abdominal viscera *from the front*

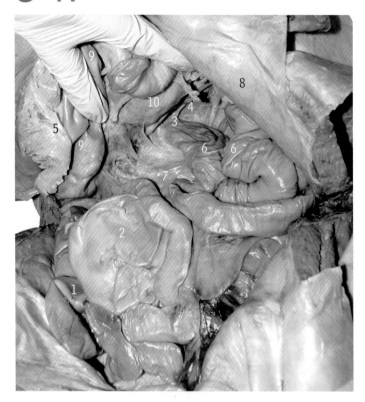

In this view the stomach, transverse colon (9) and greater omentum (5) have been lifted up to show the region of the duodenojejunal flexure (3).

1 Ascending colon
2 Coils of the small intestine
3 Duodenojejunal flexure
4 Duodenum, first part
5 Greater omentum
6 Jejunum
7 Mesentery
8 Parietal peritoneum on anterior abdominal wall, reflected superiorly
9 Transverse colon, reflected superiorly
10 Transverse mesocolon

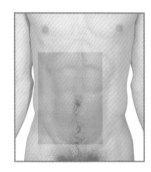

Ⓑ Lesser sac in upper abdomen

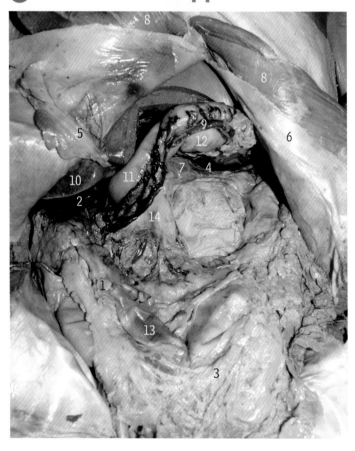

1 Appendices epiploicae
2 Gall bladder
3 Greater omentum, reflected inferiorly
4 Lesser sac (omental bursa)
5 Ligamentum teres hepatis in falciform ligament
6 Parietal peritoneum on anterior abdominal wall
7 Peritoneum of lesser sac overlying pancreas
8 Rectus abdominis muscle, reflected
9 Right and left gastro-epiploic veins
10 Right lobe of the liver
11 Stomach, greater curvature
12 Stomach, posterior surface
13 Transverse colon, reflected inferiorly
14 Transverse mesocolon

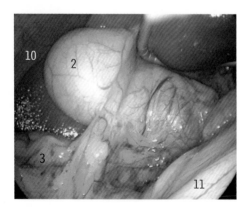

Laparoscopic view of gall bladder

Ascites, laparoscopy, see pages 280–284.

Mesentery and colon *from the front*

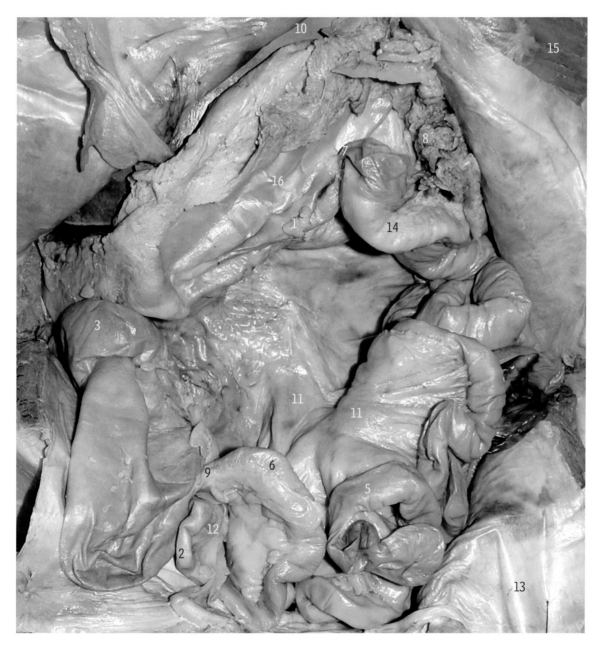

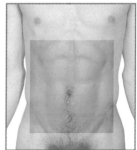

1	Appendices epiploicae	**9**	Ileocaecal junction
2	Appendix	**10**	Liver
3	Ascending colon	**11**	Mesentery of small intestine
4	Caecum	**12**	Mesoappendix
5	Coils of small intestine	**13**	Parietal peritoneum on anterior abdominal wall
6	Distal ileum	**14**	Proximal jejunum
7	Duodenojejunal junction	**15**	Rectus abdominis muscle, reflected
8	Greater omentum	**16**	Transverse colon

Diverticular disease, volvulus, see pages 280–284.

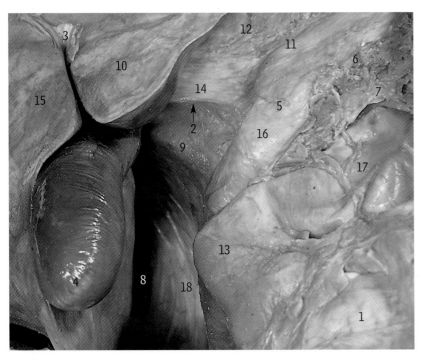

A Hepatorenal pouch of peritoneum
from the right and below

With the body lying on its back and seen from the right, the liver (15) has been turned upwards (towards the left) to open up the gap between the liver and upper pole of the right kidney (18) – the hepatorenal pouch of peritoneum (8, Morison's pouch or the right subhepatic compartment of the peritoneal cavity).

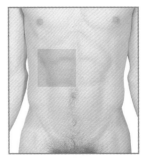

1 Ascending colon	**7** Greater omentum
2 Epiploic foramen (winslow)	**8** Hepatorenal (Morison's) pouch
3 Falciform ligament	**9** Inferior vena cava
4 Gall bladder	**10** Left lobe of liver
5 Gastroduodenal junction	**11** Lesser curvature of stomach
6 Greater curvature of stomach	**12** Lesser omentum overlying pancreas

13 Right colic (hepatic) flexure
14 Right free margin of lesser omentum
15 Right lobe of liver
16 Superior (first) part of duodenum
17 Transverse colon
18 Upper pole of right kidney

Diagrams of peritoneum *(see pages 227–232)*

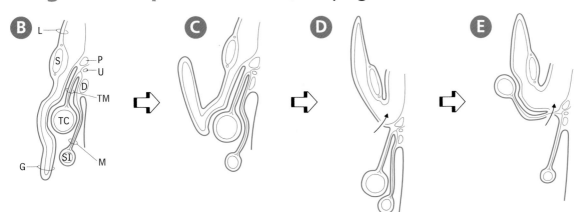

B normal position

C with the lower part of the greater omentum lifted up

D with the greater omentum lifted up and separated from the transverse mesocolon and colon, with an opening into the lesser sac

E with the greater omentum and transverse mesocolon and colon lifted up, with an opening into the lesser sac through the mesocolon

These drawings of a sagittal section through the middle of the abdomen, viewed from the left, illustrate theoretically how the peritoneum forms the lesser omentum (L, passing down to the stomach, S), greater omentum (G), transverse mesocolon (TM) passing to the transverse colon (TC), and the mesentery (M) of the small intestine (SI). The layer in blue represents the peritoneum of the lesser sac. The superior mesenteric artery passes between the head and uncinate process of the pancreas (P and U), and continues across the duodenum (D) into the mesentery (M) to the small intestine (SI), giving off the middle colic artery which runs in the transverse mesocolon (TM) to the transverse colon (TC). The greater omentum (G) is formed by four layers fused together and also fused with the front of the transverse mesocolon (TM, two layers) and transverse colon. On dissection, no separation between any layers is possible except between the greater omentum and the transverse mesocolon. The six layers between the stomach and transverse colon are sometimes collectively known as the gastrocolic omentum. B corresponds to the dissections on pages 227 and 228, C to page 229, D to page 231A, and E to page 231B. The small arrows in D and E indicate the layers cut to make artificial openings into the lesser sac.

Coeliac trunk

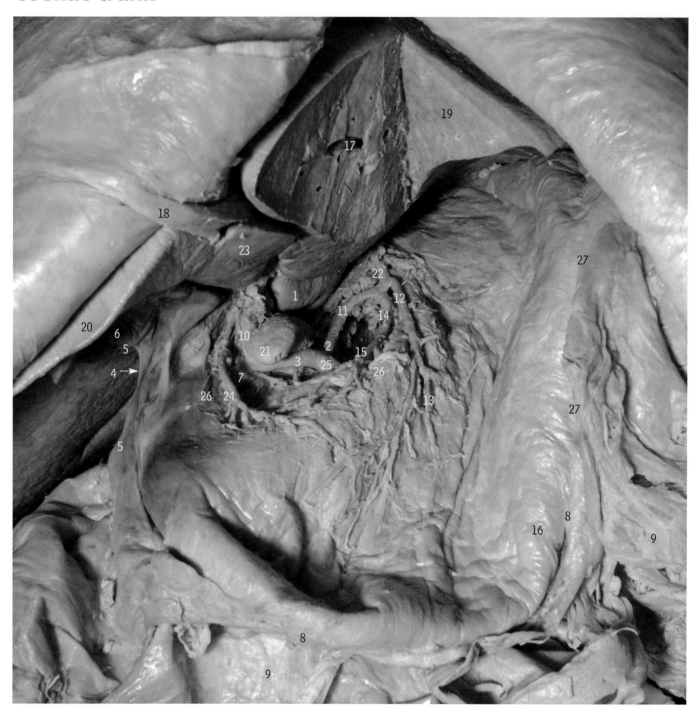

1 Caudate lobe of liver
2 Coeliac trunk
3 Common hepatic artery
4 Epiploic foramen – arrow
5 Free edge, lesser omentum
6 Gall bladder
7 Gastroduodenal artery
8 Greater curvature of stomach
9 Greater omentum
10 Hepatic artery, proper
11 Left gastric artery
12 Left gastric, anterior branch
13 Left gastric, anterior branch to body of stomach
14 Left gastric, posterior branch

15 Left gastric, posterior branch to lesser curvature of stomach
16 Left gastroepiploic vessels
17 Left portal vein
18 Ligamentum teres hepatis within falciform ligament
19 Liver, left lobe
20 Liver, right lobe
21 Lymph node, enlarged coeliac node
22 Oesophageal branch of left gastric artery
23 Quadrate lobe of liver
24 Right gastric artery, antral branch
25 Splenic artery
26 Stomach, lesser curvature
27 Visceral peritoneum, cut edge

Abdominal vasculature variations, carcinoma of the stomach, see pages 280–284.

Superior mesenteric vessels, origins

A *duodenum and pancreas in situ*
B *duodenum reflected to reveal posterior relations of vessels*

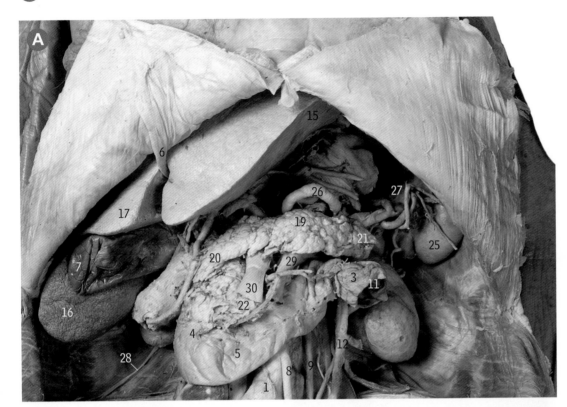

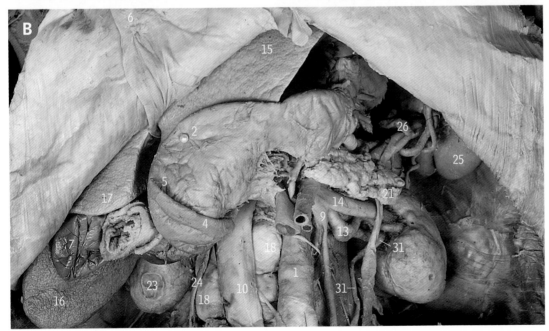

1 Aorta
2 Duodenum reflected and pinned
3 Duodenum, ascending (fourth) part
4 Duodenum, descending (second) part
5 Duodenum, horizontal (third) part
6 Falciform ligament
7 Gall bladder, fundus
8 Inferior mesenteric artery
9 Inferior mesenteric vein
10 Inferior vena cava
11 Jejunum, origin
12 Left gonadal vein
13 Left renal artery
14 Left renal vein
15 Liver, left lobe
16 Liver, Riedel's lobe
17 Liver, right lobe
18 Lymph nodes, moderately enlarged pre and para-aortic
19 Pancreas, body
20 Pancreas, head
21 Pancreas, tail
22 Pancreas, uncinate process
23 Renal cyst, benign
24 Right gonadal vein
25 Spleen
26 Splenic artery
27 Splenic vein
28 Subcostal nerve
29 Superior mesenteric artery
30 Superior mesenteric vein
31 Ureter

Inferior vena cava (IVC) obstruction, pancreatic pathology, pancreatitis, see pages 280–284.

Coeliac trunk, upper abdomen *detailed dissection*

The stomach has been sectioned to expose the dissected liver, biliary tree, pancreas, duodenum, and superior mesenteric vessels lying posterior to the stomach bed.

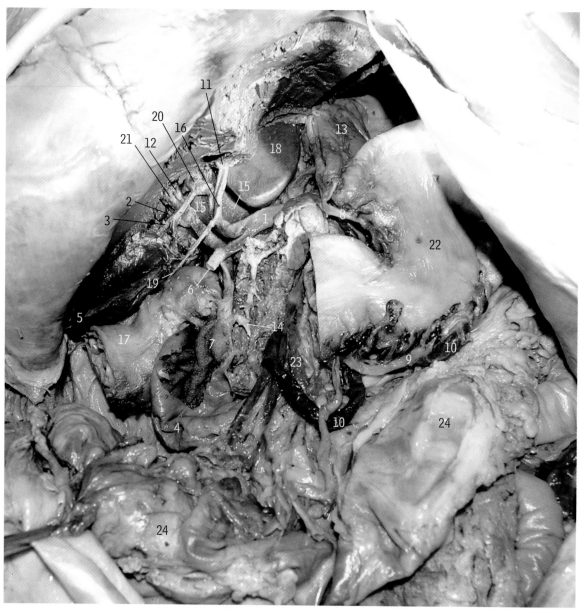

1 Common hepatic artery	**13** Oesophagus
2 Cystic artery	**14** Pancreatic duct
3 Cystic duct	**15** Portal vein
4 Duodenum	**16** Proper hepatic artery
5 Gall bladder	**17** Pylorus
6 Gastroduodenal artery	**18** Caudate lobe (liver)
7 Hepatopancreatic ampulla	**19** Right gastric artery
8 Left gastric artery	**20** Right hepatic artery
9 Left gastroepiploic artery	**21** Right hepatic duct
10 Left gastroepiploic vein	**22** Stomach
11 Left hepatic artery	**23** Superior mesenteric vein
12 Left hepatic duct	**24** Transverse colon

Pyloric stenosis (adult), see pages 280–284.

Coeliac trunk, upper abdomen *detailed dissection*

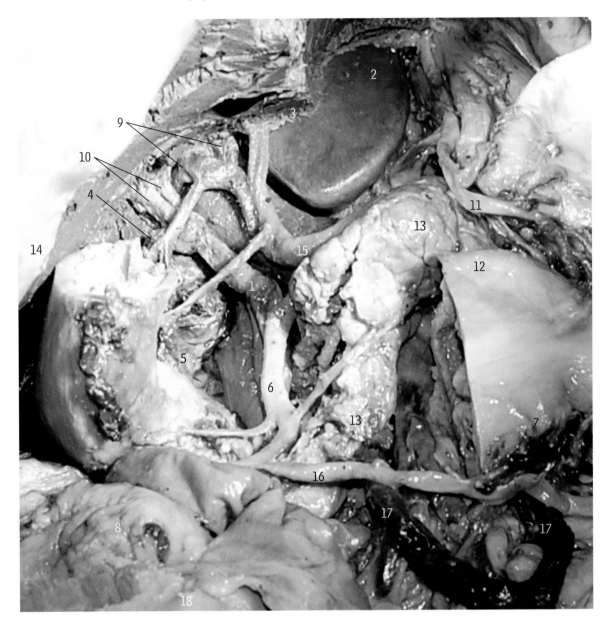

1 (Common) bile duct
2 Caudate lobe
3 Cut edge of the liver
4 Cystic duct
5 Fundus of gallbladder
6 Gastroduodenal artery
7 Greater curvature of stomach
8 Greater omentum
9 Left and right hepatic artery
10 Left and right hepatic duct

11 Left gastric artery
12 Lesser curvature of stomach
13 Pancreas
14 Parietal peritoneum on anterior abdominal
    wall, reflected laterally
15 Proper hepatic artery
16 Right gastro-omental artery
17 Right gastro-omental vein
18 Transverse colon

Superior mesenteric vessels

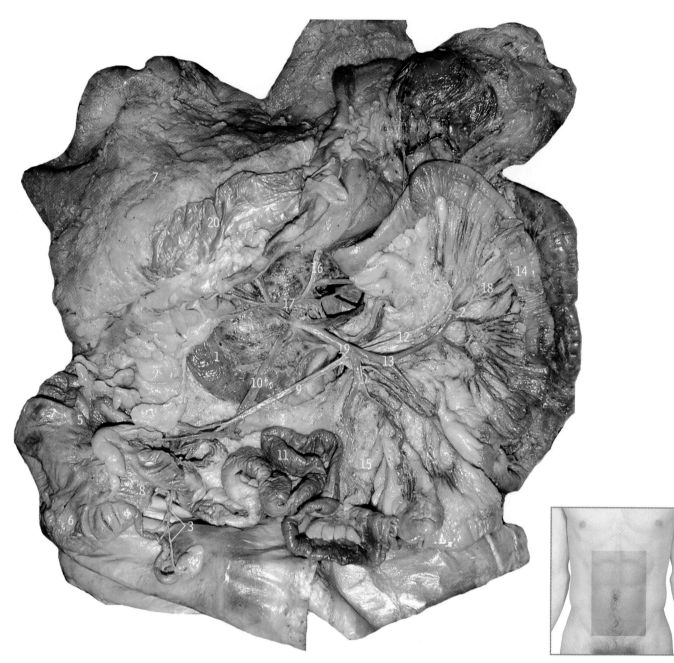

1 Third part of the duodenum	**8** Ileocaecal junction
2 Anastomotic arcades	**9** Ileocolic artery
3 Appendicular artery	**10** Ileocolic vein
4 Appendix	**11** Ileum
5 Ascending colon	**12** Jejunal artery
6 Caecum	**13** Jejunal vein
7 Greater omentum	**14** Jejunum

15 Mesentery of the ileum
16 Middle colic artery
17 Right colic artery
18 Straight arteries
19 Superior mesenteric vein
20 Transverse colon

Meckel's diverticulum, see pages 280–284.

Inferior mesenteric vessels *from the front*

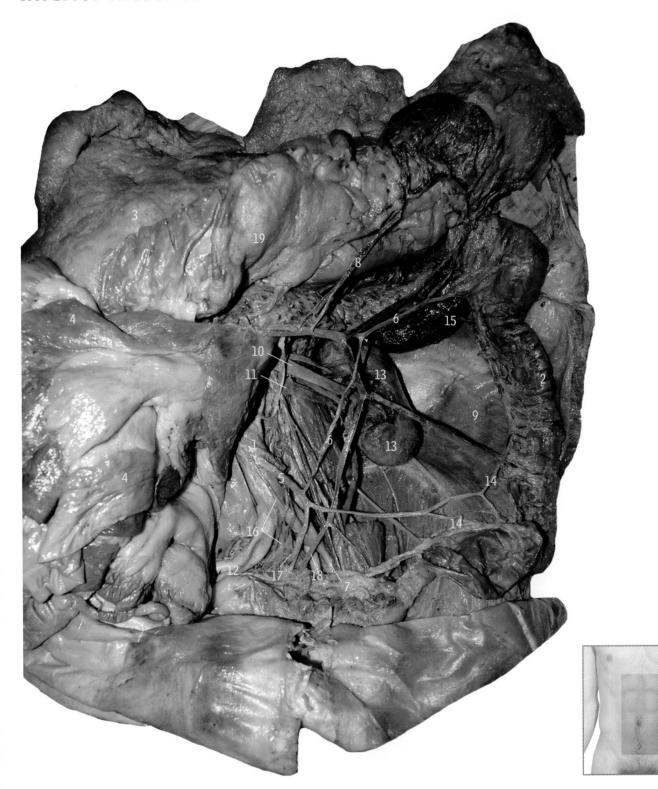

1 Abdominal aorta	**6** Left colic artery	**11** Renal vein	**16** Superior hypogastric plexus
2 Descending colon	**7** Left common iliac artery	**12** Right common iliac artery	**17** Superior rectal artery
3 Greater omentum	**8** Marginal artery	**13** Right kidney	**18** Superior rectal vein
4 Ileum and jejunum	**9** Transverse abdominis	**14** Sigmoid arteries	**19** Transverse colon
5 Inferior mesenteric artery	**10** Renal artery	**15** Spleen	

Bowel ischaemia, see pages 280–284.

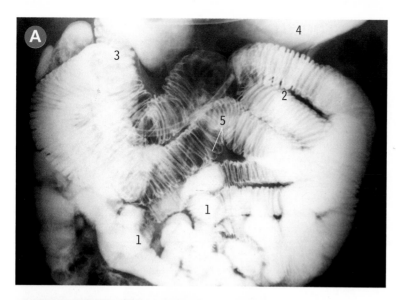

Ⓐ Small bowel radiograph

enema via a tube in the duodenum

1 Coils of ileum
2 Coils of jejunum
3 Descending (second) part of duodenum
4 Stomach
5 Valvulae conniventes

Ⓑ Large intestine radiograph

In this double-contrast barium enema (barium and air), the sacculations (haustrations, 9) of the various parts of the colon allow it to be distinguished from the narrower terminal ileum (11), which has become partly filled by barium flowing into it through this incompetent ileocaecal junction (5).

1 Ascending colon	**8** Right colic (hepatic) flexure	
2 Caecum	**9** Sacculations	
3 Descending colon	**10** Sigmoid colon	
4 Hip joint	**11** Terminal ileum	
5 Ileocaecal junction	**12** Transverse colon	
6 Left colic (splenic) flexure		
7 Rectum		

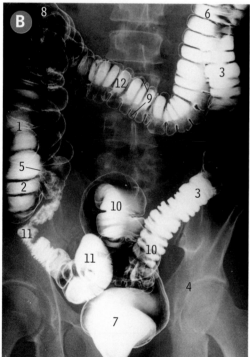

Ⓒ 3D reconstruction CT 64 slice scan "3D scout scan from virtual colonoscopy"

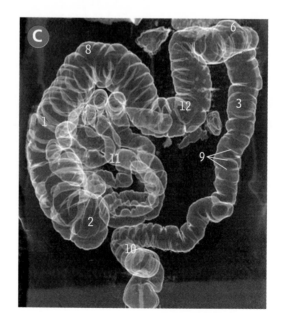

Colonic stents, colostomy, rectosigmoid foreign bodies, see pages 280–284.

Stomach *with vessels and vagus nerves, from the front*

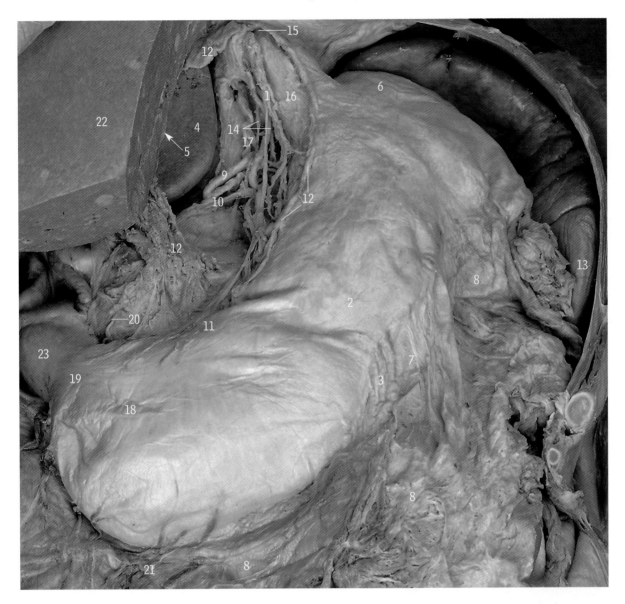

The anterior thoracic and abdominal walls and the left lobe of the liver have been removed, with part of the lesser omentum (12), to show the stomach (6, 2, 18 and 19) in its undisturbed position.

1 Anterior (left) vagal trunk	**13** Lower end of spleen
2 Body of stomach	**14** Oesophageal branches of left gastric vessels
3 Branches of left gastro-epiploic vessels	**15** Oesophageal opening in diaphragm
4 Caudate lobe of liver	**16** Oesophagus
5 Fissure for ligamentum venosum	**17** Posterior (right) vagal trunk
6 Fundus of stomach	**18** Pyloric antrum
7 Greater curvature of stomach	**19** Pyloric canal
8 Greater omentum	**20** Right gastric artery
9 Left gastric artery	**21** Right gastro-epiploic vessels and branches
10 Left gastric vein	**22** Right lobe of liver
11 Lesser curvature of stomach	**23** Superior (first) part of duodenum
12 Lesser omentum (cut edge)	

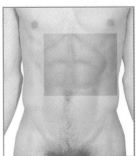

Oesophageal varices, vagotomy, see pages 280–284.

Upper abdomen ⒶA *stomach – barium meal*

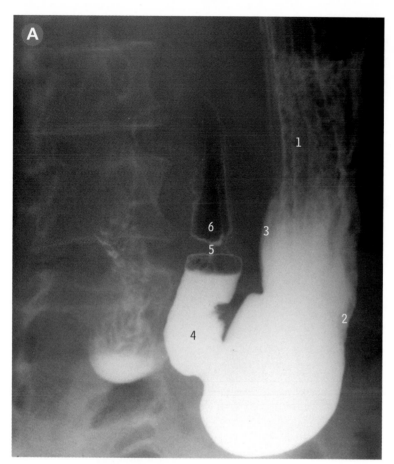

1 Body of stomach
2 Greater curvature of stomach
3 Lesser curvature of stomach
4 Pyloric antrum
5 Pyloric canal
6 Duodenal cap

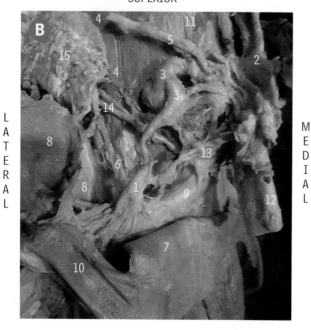

SUPERIOR

LATERAL

MEDIAL

INFERIOR

ⒷB *posterior wall – coeliac ganglion and relations*

1 Aorto-renal ganglion
2 Coeliac arterial trunk (reflected anteriorly)
3 Coeliac ganglion
4 Diaphragm
5 Inferior phrenic artery
6 Inferior suprarenal artery
7 Inferior vena cava (reflected inferiorly)

8 Kidney, right
9 Renal artery, right
10 Renal vein (reflected)
11 Right crus, diaphragm
12 Superior mesenteric artery
13 Superior mesenteric ganglion
14 Superior suprarenal artery
15 Suprarenal gland

Coeliac plexus block, gastric pacemaker, hiatus hernia, see pages 280–284.

A Pancreas, duodenum and superior mesenteric vessels

The stomach with its attached greater omentum has been lifted up.

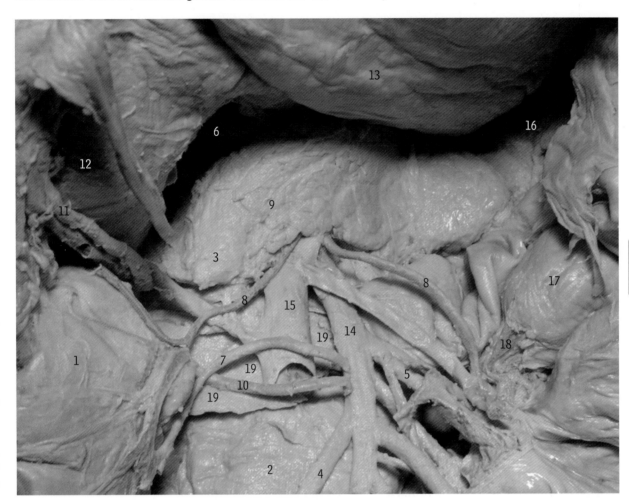

B Duodenal papilla

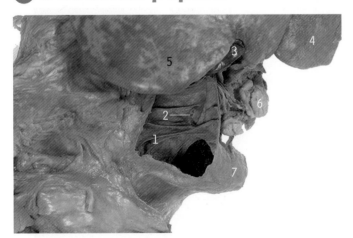

The stomach has been retracted superiorly to reveal the 'stomach bed.'

1 Ascending colon
2 Duodenum, third part
3 Head of pancreas
4 Ileocolic artery
5 Jejunal branch of superior mesenteric artery
6 Lesser sac
7 Middle colic artery
8 Middle colic artery, aberrant variation
9 Neck of pancreas
10 Right colic artery

11 Right gastroepiploic vessels
12 Stomach, antrum (reflected anteriorly)
13 Stomach, body
14 Superior mesenteric artery
15 Superior mesenteric vein
16 Tail of pancreas
17 Transverse colon
18 Transverse colon, artery and vein
19 Uncinate process of pancreas

The anterior wall of the descending (second) part of the duodenum has been removed.

1 Circular folds of mucous membrane
2 Duodenal papilla
3 Gall bladder

4 Liver, left lobe
5 Liver, right lobe
6 Pancreas
7 Third part of duodenum

Pancreatitis, see pages 280–284.

Liver *from the front*

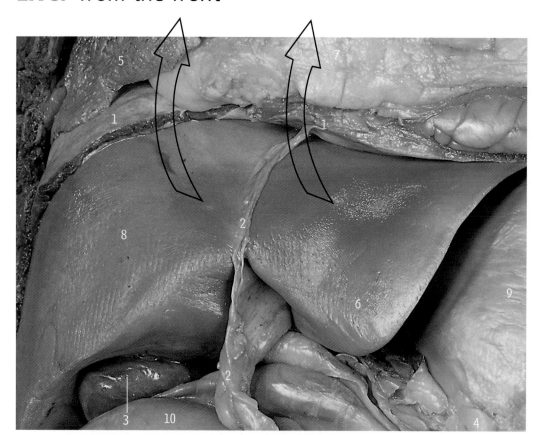

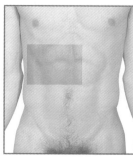

1 Diaphragm
2 Falciform ligament
3 Gall bladder, fundus
4 Greater omentum
5 Inferior lobe of right lung
6 Left lobe of liver
7 Pericardial fat
8 Right lobe of liver
9 Stomach
10 Transverse colon

For an explanation of peritoneal structures, see the diagrams on pages 220, 233.

The thoracic and abdominal walls and the anterior part of the diaphragm have been removed to show the undisturbed viscera. The liver (6 and 8) and stomach (9) are immediately below the diaphragm (1). The greater omentum (4) hangs down from the greater curvature (lower margin) of the stomach (9), overlying much of the small and large intestine but leaving some of the transverse colon (10) uncovered. The fundus (tip) of the gall bladder (3) is seen between the right lobe of the liver (8) and transverse colon (10). Arrows indicate the direction of liver reflection for the view on following page (page 245).

Coronal CT, upper abdomen

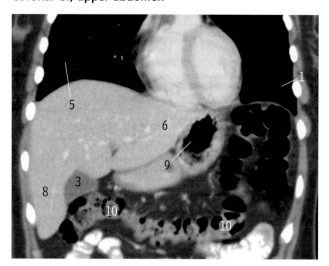

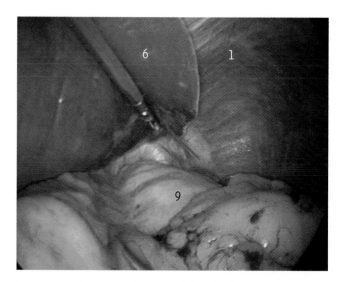

Laparoscopic view of upper abdominal viscera

 Cirrhosis of liver, liver trauma, see pages 280–284.

Liver *from below and behind*

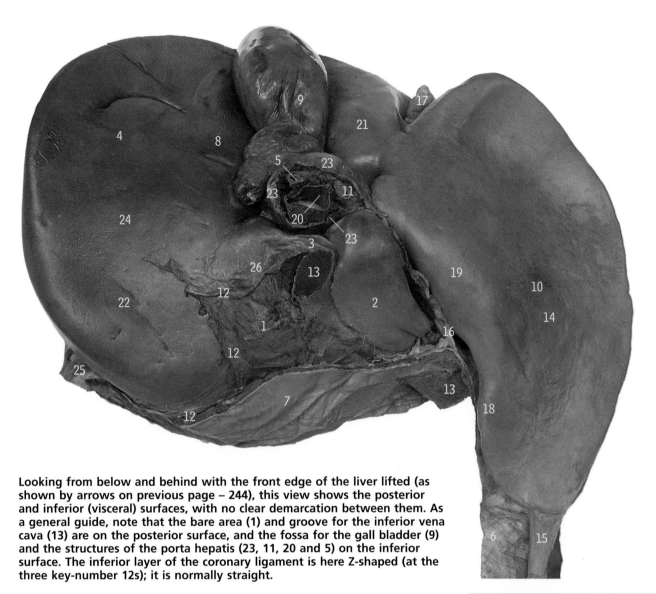

Looking from below and behind with the front edge of the liver lifted (as shown by arrows on previous page – 244), this view shows the posterior and inferior (visceral) surfaces, with no clear demarcation between them. As a general guide, note that the bare area (1) and groove for the inferior vena cava (13) are on the posterior surface, and the fossa for the gall bladder (9) and the structures of the porta hepatis (23, 11, 20 and 5) on the inferior surface. The inferior layer of the coronary ligament is here Z-shaped (at the three key-number 12s); it is normally straight.

1	Bare area	**15**	Left triangular ligament
2	Caudate lobe	**16**	Lesser omentum in fissure for ligamentum venosum
3	Caudate process		
4	Colic impression	**17**	Ligamentum teres and falciform ligament in fissure for ligamentum teres
5	Common hepatic duct		
6	Diaphragm		
7	Diaphragm on part of bare area (obstructing view of superior layer of coronary ligament)	**18**	Oesophageal groove
		19	Omental tuberosity
		20	Portal vein
8	Duodenal impression	**21**	Quadrate lobe
9	Gall bladder	**22**	Renal impression
10	Gastric impression	**23**	Right free margin of lesser omentum in porta hepatis
11	Hepatic artery		
12	Inferior layer of coronary ligament	**24**	Right lobe
13	Inferior vena cava	**25**	Right triangular ligament
14	Left lobe	**26**	Suprarenal impression

The caudate (2) and quadrate (21) lobes are classified anatomically as part of the right lobe (24), but functionally they belong to the left lobe (14), since they receive blood from the left branches of the hepatic artery and portal vein, and drain bile to the left hepatic duct.

Liver abscess, Riedel's lobe, see pages 280–284.

Cast of the liver, extrahepatic biliary tract and associated vessels *from below and behind*

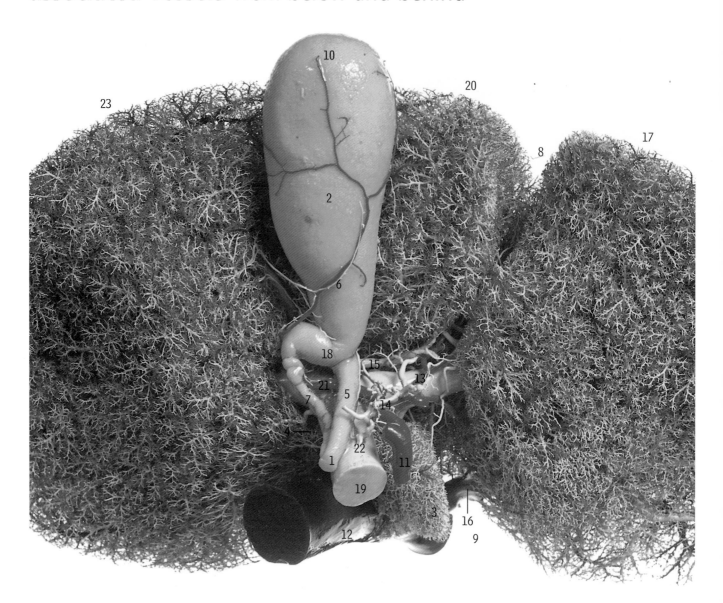

Yellow, gall bladder and biliary tract
Red, hepatic artery and branches
Light blue, portal vein and tributaries
Dark blue, inferior vena cava, hepatic veins and tributaries

This view, like the one on page 245, shows the inferior and posterior surfaces, as looking into the abdomen from below with the lower border of the liver pushed up towards the thorax.

1	Bile duct	**14**	Left gastric vein
2	Body of gall bladder	**15**	Left hepatic duct
3	Caudate lobe	**16**	Left hepatic vein
4	Caudate process	**17**	Left lobe
5	Common hepatic duct	**18**	Neck of gall bladder
6	Cystic artery and veins	**19**	Portal vein
7	Cystic duct	**20**	Quadrate lobe
8	Fissure for ligamentum teres	**21**	Right branch of hepatic artery overlying right branch of portal vein
9	Fissure for ligamentum venosum		
10	Fundus of gall bladder	**22**	Right gastric vein
11	Hepatic artery	**23**	Right lobe
12	Inferior vena cava		
13	Left branch of hepatic artery overlying left branch of portal vein		

Ⓐ Endoscopic retrograde cholangiopancreatogram *ERCP*

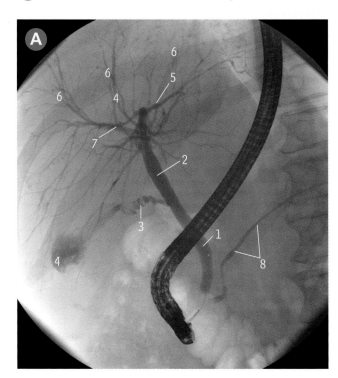

During an ERCP, an endoscope is passed through the mouth, pharynx, oesophagus and stomach into the duodenum, and through it, a cannula is introduced into the major duodenal papilla (page 243B) and bile duct so that contrast medium can be injected up the biliary tract. (The pancreatic duct can also be cannulated in this way.)

1 Common bile duct
2 Common hepatic duct
3 Cystic duct
4 Gall bladder
5 Left hepatic duct
6 Liver shadow and tributaries of hepatic ducts
7 Right hepatic duct
8 Pancreatic duct

Ⓒ Magnetic resonance cholangiopancreatogram *MRCP*

Ⓑ Pancreatic duct *ERCP*

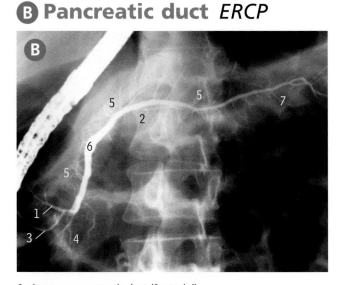

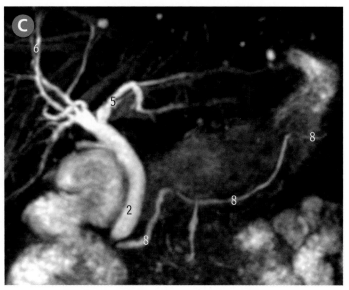

1 Accessory pancreatic duct (Santorini)
2 Body of pancreas
3 Cannula in ampulla (Vater)
4 Head of pancreas
5 Intralobular ducts of the pancreas
6 Pancreatic duct (Wirsung)
7 Tail of pancreas

See label list for A.

Carcinoma of the pancreas, cholecystectomy, gallstones, see pages 280–284.

Cast of the portal vein and tributaries, and the mesenteric vessels *from behind*

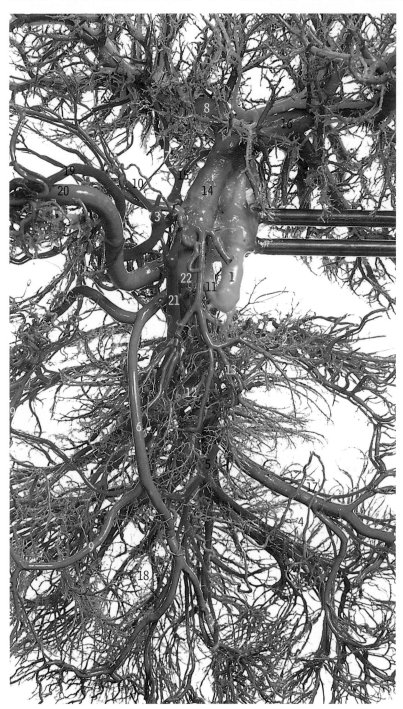

1 Bile duct
2 Branches of middle colic vessels
3 Coeliac trunk
4 Ileocolic vessels
5 Inferior mesenteric artery
6 Inferior mesenteric vein
7 Left branch of hepatic artery
8 Left branch of portal vein
9 Left colic vessels
10 Left gastric artery and vein
11 Pancreatic duct
12 Pancreatic ducts in head of pancreas
13 Pancreaticoduodenal vessels
14 Portal vein
15 Right branch of hepatic artery
16 Right branch of portal vein
17 Right colic vessels
18 Sigmoid vessels
19 Splenic artery
20 Splenic vein
21 Superior mesenteric artery
22 Superior mesenteric vein

Coronal CT, abdomen

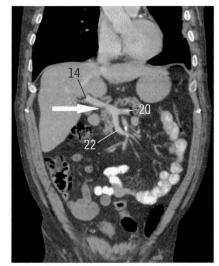

Yellow, biliary tract and pancreatic ducts; red, arteries; blue, portal venous system

In this posterior view (chosen in preference to the anterior view, where the many very small vessels to the intestines would have obscured the larger branches), the superior mesenteric vein (22) is seen continuing upwards to become the portal vein (14) after it has been joined by the splenic vein (20). In the porta hepatis, the portal vein divides into the left and right branches (8 and 16). Owing to removal of the aorta, the upper part of the inferior mesenteric artery (5) has become displaced slightly to the right and appears to have given origin to the ileocolic artery (4), but this is simply an overlap of the vessels; the origin of the ileocolic from the superior mesenteric is not seen in this view.

A Spleen *from the front*

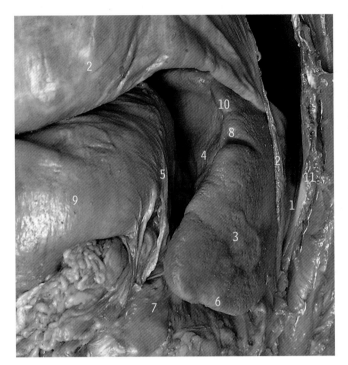

The left upper anterior abdominal and lower anterior thoracic walls have been removed and part of the diaphragm (2) turned upwards to show the spleen in its normal position, lying adjacent to the stomach (9) and colon (7), with the lower part against the kidney (D16 and 9, opposite).

The gastrosplenic ligament contains the short gastric and left gastro-epiploic branches of the splenic vessels.

The lienorenal ligament contains the tail of the pancreas and the splenic vessels.

Coronal CT

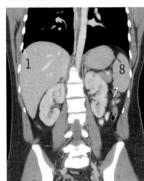

1 Costodiaphragmatic recess
2 Diaphragm
3 Diaphragmatic surface
4 Gastric impression
5 Gastrosplenic ligament
6 Inferior border
7 Left colic flexure
8 Splenic notch
9 Stomach
10 Superior border
11 Thoracic wall

B Spleen *visceral surface*

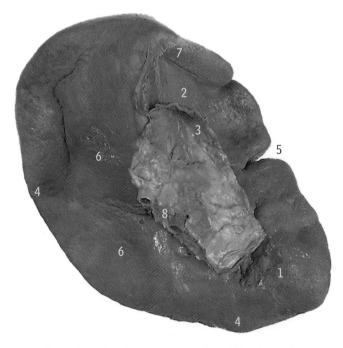

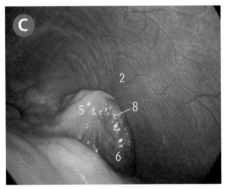

C Spleen *Laparoscopic view*

Labels refer to key in A.

1 Colic impression
2 Gastric impression
3 Gastrosplenic ligament containing short gastric and left gastro-epiploic vessels
4 Inferior border
5 Splenic notch
6 Renal impression
7 Superior border
8 Tail of pancreas and splenic vessels in lienorenal ligament

In B, the spleen has been removed and its visceral or medial surface is shown, with a small part of the gastrosplenic (3) and lienorenal (8) ligaments remaining attached.

Ruptured spleen, splenic cysts, splenic infarct, splenectomy, splenomegaly, splenunculi, see pages 280–284.

D Spleen *in a transverse section of the left upper abdomen*

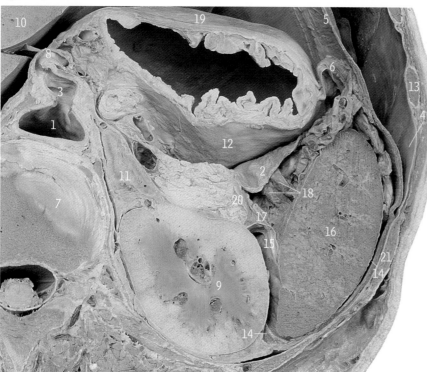

The section is at the level of the disc (7) between the twelfth thoracic and first lumbar vertebrae, and is viewed from below looking towards the thorax.

1 Abdominal aorta
2 Anterior layer of lienorenal ligament
3 Coeliac trunk
4 Costodiaphragmatic recess of pleura
5 Diaphragm
6 Gastrosplenic ligament
7 Intervertebral disc
8 Left gastric artery
9 Left kidney
10 Left lobe of liver
11 Left suprarenal gland
12 Lesser sac
13 Ninth rib
14 Peritoneum of greater sac
15 Posterior layer of lienorenal ligament
16 Spleen
17 Splenic artery
18 Splenic vein
19 Stomach
20 Tail of pancreas
21 Tenth rib

E Caecum *in sagittal section, interior view*

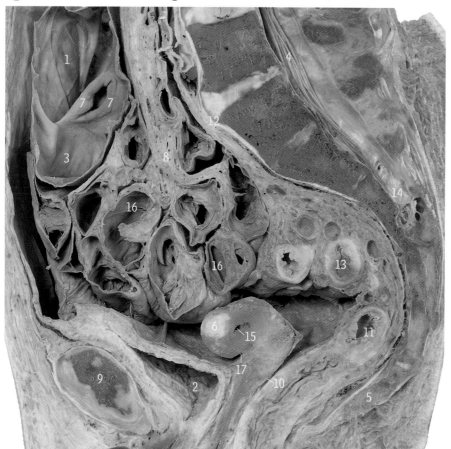

This is a median section of the female pelvis, right side viewed from the left. The caecal anterior wall has been cut open and reflected to show the lips of the ileocaecal valve (7).

1 Ascending colon
2 Bladder
3 Caecum
4 Cauda equina
5 Coccyx
6 Fibroid in uterine fundus
7 Lips of ileocaecal valve
8 Mesentery of small intestine
9 Pubic symphysis
10 Recto-uterine pouch (of Douglas)
11 Rectum
12 Sacral promontory
13 Sigmoid colon
14 Thecal sac termination
15 Uterine cavity
16 Valvulae conniventes
17 Vesico-uterine pouch

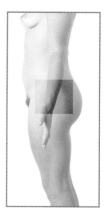

Carcinoma of the bladder, intussusception, see pages 280–284.

A Appendix, ileocolic artery and related structures
from the front

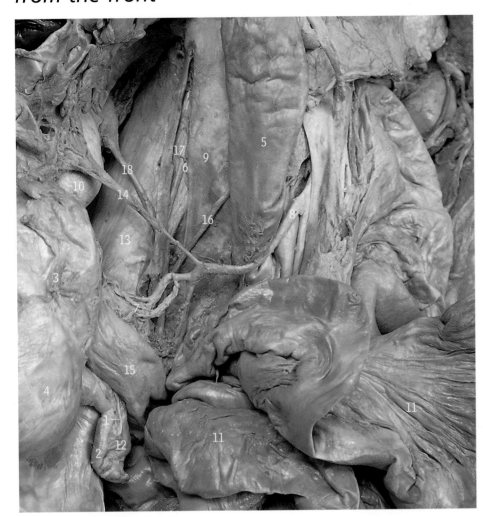

Most of the peritoneum of the mesentery and posterior abdominal wall has been removed, and coils of small intestine (11) have been displaced to the right of the picture, to show the ileocolic artery (8), terminal ileum (15) and appendix (2) with its appendicular artery (1).

1 Appendicular artery in mesoappendix
2 Appendix
3 Ascending colon
4 Caecum
5 Descending (second) part of duodenum
6 Genitofemoral nerve
7 Ileal and caecal vessels
8 Ileocolic artery
9 Inferior vena cava
10 Lower pole of kidney
11 Mesentery and coils of jejunum and ileum
12 Mesoappendix
13 Psoas major
14 Right colic artery
15 Terminal part of ileum
16 Testicular artery
17 Testicular vein
18 Ureter

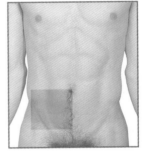

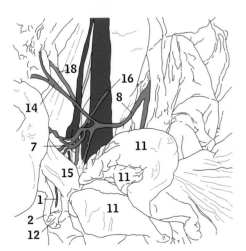

B Caecum and appendix *from the front*

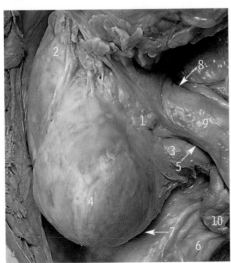

The terminal ileum (9) is seen joining the large intestine at the junction of the caecum (4) and ascending colon (2), and the appendix (3) joins the caecum just below the ileocaecal junction.

1 Anterior taenia coli
2 Ascending colon
3 Base of appendix
4 Caecum
5 Inferior ileocaecal recess
6 Peritoneum overlying external iliac vessels
7 Retrocaecal recess
8 Superior ileocaecal recess
9 Terminal ileum
10 Tip of appendix

Appendicitis, see pages 280–284.

Small intestine

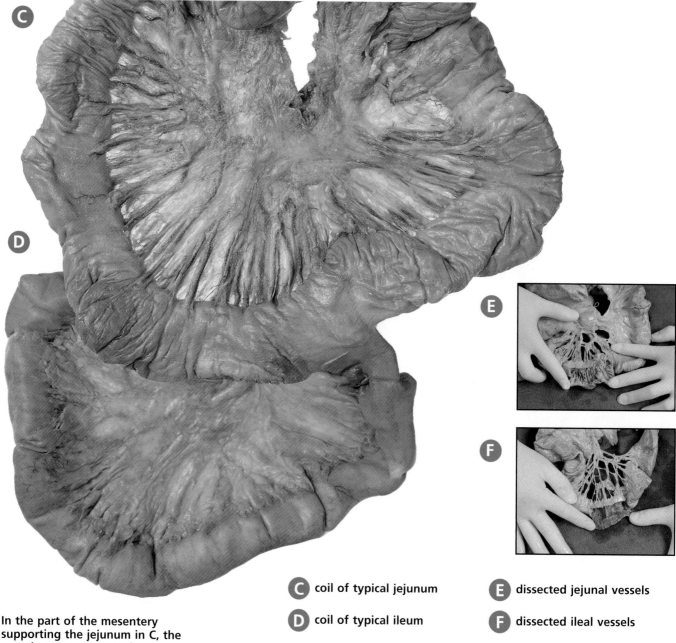

In the part of the mesentery supporting the jejunum in C, the vessels anastomose to form one or perhaps two vascular arcades (E) which give off long straight branches that run to the intestinal wall. The fat in the mesentery tends to be concentrated near the root, leaving areas or 'windows' near the gut wall that are devoid of fat. In the mesentery supporting the ileum in D, the vessels form several arcades with shorter branches (F), and there are no fat-free areas. The jejunal wall (C) is thicker than that of the ileum (D) and has a larger lumen. The jejunum also feels thicker, because the folds of its mucous membrane are more numerous than in the ileum.

C coil of typical jejunum

D coil of typical ileum

E dissected jejunal vessels

F dissected ileal vessels

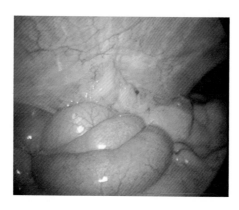

Laparoscopic view of small intestine

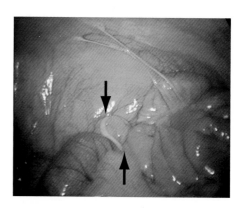

Laparoscopic view of appendix

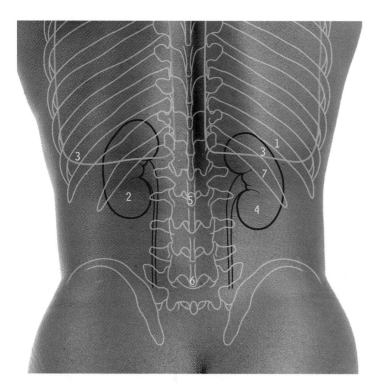

A Kidneys and ureters
surface markings, from behind

The upper pole of the left kidney rises to the level of the eleventh rib, but the right kidney is slightly lower (due to the bulk of the liver on the right). The hilum of each kidney is 5 cm (2 in) from the midline. The lower edge of the costodiaphragmatic recess of the pleura crosses the twelfth rib; compare with the dissection below (B6).

1 Eleventh rib
2 Left kidney
3 Lower edge of pleura
4 Right kidney
5 Spinous process of first lumbar vertebra
6 Spinous process of fourth lumbar vertebra
7 Twelfth rib

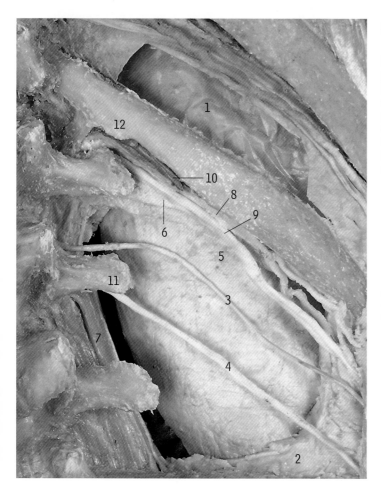

B Right kidney *from behind*

Most thoracic and abdominal muscles have been removed to show the three nerves (9, 3 and 4) that lie behind the kidney (5). Much more important is the relationship of the upper part of the kidney to the pleura. A window has been cut in the parietal pleura above the twelfth rib (12) to open into the costodiaphragmatic recess (1), whose lower limit (6) runs transversely behind the kidney and in front of the obliquely placed twelfth rib.

1 Costodiaphragmatic recess of pleura
2 Extraperitoneal tissue
3 Iliohypogastric nerve
4 Ilio-inguinal nerve
5 Kidney
6 Lower edge of pleura
7 Psoas major
8 Subcostal artery
9 Subcostal nerve
10 Subcostal vein
11 Transverse process of second lumbar vertebra
12 Twelfth rib

Lumbar hernia, renal biopsy, see pages 280–284.

C Left kidney, suprarenal gland and related vessels *from the front*

D Right kidney, suprarenal gland and related vessels *from behind*

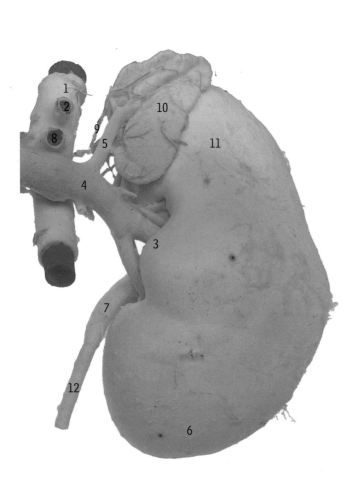

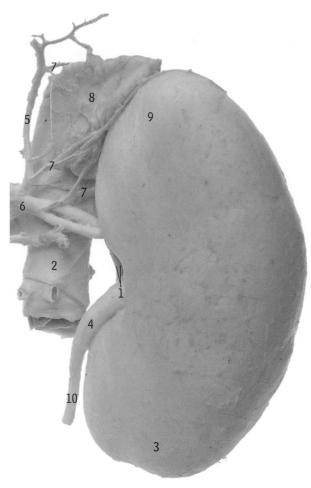

The vessels have been distended by injection of resin, and all fascia has been removed, but the suprarenal gland (10) has been retained in its normal position, lying against the medial side of the upper pole of the kidney (11).

1 Abdominal aorta	**7** Pelvis of kidney
2 Coeliac trunk	**8** Superior mesenteric artery
3 Hilum of kidney	**9** Suprarenal arteries
4 Left renal vein overlying renal artery	**10** Suprarenal gland
	11 Upper pole of kidney
5 Left suprarenal vein	**12** Ureter
6 Lower pole of kidney	

Similar to B, but note that this is the right kidney from behind, not the left; the hilum of each kidney faces medially.

1 Hilum of kidney	**6** Right renal artery
2 Inferior vena cava	**7** Suprarenal arteries
3 Lower pole of kidney	**8** Suprarenal gland
4 Pelvis of kidney	**9** Upper pole of kidney
5 Right inferior phrenic artery	**10** Ureter

Adrenal gland pathology, see pages 280–284.

Ⓐ Kidney *internal structure in longitudinal section*

The section is through the centre of the kidney and has included the renal pelvis (9) and beginning of the ureter (10). The major vessels in the hilum (2) have been removed.

1 Cortex
2 Hilum
3 Major calix
4 Medulla
5 Medullary pyramid

6 Minor calix
7 Renal column
8 Renal papilla
9 Renal pelvis
10 Ureter

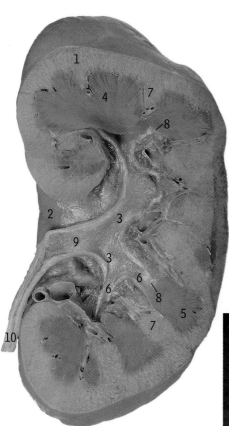

The two or three major calices (3) unite to form the renal pelvis (9) which passes out through the hilum (2) to become the ureter (10), often with a slight narrowing at the junction. This is known as the pelvi-ureteric junction (PUJ) and is a site of renal stone obstruction.

Laparoscopic view of right kidney (NB peritoneal covering)

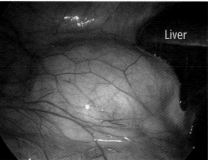

Liver

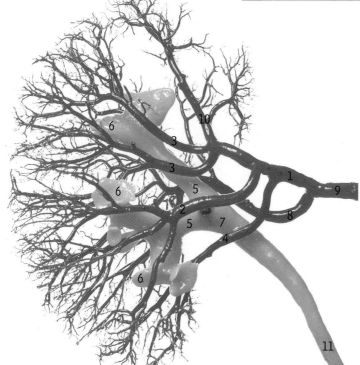

Ⓑ Cast of the right kidney *from the front*

Red, renal artery
Yellow, urinary tract

The posterior division (8) of the renal artery (9) here passes behind the pelvis (7) and upper calix (upper 5), but all other vessels are in front of the urinary tract; hence this is a right kidney seen from the front (vein, artery, ureter from front to back, and the hilum on the medial side – see page 254), not a left kidney from behind.

1 Anterior division of the renal artery
2 Anterior inferior segment artery
3 Anterior superior segment artery (double)
4 Inferior segment artery
5 Major calix
6 Minor calix
7 Pelvis of kidney
8 Posterior division (forming posterior segment artery)
9 Renal artery
10 Superior segment artery
11 Ureter

C Cast of the aorta and kidneys *from the front*

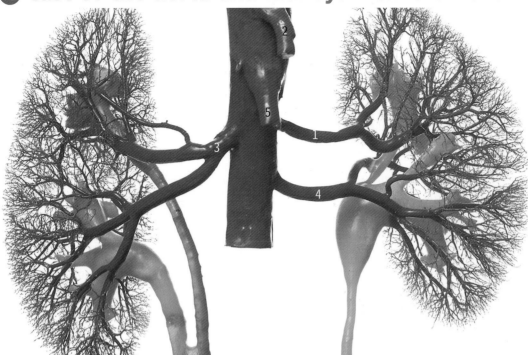

Red, arteries
Yellow, urinary tracts

1 Accessory left renal artery
2 Coeliac trunk
3 Early branching of right renal artery
4 Left renal artery
5 Superior mesenteric artery

Accessory renal arteries represent segmental vessels that arise directly from the aorta. In this specimen, the left accessory vessel (C1) supplies the superior and anterior superior segments, leaving the 'normal' vessel to supply the posterior, anterior inferior and inferior segments.

On the right side, the ureters (unlabelled) are double, each arising from a separate set of calices. On the left, the arteries are double (1 and 4).

D Cast of the kidneys and great vessels *from the front*

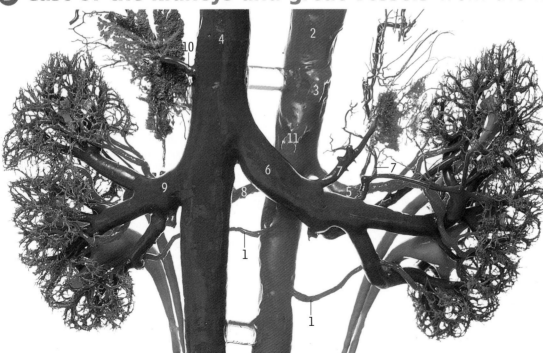

Red, arteries
Blue, veins
Yellow, urinary tracts

1 Accessory renal arteries
2 Aorta
3 Coeliac trunk
4 Inferior vena cava
5 Left renal artery
6 Left renal vein
7 Left suprarenal veins
8 Right renal artery
9 Right renal vein
10 Right suprarenal vein
11 Superior mesenteric artery

Here both kidneys show double ureters (unlabelled), and there are accessory renal arteries (1) to the lower poles of both kidneys. The suprarenal glands (also unlabelled) are outlined by their venous patterns, and the short right suprarenal vein (10) is shown draining directly to the inferior vena cava (4). On the left, there are two suprarenal veins (7), both draining to the left renal vein (6). See also page 257, A14, A9, A12.

Congenital kidney variants, see pages 280–284.

A Left kidney and suprarenal gland *from the front*

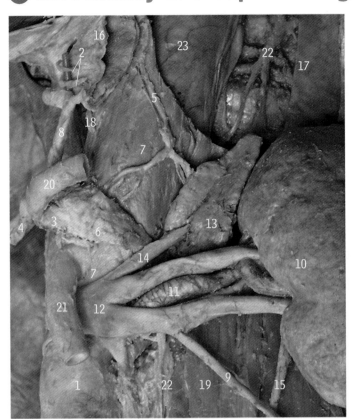

The left kidney (10) and suprarenal gland (13) are seen on the posterior abdominal wall. Much of the diaphragm has been removed but the oesophageal opening remains, with the end of the oesophagus (16) opening out into the cardiac part of the stomach and a (double) anterior vagal trunk (2) overlying the red marker. The posterior vagal trunk (18) is behind and to the right of the oesophagus. Part of the pleura has been cut away (17) to show the sympathetic trunk (22) on the side of the lower thoracic vertebrae. The left coeliac ganglion and the coeliac plexus (6) are at the root of the coeliac trunk (3).

1 Abdominal aorta
2 Anterior vagal trunk (double, over marker)
3 Coeliac trunk
4 Common hepatic artery
5 Inferior phrenic vessels
6 Left coeliac ganglion and coeliac plexus
7 Left crus of diaphragm
8 Left gastric artery
9 Left gonadal vein
10 Left kidney
11 Left renal artery
12 Left renal vein
13 Left suprarenal gland
14 Left suprarenal vein
15 Left ureter
16 Lower end of oesophagus
17 Pleura (cut edge)
18 Posterior vagal trunk
19 Psoas major
20 Splenic artery
21 Superior mesenteric artery
22 Sympathetic trunk
23 Thoracic aorta

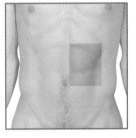

B Right kidney and renal fascia *in transverse section from below*

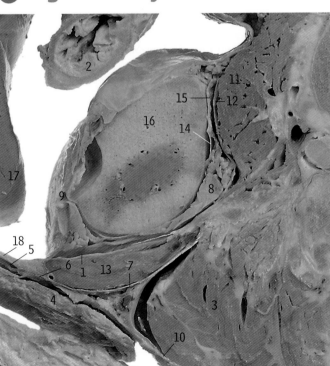

In the transverse section of the lower part of the right kidney (16), seen from below looking towards the thorax, the renal fascia (15) has been dissected out from the perirenal fat (8) and the kidney's own capsule (14). (There was a small cyst on the surface of this kidney.) The section also displays the three layers (10, 7 and 1) of the lumbar fascia (6).

1 Anterior layer of lumbar fascia
2 Coil of small intestine
3 Erector spinae
4 External oblique
5 Internal oblique
6 Lumbar fascia
7 Middle layer of lumbar fascia
8 Perirenal fat
9 Peritoneum
10 Posterior layer of lumbar fascia
11 Psoas major
12 Psoas sheath
13 Quadratus lumborum
14 Renal capsule
15 Renal fascia
16 Right kidney
17 Right lobe of liver
18 Transversus abdominis

Outside the kidney's own capsule (renal capsule, 14), there is a variable amount of fat (perirenal fat, 8) and outside this is a condensation of connective tissue forming the renal fascia (15).

Haemoperitoneum, nephrectomy, pneumoretroperitoneum, superior mesenteric artery syndrome, see pages 280–284.

Kidneys and suprarenal glands

Ⓐ dissection Ⓑ right kidney and suprarenal gland, laparoscopic view

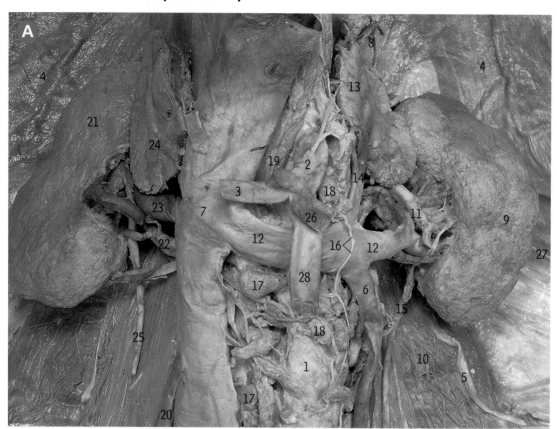

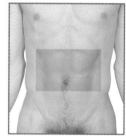

The kidneys (9 and 21) and suprarenal glands (13 and 24) are displayed on the posterior abdominal wall after the removal of all other viscera. The left renal vein (12) receives the left suprarenal (14) and gonadal (6) veins and then passes over the aorta (1) and deep to the superior mesenteric artery (28) to reach the inferior vena cava (7). In the hilum of the right kidney (21) a large branch of the renal artery (22) passes in front of the renal vein (23). The origins of the renal arteries from the aorta are not seen because they underlie the left renal vein (12) and inferior vena cava (7).

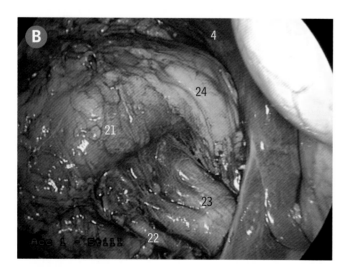

1	Abdominal aorta and aortic plexus	**15**	Left ureter
2	Coeliac trunk	**16**	Lymphatic vessels
3	Common hepatic artery	**17**	Para-aortic lymph nodes
4	Diaphragm	**18**	Pre-aortic lymph nodes
5	First lumbar spinal nerve	**19**	Right crus of diaphragm
6	Gonadal vein, left	**20**	Right gonadal vein
7	Inferior vena cava	**21**	Right kidney
8	Left inferior phrenic vessels	**22**	Right renal artery
9	Left kidney	**23**	Right renal vein
10	Left psoas major	**24**	Right suprarenal gland
11	Left renal artery	**25**	Right ureter
12	Left renal vein	**26**	Splenic artery
13	Left suprarenal gland	**27**	Subcostal nerve, left
14	Left suprarenal vein	**28**	Superior mesenteric artery

Aortic bruits, IVC duplication, renal carcinoma, retroperitoneal fibrosis, see pages 280–284.

C Intravenous urogram *IVU – 3D CT reconstruction*

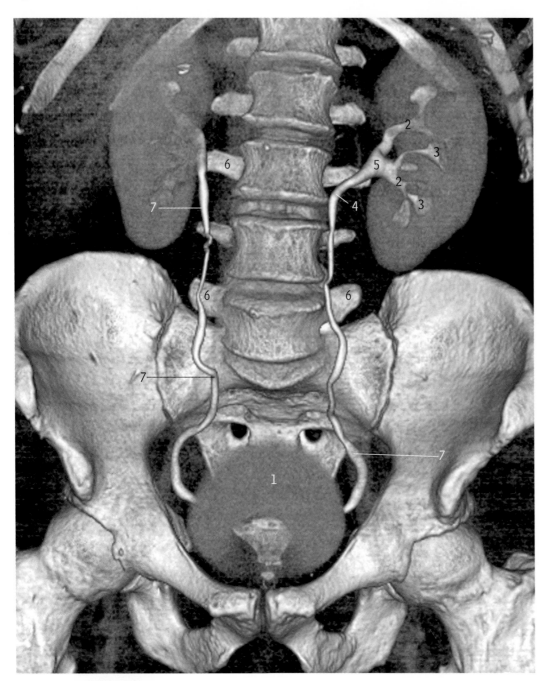

Contrast medium injected intravenously is excreted by the kidneys to outline the calices (3 and 2), renal pelvis (5) and the ureters (7) which enter the bladder (1) in the pelvis.

1 Bladder
2 Major calix
3 Minor calix
4 Pelvic-ureteric junction
5 Renal pelvis
6 Transverse processes of lumbar vertebrae
7 Ureter

The ureters normally lie near the tips of the transverse processes of the lumbar vertebrae and may kink over the psoas when the muscle is hypertrophied (e.g., in rowers and professional cyclists).

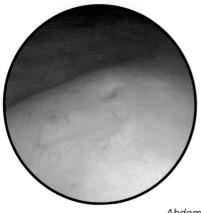

Cytoscopic view of the ureteric orifice

Abdominal aortic aneurysm, renal trauma, uretocele, urinary tract calculi, see pages 280–284.

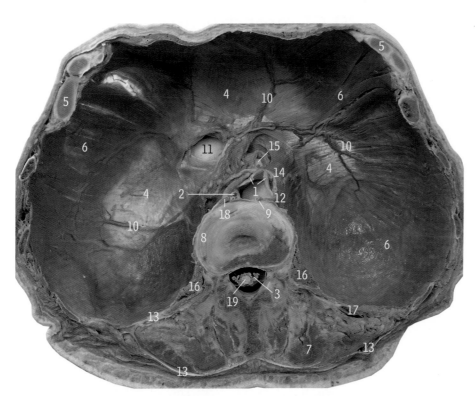

A Diaphragm
from below

1 Aorta
2 Azygos vein
3 Cauda equina
4 Central tendon of diaphragm
5 Costal margin
6 Diaphragm
7 Erector spinae muscles
8 First lumbar intervertebral disc
9 Hemi-azygos vein
10 Inferior phrenic vessels
11 Inferior vena caval opening
12 Left crus
13 Lumbar fascia
14 Median arcuate ligament
15 Oesophageal opening (hiatus)
16 Psoas major
17 Quadratus lumborum
18 Right crus
19 Spinal cord

Fibres of the right crus (A18) form the
right and left boundaries of the
oesophageal opening or hiatus (A15).

B Posterior abdominal wall
left side

The structures on the posterior abdominal wall are here
viewed from the front. The body of the pancreas (2) has
been turned upwards to expose the splenic vein (21). The
suprarenal gland (23) appears detached from the superior
pole of the kidney (compared with A13 and 10, page 256).

1 Aorta and aortic plexus
2 Body of pancreas
3 First lumbar spinal nerve
4 Greater omentum
5 Hypogastric plexus
6 Ilio-inguinal nerve
7 Iliohypogastric nerve
8 Inferior mesenteric vein
9 Inferior vena cava
10 Left colic vein
11 Liver
12 Lower pole of kidney
13 Lumbar part of
   thoracolumbar fascia
14 Ovarian vein
15 Para-aortic lymph node
16 Psoas major
17 Quadratus lumborum

18 Renal artery
19 Renal vein
20 Spleen
21 Splenic vein
22 Stomach
23 Suprarenal gland
24 Suprarenal vein
25 Transversus abdominis
26 Ureter

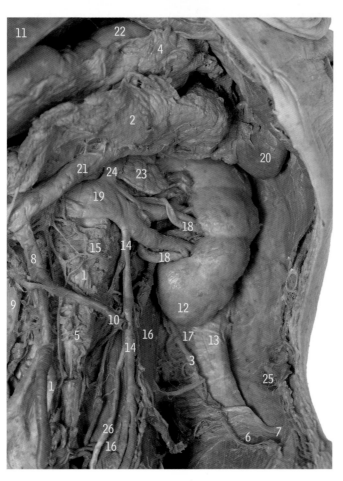

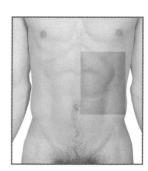

Nephrocalcinosis, retroperitoneal bleed, see pages 280–284.

Posterior abdominal and pelvic walls

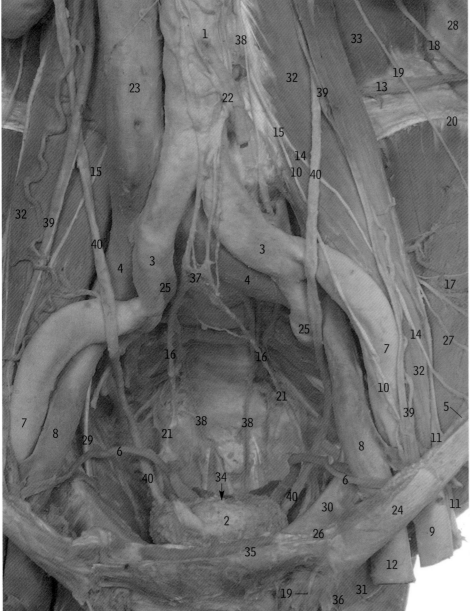

All peritoneum and viscera (except for the bladder, 2, ureter, 40, and ductus deferens or vas deferens, 6) have been removed, to display vessels and nerves.

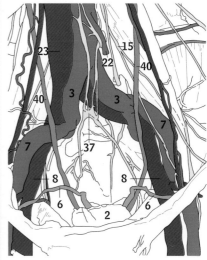

Pelvic arteriogram

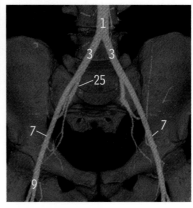

1 Aorta and aortic plexus	**16** Hypogastric nerve	**28** Lumbar part of thoracolumbar fascia
2 Bladder	**17** Iliacus and branches from femoral nerve and iliolumbar artery	**29** Obturator nerve and vessels
3 Common iliac artery	**18** Iliohypogastric nerve	**30** Pectineal ligament
4 Common iliac vein	**19** Ilio-inguinal nerve	**31** Position of femoral canal
5 Deep circumflex iliac artery	**20** Iliolumbar ligament	**32** Psoas major
6 Ductus deferens	**21** Inferior hypogastric (pelvic) plexus and pelvic splanchnic nerves	**33** Quadratus lumborum
7 External iliac artery	**22** Inferior mesenteric artery and plexus	**34** Rectum (cut edge)
8 External iliac vein	**23** Inferior vena cava	**35** Rectus abdominis
9 Femoral artery	**24** Inguinal ligament	**36** Spermatic cord
10 Femoral branch of genitofemoral nerve	**25** Internal iliac artery	**37** Superior hypogastric plexus
11 Femoral nerve	**26** Lacunar ligament	**38** Sympathetic trunk and ganglia
12 Femoral vein	**27** Lateral femoral cutaneous nerve arising from femoral nerve	**39** Testicular vessels
13 Fourth lumbar artery		**40** Ureter
14 Genital branch of genitofemoral nerve		
15 Genitofemoral nerve		

Psoas abscess, see pages 280–284.

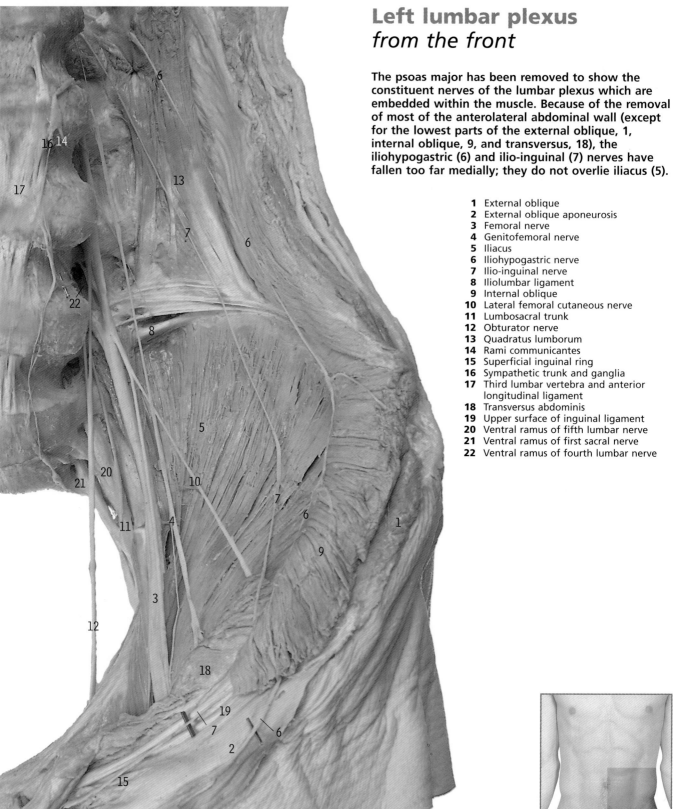

Left lumbar plexus
from the front

The psoas major has been removed to show the constituent nerves of the lumbar plexus which are embedded within the muscle. Because of the removal of most of the anterolateral abdominal wall (except for the lowest parts of the external oblique, 1, internal oblique, 9, and transversus, 18), the iliohypogastric (6) and ilio-inguinal (7) nerves have fallen too far medially; they do not overlie iliacus (5).

1 External oblique
2 External oblique aponeurosis
3 Femoral nerve
4 Genitofemoral nerve
5 Iliacus
6 Iliohypogastric nerve
7 Ilio-inguinal nerve
8 Iliolumbar ligament
9 Internal oblique
10 Lateral femoral cutaneous nerve
11 Lumbosacral trunk
12 Obturator nerve
13 Quadratus lumborum
14 Rami communicantes
15 Superficial inguinal ring
16 Sympathetic trunk and ganglia
17 Third lumbar vertebra and anterior longitudinal ligament
18 Transversus abdominis
19 Upper surface of inguinal ligament
20 Ventral ramus of fifth lumbar nerve
21 Ventral ramus of first sacral nerve
22 Ventral ramus of fourth lumbar nerve

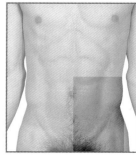

Lumbar sympathectomy, see pages 280–284.

Ⓐ Muscles of the left pelvis and proximal thigh
slightly oblique anterior view

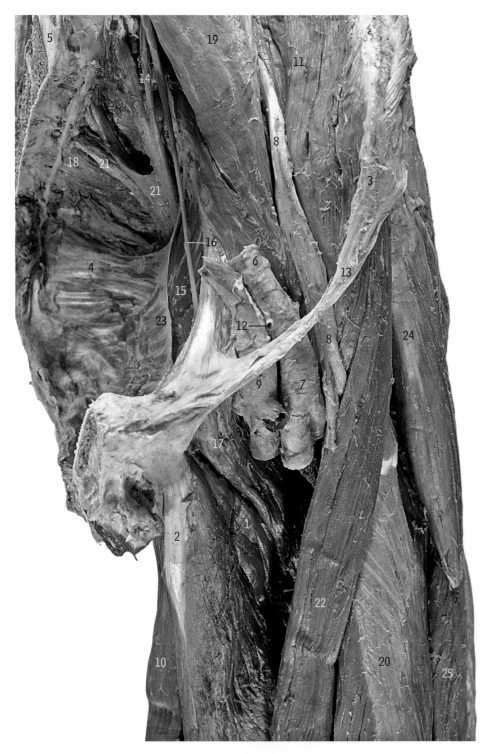

1	Adductor brevis
2	Adductor longus
3	Anterior superior iliac spine
4	Coccygeus
5	Disc, fifth lumbar
6	External iliac artery
7	Femoral artery
8	Femoral nerve
9	Femoral vein
10	Gracilis
11	Iliacus
12	Inferior epigastric artery, origin
13	Inguinal ligament
14	Lumbosacral trunk
15	Obturator internus
16	Obturator nerve
17	Pectineus
18	Piriformis
19	Psoas major
20	Rectus femoris
21	Sacral plexus
22	Sartorius
23	Tendinous arch of levator ani
24	Tensor fasciae latae
25	Vastus lateralis

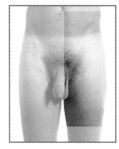

The anterior superior iliac spine (3) and the pubic tubercle, which give attachment to the ends of the inguinal ligament (13), are important palpable landmarks in the inguinal region (see page 224).

The part of obturator internus (15) *above* the attachment of levator ani is part of the lateral wall of the pelvic cavity, while the part *below* the attachment is in the perineum and forms part of the lateral wall of the ischio-anal (ischiorectal) fossa (pages 277 and 279).

Piriformis (18) passes out of the pelvis into the gluteal region through the *greater* sciatic foramen *above* the ischial spine, while obturator internus (15) passes out through the *lesser* sciatic foramen *below* the ischial spine.

The anterior abdominal wall, most viscera and fasciae have been removed. Segments of the external iliac/femoral vessels and the inferior margin of the external oblique aponeurosis (inguinal ligament) have been retained to assist orientation.

Muscles of the left half of the pelvis

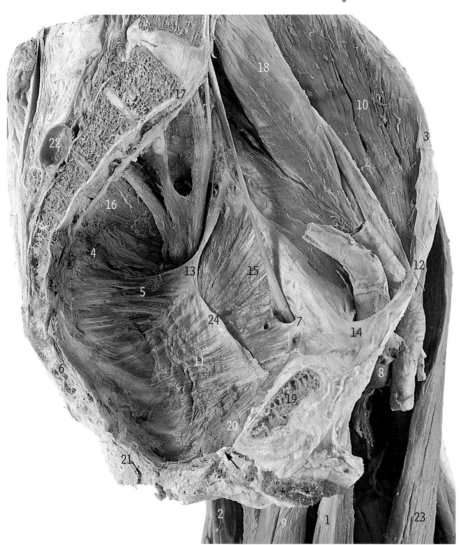

B *Male pelvis*

The fascia overlying the obturator internus (15) has been removed down to the tendinous origin of the levator ani (11 and 20), a urethral catheter (arrow) indicates the position of the sphincter urethrae, and the plane of section passes through the bulbocavernosus (asterisks).

1 Adductor longus
2 Adductor magnus
3 Anterior superior iliac spine
4 Branch of fourth sacral nerve
5 Coccygeus
6 Coccyx
7 Fascia over obturator internus
8 Femoral vein
9 Gracilis
10 Iliacus
11 Iliococcygeus part of levator ani
12 Inguinal ligament
13 Ischial spine
14 Lacunar ligament
15 Obturator internus, pierced by obturator nerve
16 Piriformis
17 Promontory of sacrum
18 Psoas major
19 Pubic symphysis
20 Pubococcygeus part of levator ani
21 Rectum
22 Sacral canal with cyst
23 Sartorius
24 Tendinous arch of levator ani

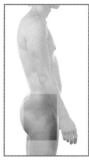

Left parasagittal CT of abdomen and pelvis

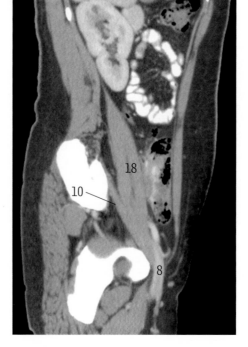

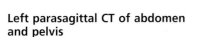

Inguinal lymphadenopathy, see pages 280–284.

Ⓐ Right spermatic cord and testis

Ⓑ Right testis, epididymis and penis *from the right*

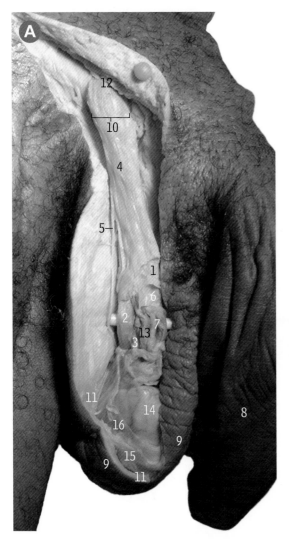

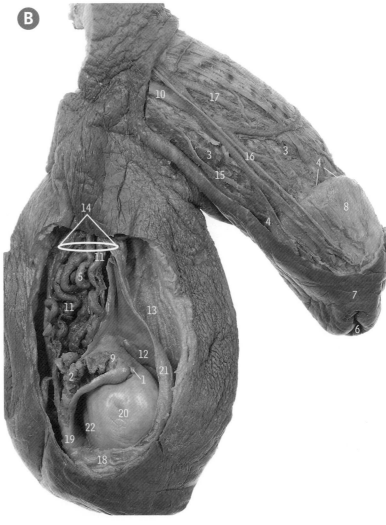

1 Cremasteric fascia	
2 Ductus deferens	
3 Ductus deferens, artery	
4 External spermatic fascia	
5 Ilio-inguinal nerve	
6 Internal spermatic fascia	
7 Pampiniform venous plexus	
8 Penis	
9 Scrotal sac	
10 Spermatic cord	
11 Superficial fascia with dartos muscle fibres	
12 Superficial inguinal ring	
13 Testicular artery	
14 Tunica albuginea	
15 Tunica vaginalis, parietal layer	
16 Tunica vaginalis, visceral layer	

1 Appendix epididymis	**13** Scrotal sac
2 Body of epididymis	**14** Spermatic cord
3 Body of penis	**15** Superficial dorsal artery
4 Corona of glans	**16** Superficial dorsal nerve
5 Ductus deferens	**17** Superficial dorsal vein
6 External urethral orifice	**18** Superficial scrotal (dartos) fascia
7 Foreskin	**19** Tail of epididymis
8 Glans penis	**20** Testis
9 Head of epididymis	**21** Tunica vaginalis, parietal
10 Lateral superficial vein	**22** Tunica vaginalis, visceral, overlying
11 Pampiniform venous plexus	tunica albuginea
12 Sac of tunica vaginalis	

Circumcision, Fournier's gangrene, hydrocele, phimosis and paraphimosis, scrotal swellings, varicoceles, vasectomy, see pages 280–284.

Male pelvis *left half of a midline sagittal section*

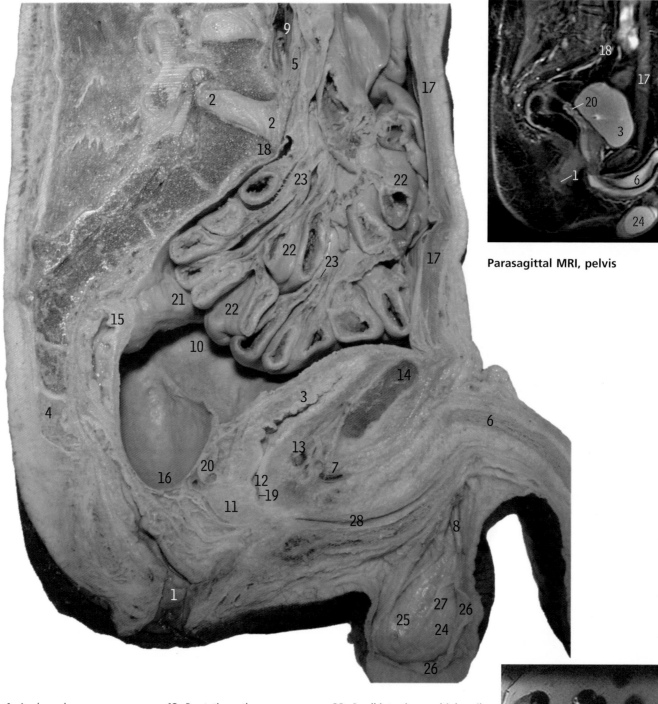

Parasagittal MRI, pelvis

Sagittal MR imaging, pelvis

1 Anal canal	**12** Prostatic urethra	**22** Small intestine, multiple coils
2 Annulus fibrosus	**13** Prostatic venous plexus	**23** Superior mesenteric vessels, jejunal and ileal branches
3 Bladder	**14** Pubic symphysis	**24** Testis
4 Coccyx	**15** Rectosigmoid junction	**25** Tunica albuginea
5 Common iliac artery	**16** Rectovesical pouch of pelvic peritoneum	**26** Tunica vaginalis, parietal layer
6 Corpus cavernosum	**17** Rectus abdominis	**27** Tunica vaginalis, visceral layer
7 Deep dorsal vein of penis	**18** Sacral promontory	**28** Urethra, bulbous
8 Ductus deferens	**19** Seminal colliculus	
9 Inferior vena cava	**20** Seminal vesicle	
10 Parietal peritoneum	**21** Sigmoid colon	
11 Prostate		

Extravasation of urine, proctoscopy and sigmoidoscopy, testicular torsion, see pages 280–284.

Pelvis, right inguinal region and penis *from above*

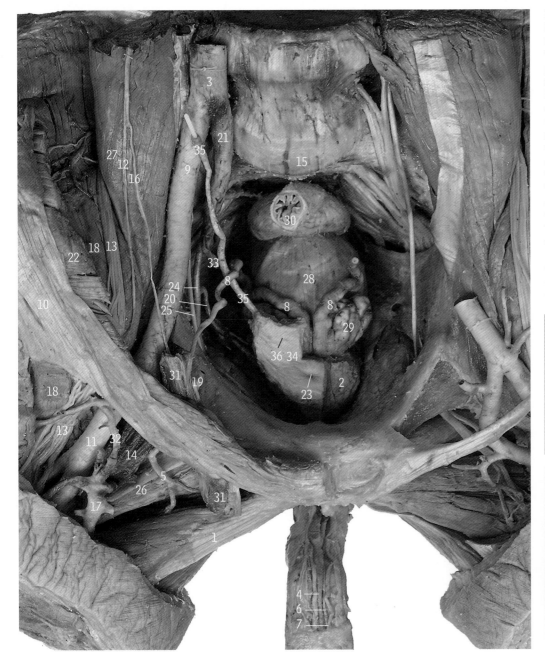

In the pelvis, most of the bladder (34) has been removed to show part of the basal surface of the prostate (2), and the left seminal vesicle (29) lying lateral to the ductus deferens (8). The ductus in the pelvis crosses superficial to the ureter (35). The external iliac artery (9) passes under the inguinal ligament (10) to become the femoral artery (11). On the dorsum of the penis, the fascia has been removed, showing the single midline deep dorsal vein (4) with a dorsal artery (6) and dorsal nerve (7) on each side.

The trigone of the bladder (34), at the lower part of the base or posterior surface, is the relatively fixed area with smooth mucous membrane between the internal urethral orifice (23) and the two ureteral openings (36 on the right side).

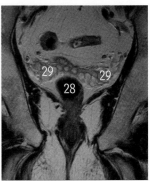

Coronal MR imaging, pelvis

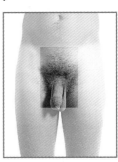

1 Adductor longus	**13** Femoral nerve	**25** Obturator nerve
2 Base of prostate	**14** Femoral vein	**26** Pectineus
3 Common iliac artery	**15** Fifth lumbar intervertebral	**27** Psoas major
4 Deep dorsal vein of penis	disc	**28** Rectum
5 Deep external pudendal artery	**16** Genital branch of	**29** Seminal vesicle
6 Dorsal artery of penis	genitofemoral nerve	**30** Sigmoid colon (cut lower end)
7 Dorsal nerve of penis	**17** Great saphenous vein	**31** Spermatic cord
8 Ductus deferens	**18** Iliacus	**32** Superficial circumflex iliac vein
9 External iliac artery	**19** Inferior epigastric artery	**33** Superior vesical artery
10 External oblique aponeurosis	**20** Inferior vesical artery	**34** Trigone of bladder
and inguinal ligament	**21** Internal iliac artery	**35** Ureter
11 Femoral artery	**22** Internal oblique	**36** Ureteral orifice
12 Femoral branch of	**23** Internal urethral orifice	
genitofemoral nerve	**24** Obturator artery	

Carcinoma of the large bowel, cystitis, cystoscopy, ureteric variants, see pages 280–284.

Ⓐ Bladder and prostate *from behind*

1 Base of bladder
2 Ductus deferens
3 Left ejaculatory duct
4 Posterior surface of prostate
5 Seminal vesicle
6 Ureter

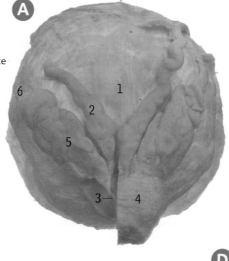

Ⓑ Left side of the male pelvis *from the right*

In this midline sagittal section, the prostate (24) is enlarged, lengthening the prostatic urethra (25) and accentuating the trabeculae of the bladder. The mucous membrane of the bladder (whose trigone is labelled at 36) has been removed to show muscular trabeculae in the wall. Variations in the branches of the internal iliac artery (14) are common, and here the obturator artery (22) gives origin to the superior vesical (34) and inferior vesical (13) as well as the middle rectal (20) arteries.

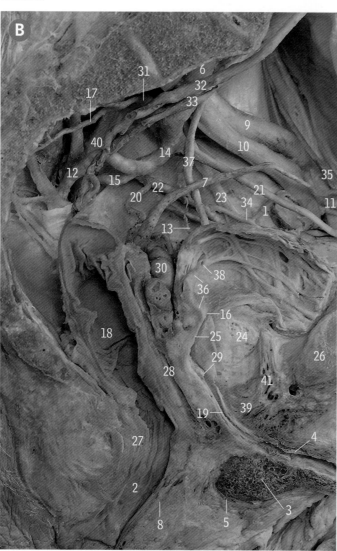

Ⓒ Cytoscopy of bladder

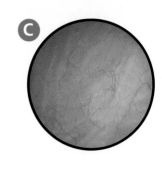

Ⓓ Cytoscopy of prostate (TURP)

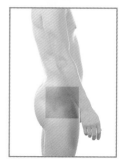

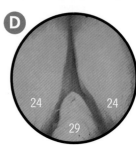

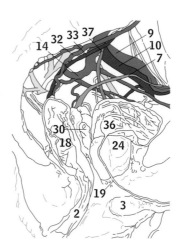

1 Accessory obturator vein
2 Anal canal
3 Bulb of penis
4 Bulbar part of spongy urethra
5 Bulbospongiosus
6 Common iliac artery
7 Ductus deferens
8 External anal sphincter
9 External iliac artery
10 External iliac vein
11 Inferior epigastric vessels
12 Inferior gluteal artery
13 Inferior vesical artery
14 Internal iliac artery
15 Internal pudendal artery
16 Internal urethral orifice
17 Lateral sacral artery
18 Lower end of rectum
19 Membranous part of urethra
20 Middle rectal artery
21 Obliterated umbilical artery
22 Obturator artery
23 Obturator nerve
24 Prostate (enlarged)
25 Prostatic part of urethra
26 Pubic symphysis
27 Puborectalis part of levator ani
28 Rectovesical fascia
29 Seminal colliculus
30 Seminal vesicle
31 Superior gluteal artery
32 Superior rectal artery
33 Superior rectal vein
34 Superior vesical artery
35 Testicular vessels and deep inguinal ring
36 Trigone of bladder
37 Ureter
38 Ureteral orifice
39 Urogenital diaphragm
40 Ventral ramus of first sacral nerve
41 Vesicoprostatic venous plexus

Benign prostatic hyperplasia, carcinoma of the prostate, transurethral resection of the prostate (TURP), urethral stricture, see pages 280–284.

A Arteries and nerves of the pelvis *from the right*

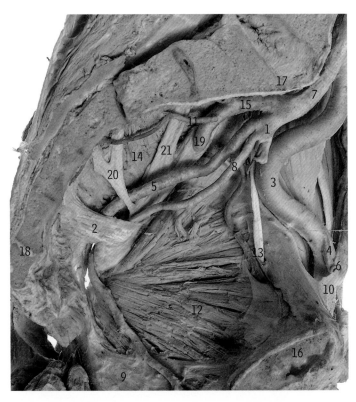
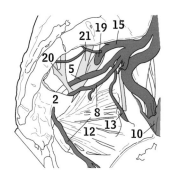
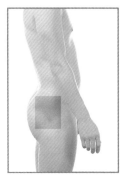

1 Anterior trunk of internal iliac artery
2 Coccygeus and sacrospinous ligament
3 External iliac artery
4 Inferior epigastric artery
5 Inferior gluteal artery
6 Inguinal ligament
7 Internal iliac artery
8 Internal pudendal artery
9 Ischial tuberosity
10 Lacunar ligament
11 Lateral sacral artery
12 Obturator internus
13 Obturator nerve and artery
14 Piriformis
15 Posterior trunk of internal iliac artery
16 Pubic symphysis
17 Sacral promontory
18 Sacrococcygeal joint
19 Superior gluteal artery piercing lumbosacral trunk
20 Union of ventral rami of second and third sacral nerves
21 Ventral ramus of first sacral nerve

In this left half section of the pelvis, all peritoneum, fascia, veins and visceral arteries have been removed together with the left levator ani, so displaying the whole of the internal surface of obturator internus (12). On the posterior pelvic wall, the vessels in general lie superficial to the nerves.

In this specimen, the external iliac artery (3) is unusually tortuous, and the anterior trunk of the internal iliac artery (1) has divided unusually high up into its terminal branches, the internal pudendal (8) and the inferior gluteal (5). The superior gluteal artery (19) has perforated the lumbosacral trunk.

B Left inferior hypogastric plexus *from the right*

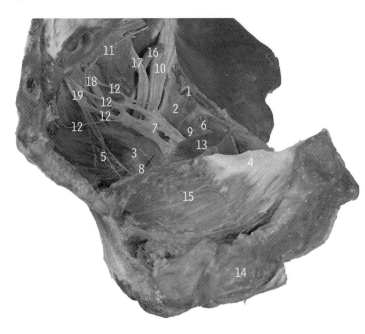
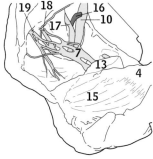

1 Arcuate line of ilium
2 Fascia overlying obturator internus
3 Ischial spine
4 Lateral surface of fascia overlying right obturator internus
5 Left coccygeus and nerves to levator ani
6 Left ductus deferens
7 Left inferior hypogastric plexus
8 Left levator ani
9 Left seminal vesicle
10 Lumbosacral trunk
11 Part of left sympathetic trunk
12 Pelvic splanchnic nerves (nervi erigentes)
13 Rectum
14 Right ischiopubic ramus
15 Right levator ani and ischio-anal (ischiorectal) fossa
16 Superior gluteal artery
17 Ventral ramus of first sacral nerve
18 Ventral ramus of second sacral nerve
19 Ventral ramus of third sacral nerve

In this view of the left side of the pelvis from the right, the right pelvic wall has been removed but the right levator ani (15) forming part of the pelvic floor (pelvic diaphragm) has been preserved and is seen from its right (perineal) side. Pelvic splanchnic nerves (12) arise from the ventral rami of the second and third sacral nerves (18 and 19) and contribute to the inferior hypogastric plexus (7).

Internal iliac artery *branches and relationships, left side female pelvis*

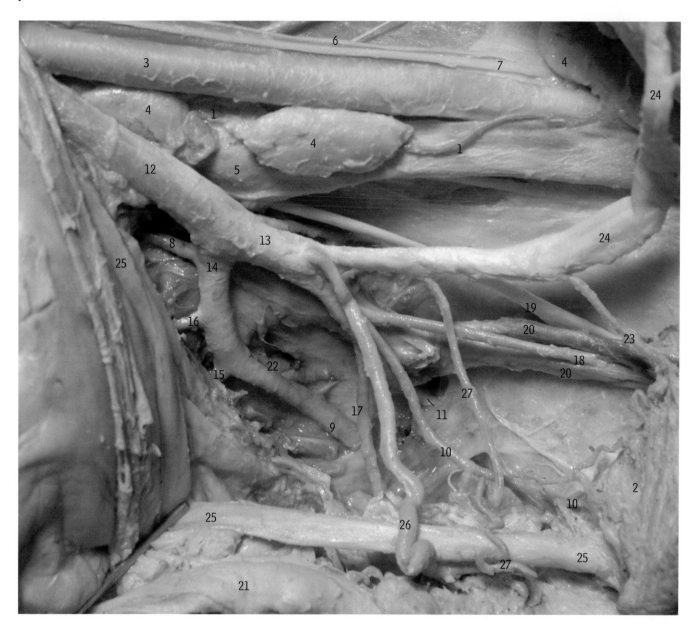

1 Artery to iliac nodes	**10** Inferior vesical artery	**19** Obturator nerve
2 Bladder	**11** Internal pudendal artery	**20** Obturator veins
3 External iliac artery	**12** Internal iliac artery	**21** Round ligament of the uterus (reflected)
4 External iliac lymph nodes (enlarged)	**13** Internal iliac artery, anterior division	**22** Superior gluteal artery
5 External iliac vein	**14** Internal iliac artery, posterior division	**23** Superior vesical artery
6 Genitofemoral nerve, femoral branch	**15** Lateral sacral artery, inferior	**24** Umbilical artery remnant
7 Genitofemoral nerve, genital branch	**16** Lateral sacral artery, superior	**25** Ureter (retracted)
8 Iliolumbar artery	**17** Middle rectal artery	**26** Uterine artery
9 Inferior gluteal artery	**18** Obturator artery	**27** Vaginal artery

Internal iliac embolisation, see pages 280–284.

A Pelvic skeleton and ligaments *left side*

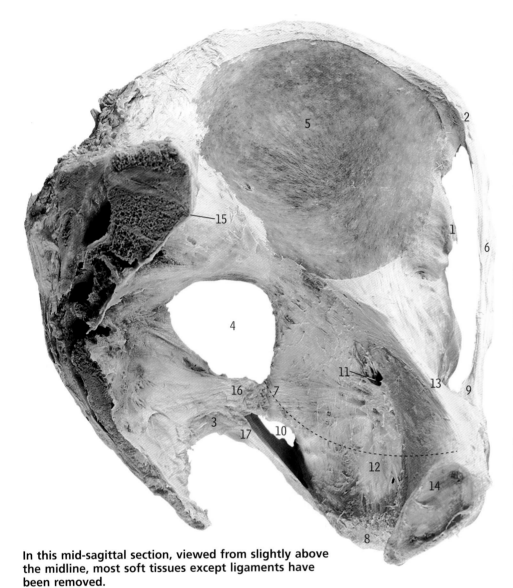

In this mid-sagittal section, viewed from slightly above the midline, most soft tissues except ligaments have been removed.

1 Anterior inferior iliac spine and origin of straight head of rectus femoris
2 Anterior superior iliac spine
3 Falciform process of sacrotuberous ligament
4 Greater sciatic foramen
5 Iliac fossa
6 Inguinal ligament
7 Ischial spine
8 Ischial tuberosity
9 Lacunar ligament
10 Lesser sciatic foramen
11 Obturator foramen with obturator nerve and vessels
12 Obturator membrane
13 Pectineal ligament
14 Pubic symphysis
15 Sacral promontory
16 Sacrospinous ligament
17 Sacrotuberous ligament

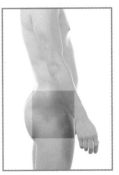

The ligaments classified as 'the ligaments of the pelvis' (vertebropelvic ligaments) are the sacrotuberous (17), sacrospinous (16) and iliolumbar (seen in the posterior view on page 325, C7).

The lacunar ligament (9) passes backwards from the medial end of the inguinal ligament (6) to the medial end of the pectineal line of the pubis, to which the pectineal ligament (13) is attached.

B Greater sciatic foramen, sacral plexus and levator ani *left side*

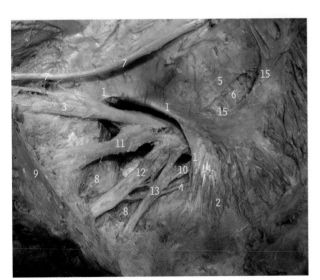

1 Greater sciatic foramen
2 Levator ani
3 Lumbosacral trunk (with S1)
4 Nerve to levator ani
5 Obturator internus fascia
6 Obturator internus muscle
7 Obturator nerve
8 Piriformis muscle fibres (muscle bulk removed)
9 Posterior longitudinal ligament, overlying sacrum
10 Pudendal nerve
11 Sacral nerve, S2
12 Sacral nerve, S3 and S4
13 Sacral nerve, S5
14 Sacrospinous ligament
15 Tendinous arch of levator ani, an origin of levator

Bone marrow aspiration, obturator hernia, sacral nerve stimulation, see pages 280–284.

Female pelvis *left half with arterial injection, viewed from right*

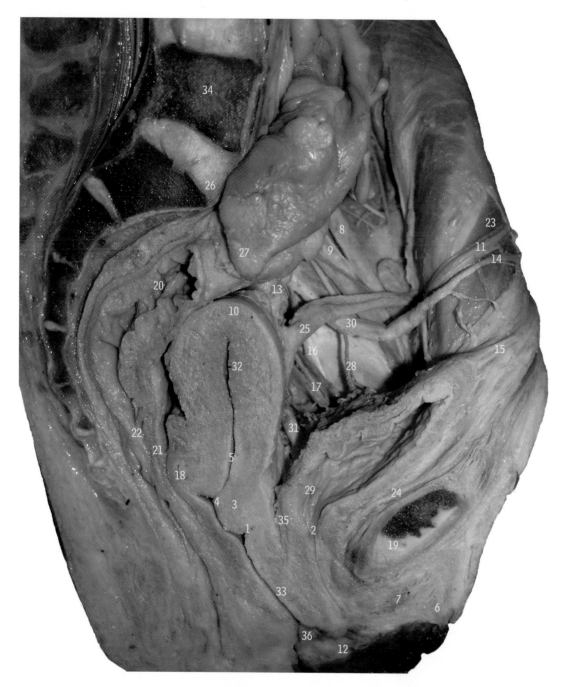

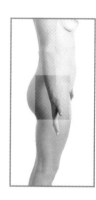

1 Anterior vaginal fornix	**15** Median umbilical ligament (urachus)	**28** Superior vesical artery
2 Bladder neck	**16** Obturator nerve	**29** Trigone of bladder
3 Cervix	**17** Obturator vessels	**30** Umbilical artery (remnant)
4 Cervix, external os	**18** Posterior vaginal fornix	**31** Ureter
5 Cervix, internal os	**19** Pubic symphysis	**32** Uterine cavity
6 Clitoris	**20** Rectosigmoid junction	**33** Vagina
7 Crus of clitoris	**21** Rectouterine peritoneal space	**34** Vertebral body, L5
8 External iliac artery	**22** Rectum	**35** Vesicouterine peritoneal pouch
9 External iliac vein	**23** Rectus abdominis	**36** Vestibule of vagina
10 Fundus of uterus	**24** Retropubic space	
11 Inferior epigastric vessels	**25** Round ligament of uterus	**NB: retroverted uterus – a**
12 Labium minus	**26** Sacral promontory	**common normal variant.**
13 Ligament of ovary	**27** Sigmoid colon	
14 Medial umbilical ligament		

Faecal continence, haemorrhoids, ligation–uterine tubes, rectal (PR) examination, rectal prolapse, uterine fibroids, uterine variants, see pages 280–284.

Female pelvis

A *sagittal MR image during menstruation*   B *coronal MR image*

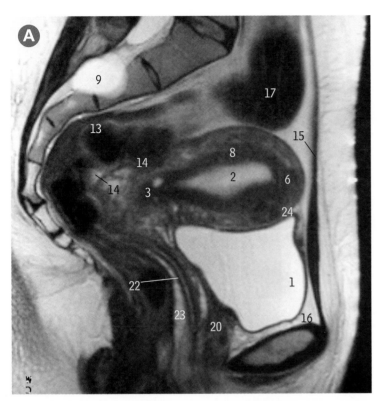

1 Bladder
2 Blood clot in endometrial cavity
3 Cervix of uterus
4 Corpus luteum
5 Endometrial cavity
6 Fundus of uterus
7 Levator ani
8 Myometrium
9 Nerve root cyst (Tarlov)
10 Ovary
11 Perineal muscles
12 Posterior fornix of vagina
13 Rectosigmoid junction
14 Recto-uterine pouch (Douglas)
15 Rectus abdominis muscle
16 Retropubic space (Retzius)
17 Sigmoid colon
18 Small intestine
19 Trigone
20 Urethra
21 Uterine (Fallopian) tube
22 Vaginal cavity
23 Vaginal wall
24 Vesico-uterine pouch

Looking down into the pelvis from the front, the fundus of the uterus (6) overlies the bladder (1) with the peritoneum of the vesico-uterine pouch (24) intervening. These relationships are seen in this MR image B.

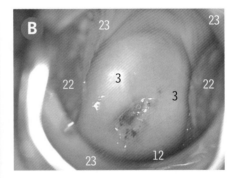

Speculum examination of cervix

Cervical smear, cystitis, ovarian dermoid, vaginal examination, see pages 280–284.

Female pelvis

Ⓐ uterus and ovaries, from above and in front   Ⓑ hysterosalpingogram (HSG)

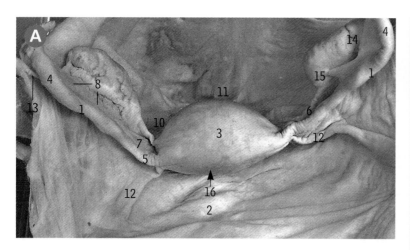

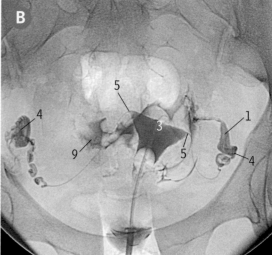

1 Ampulla of uterine tube	**10** Posterior surface of broad
2 Bladder	ligament
3 Fundus of uterus	**11** Recto-uterine space
4 Infundibulum of uterine tube	**12** Round ligament of uterus
5 Isthmus of uterine tube	**13** Suspensory ligament of ovary
6 Ligament of ovary	with ovarian vessels
7 Mesosalpinx	**14** Tubal extremity of ovary
8 Mesovarium	**15** Uterine extremity of ovary
9 Overspill of contrast into the	**16** Vesico-uterine pouch
peritoneal cavity	

Looking down into the pelvis from the front in A, the fundus of the uterus (3) overlies the bladder (2) with the peritoneum of the vesico-uterine pouch (16) intervening. In B, contrast medium has filled the uterus and tubes (3, 5, 1 and 4) and spilled out into the peritoneal cavity (9).

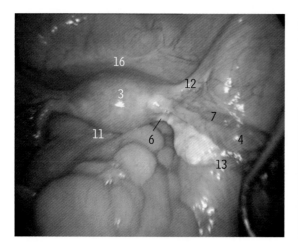

Laparoscopic view of female pelvis

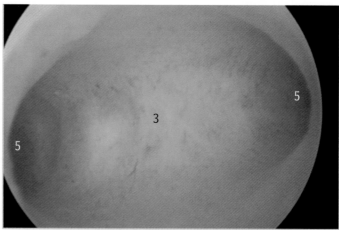

Hysteroscopic view of uterine cavity and uterine tubes

Acute salpingitis, carcinoma of the ovary, ectopic pregnancy rupture, intrauterine contraceptive devices (IUCDs), ligation–uterine tubes, see pages 280–284.

Female pelvis *left half, obliquely from the front*

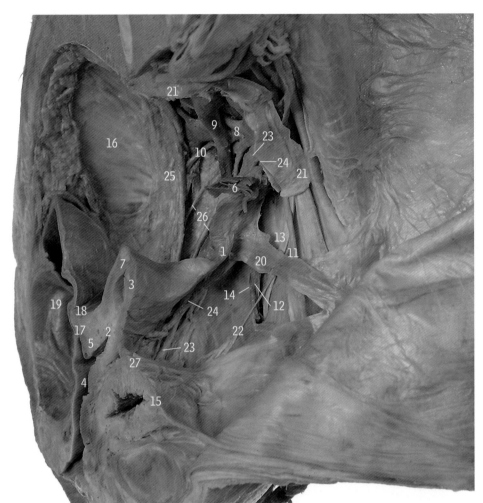

1 Ampulla of uterine tube
2 Anterior fornix of vagina
3 Body of uterus
4 Cavity of vagina
5 Cervix of uterus
6 Fimbriated end of uterine tube
7 Fundus of uterus
8 Internal iliac artery
9 Internal iliac vein
10 Middle rectal artery
11 Obliterated umbilical artery
12 Obturator artery
13 Obturator nerve
14 Obturator vein
15 Peritoneum overlying bladder
16 Peritoneum overlying piriformis
17 Posterior fornix of vagina
18 Recto-vaginal pouch
19 Rectum
20 Round ligament of uterus
21 Sigmoid mesocolon
22 Superior vesical artery
23 Ureter
24 Uterine artery
25 Uterosacral ligament
26 Vaginal artery (double)
27 Vesico-uterine pouch

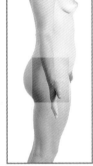

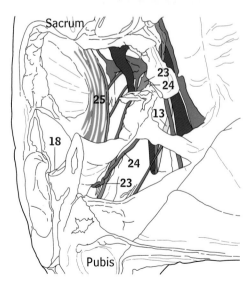

Looking obliquely into the left half of the pelvis from the front, with the anterior abdominal wall turned forwards, the peritoneum of the vesico-uterine pouch (27) has been incised and the uterus (3) displaced backwards. This shows the ureter (23) running towards the bladder and being crossed by the uterine artery (24). The uterosacral ligament (25) passes backwards at the side of the rectum (19) towards the pelvic surface of the sacrum. The root of the sigmoid mesocolon (21) has been left in place to emphasise that the left ureter (23) passes from the abdomen into the pelvis beneath it.

Anorectal abscesses, carcinoma of the uterus, hysterectomy, support of the pelvic viscera, unsafe abortion, see pages 280–284.

Female perineum   Ⓐ *Surface features*

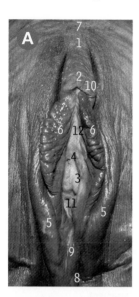

1 Anterior commissure of labia majora	**7** Mons pubis
2 Clitoris	**8** Perineal body
3 Cystocele (prolapse of bladder)	**9** Posterior commissure of labia majora
4 External urethral orifice (urinary meatus)	**10** Prepuce of clitoris
5 Labium majus	**11** Vaginal orifice (introitus)
6 Labium minus	**12** Vestibule

Ⓑ *Ischio-anal fossae from behind*

1 Anal margin	**12** Ischial tuberosity	**22** Quadratus femoris
2 Anococcygeal body	**13** Ischio-anal fossa, fat removed	**23** Sacrotuberous ligament
3 Biceps femoris, long head	**14** Levator ani	**24** Sacrum
4 Coccyx	**15** Obturator internus and fascia	**25** Sciatic nerve
5 External anal sphincter	**16** Obturator internus tendon	**26** Semimembranosus and semitendinosus
6 Gluteal maximus	**17** Piriformis	**27** Superficial transverse perineal muscle
7 Gluteus medius	**18** Posterior femoral cutaneous nerve, perineal branch	**28** Superior gluteal artery
8 Gracilis	**19** Posterior labial nerve	
9 Inferior gemellus	**20** Pudendal artery	
10 Inferior gluteal artery	**21** Pudendal nerve	
11 Inferior rectal nerve		

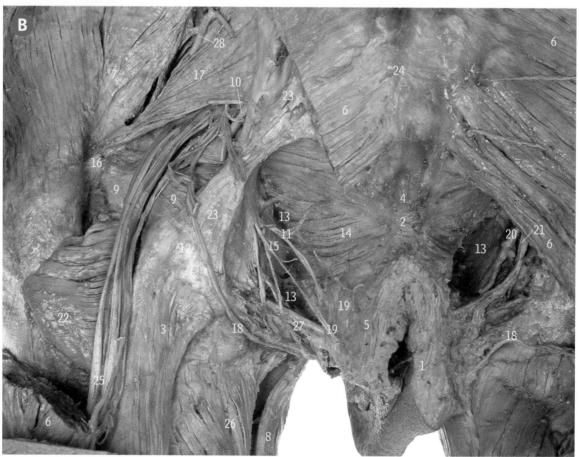

The ischiorectal fossa is now properly and more correctly called the ischio-anal fossa; the anal canal, not the rectum, is its lower medial boundary. The walls and contents are similar in both sexes.

Bartholin's abscess, episiotomy, female genital circumcision, pudendal block, see pages 280–284.

Female perineum and ischio-anal fossae *from below (lithotomy position)*

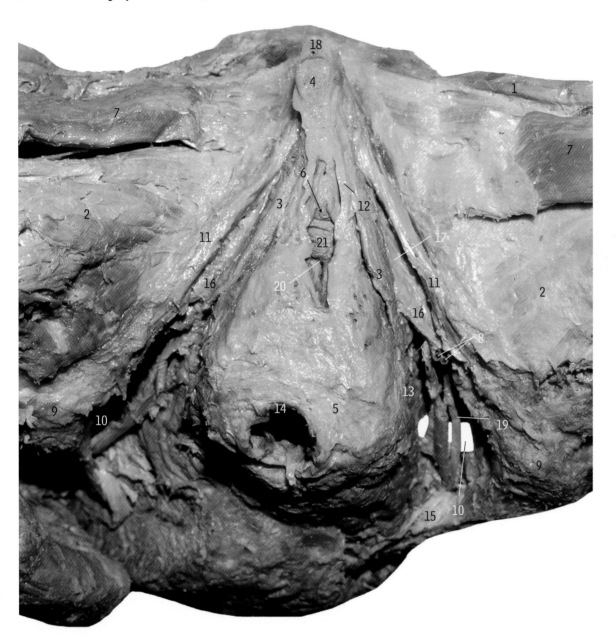

1 Adductor longus muscle
2 Adductor magnus muscle
3 Bulbspongiosus muscle
4 Clitoris (transected)
5 External anal sphincter
6 External urethral orifice (urinary meatus)
7 Gracilis
8 Internal pudendal artery passing superior to perineal membrane
9 Ischial tuberosity
10 Ischio-anal fossa
11 Ischiocavernosus muscle
12 Labium minus
13 Levator ani muscle
14 Margin of anus
15 Sacrotuberous ligament
16 Superficial transverse perineal muscle overlying posterior border of perineal membrane
17 Perineal membrane
18 Pubic symphysis
19 Pudendal nerve
20 Vaginal opening (introitus)
21 Vestibule of vagina (space between labium minus)

Gartner duct cyst in vaginal wall, genital ambiguous development, see pages 280–284.

Ⓐ Male perineum

The central area is shown, with the scrotum (5) pulled upwards and forwards.

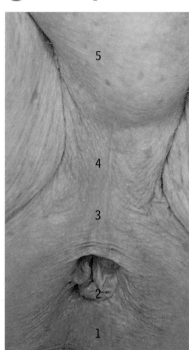

1 Anococcygeal body
2 Margin of anus, with skin tags
3 Perineal body
4 Raphe overlying bulb of penis
5 Scrotum overlying right testis

Skin tags are often the remnants of previous haemorrhoids.

Ⓑ Root of the penis *from below and in front*

The front part of the penis has been removed to show the root, formed by the two corpora cavernosa dorsally (2) and the single corpus spongiosum ventrally (3) containing the urethra (14).

1 Bulbospongiosus
2 Corpus cavernosum
3 Corpus spongiosum
4 Deep dorsal vein of penis
5 Dorsal artery of penis
6 Dorsal nerve of penis
7 External anal sphincter
8 Inferior rectal vessels and nerve crossing ischio-anal fossa
9 Ischiocavernosus
10 Ischiopubic ramus
11 Perineal body
12 Pubic symphysis
13 Superficial transverse perineal muscle overlying perineal membrane
14 Urethra

Cytoscopic view of urethra

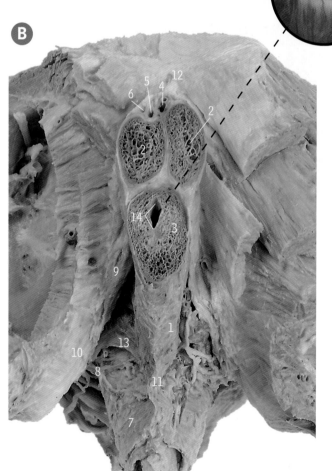

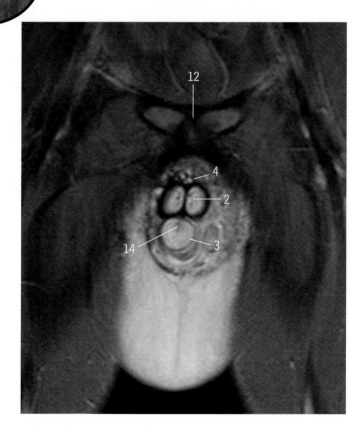

MR, penis

Bulbourethral glands, carcinoma of the anus, hydrocoele, hypospadias, imperforate anus, see pages 280–284.

Male perineum and ischio-anal (ischiorectal) fossae from below

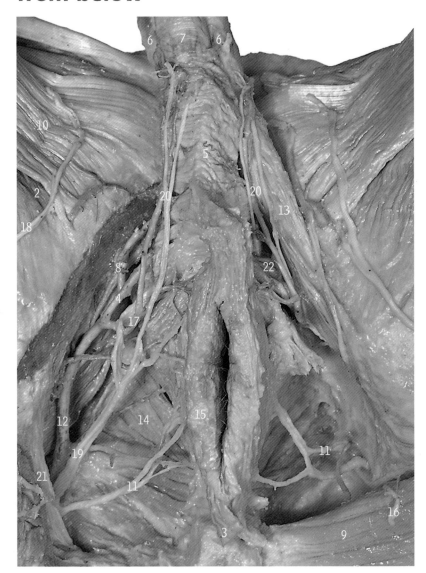

All the fat has been removed from the ischio-anal fossae so that a clear view is obtained of the perineal surface of levator ani (14) and of the vessels and nerves within the fossae. On the left side (right of the picture) the perineal membrane (22) is intact but on the right side it, and the underlying muscle (urogenital diaphragm), have been removed.

1 Adductor longus
2 Adductor magnus
3 Anococcygeal body
4 Artery to bulb
5 Bulbospongiosus overlying bulb of penis
6 Corpus cavernosum of penis
7 Corpus spongiosum of penis
8 Dorsal nerve and artery of penis
9 Gluteus maximus
10 Gracilis
11 Inferior rectal vessels and nerve in ischio-anal fossa
12 Internal pudendal artery
13 Ischiocavernosus overlying crus of penis
14 Levator ani
15 Margin of anus
16 Perforating cutaneous nerve
17 Perineal artery
18 Perineal branch of posterior femoral cutaneous nerve
19 Perineal nerve
20 Posterior scrotal vessels and nerves
21 Sacrotuberous ligament
22 Superficial transverse perineal muscle overlying posterior border of perineal membrane

In both sexes, the ischio-anal (ischiorectal) fossa has the pudendal canal in its lateral wall. The canal has been opened up to display its contents: the internal pudendal artery (12) and the terminal branches of the pudendal nerve – the perineal nerve (19) and the dorsal nerve of the penis (8) or clitoris.

Lithotomy position

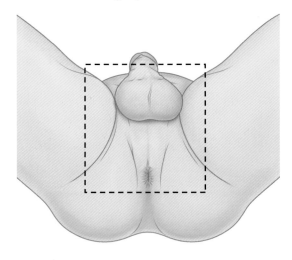

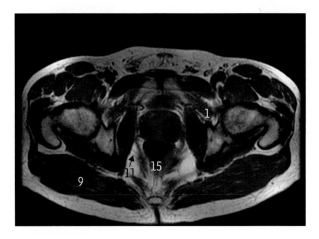

Axial MR, pelvis

Priapism, see pages 280–284.

Abdomen and pelvis

Clinical thumbnails, see website for details and further clinical images to download into your own notes.

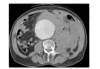
Abdominal aortic aneurysm

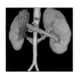
Abdominal vasculature variations

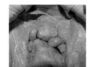
Acute salpingitis

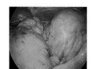
Adrenal gland pathology

Anorectal abscesses

Aortic bruits

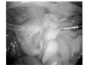
Appendicitis

Ascites

Bartholin's abscess

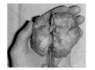
Benign prostatic hyperplasia

Bone marrow aspiration

Bowel ischaemia

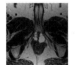
Bulbourethral glands

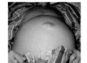
Caput medusae

Carcinoma of the anus

Carcinoma of the bladder

Carcinoma of the large bowel

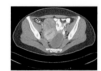
Carcinoma of the ovary

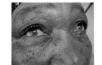
Carcinoma of the pancreas

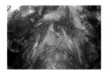
Carcinoma of the prostate

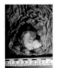
Carcinoma of the stomach

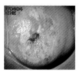
Carcinoma of the uterus

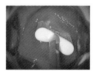
Cervical smear

Cholecystectomy

Circumcision

Cirrhosis of liver

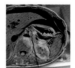
Coeliac plexus block

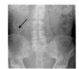
Colonic stents

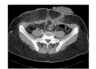
Colostomy

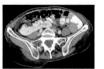
Congenital kidney variants

Cushing striations

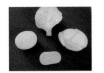
Cystitis

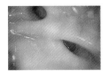
Cystoscopy

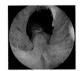
Diverticular disease

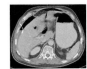
Drainage of subphrenic abscesses

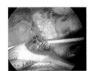
Ectopic pregnancy rupture

Episiotomy

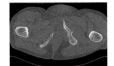
Extravasation of urine

Faecal continence

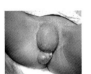
Female genital circumcision

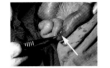
Femoral hernia

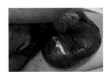
Fournier's gangrene

Gallstones

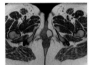
Gartner's duct cyst in vaginal wall

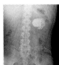
Gastric pacemaker

Genital ambiguous development

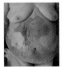
Haematoma of the rectus sheath

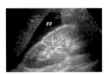
Haemoperitoneum

Haemorrhoids

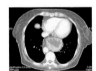
Hiatus hernia

Hydrocele

Hypospadias

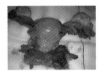
Hysterectomy

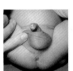
Imperforate anus

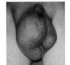
Indirect inguinal hernia

Inferior vena cava (IVC) obstruction

Inguinal hernia

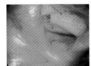
Inguinal hernia repair

Inguinal lymphadenopathy

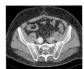
Internal Iliac embolisation

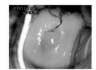

Intrauterine contraceptive devices (IUCDs)

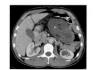

Intussusception

IVC duplication

Laparoscopy

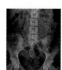

Ligation–uterine tubes

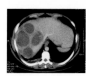

Liver abscess

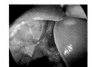

Liver biopsy

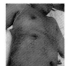

Liver trauma

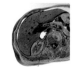

Lumbar hernia

Lumbar sympathectomy

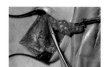

McBurney's point

Meckel's diverticulum

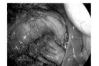

Nephrectomy

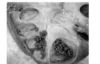

Nephrocalcinosis

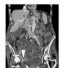

Obturator hernia

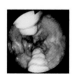

Oesophageal varices

Omental cake

Omphalocele

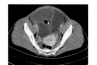

Ovarian dermoid

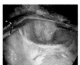

Pancreatic pathology

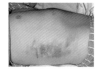

Pancreatitis

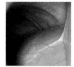

Peritoneal lavage

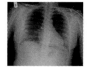

Peritonitis

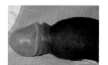

Phimosis and paraphimosis

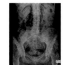

Pneumoretroperitoneum

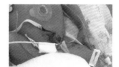

Postnatal umbilical vein catheter

Priapism

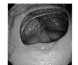

Proctoscopy and sigmoidoscopy

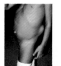

Psoas abscess

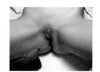

Pudendal block

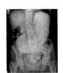 Pyloric stenosis (adult)

 Rectal (PR) examination

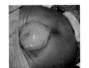 Rectal prolapse

 Rectosigmoid foreign bodies

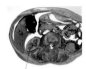 Renal biopsy

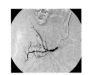 Renal carcinoma

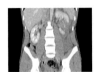 Renal trauma

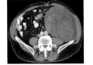 Retroperitoneal bleed

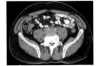 Retroperitoneal fibrosis

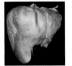 Riedel's lobe

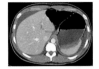 Ruptured spleen

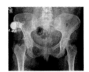 Sacral nerve stimulation

 Scrotal swellings

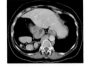 Situs inversus totalis

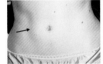 Spigelian hernia

 Splenectomy

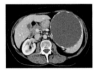 Splenic cysts

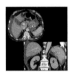 Splenic infarct

 Splenomegaly

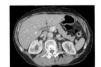 Splenunculi

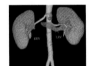 Superior mesenteric artery syndrome

 Support of the pelvic viscera

 Testicular torsion

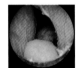 Transurethral resection of the prostate (TURP)

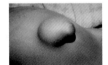 Umbilical and paraumbilical hernia

 Unsafe abortion

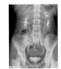 Ureteric variants

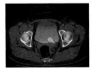 Ureterocele

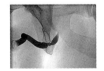 Urethral stricture

 Urinary tract calculi

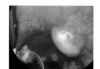

Uterine fibroids

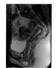

Uterine variants

Vaginal examination

Vagotomy

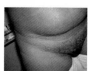

Varicella-zoster virus infection – abdominal wall

Varicocele

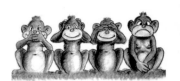

Vasectomy

Volvulus

Lower limb

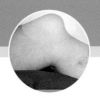

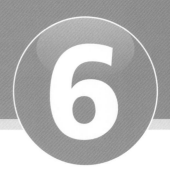

Lower limb (A) *surface anatomy, from the front*
(B) *dissection, from the front* (C) *dissection, from behind*
(D) *dissection, from the lateral side* (E) *skeleton, from the lateral side*

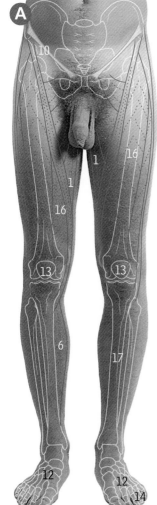
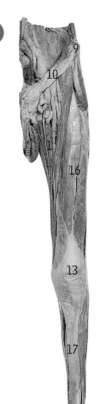

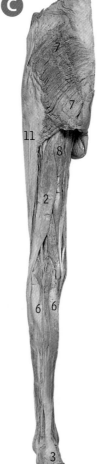
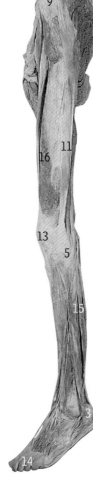
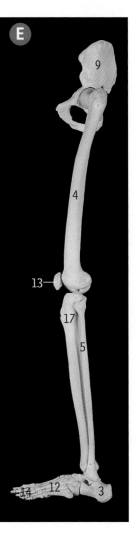

1 Adductors	**5** Fibula	**9** Hip bone	**12** Metatarsal bones	**15** Peroneus (fibularis)
2 Biceps femoris	**6** Gastrocnemius	**10** Inguinal ligament	**13** Patella	**16** Quadriceps
3 Calcaneus	**7** Gluteus maximus	**11** Iliotibial tract	**14** Phalanges of toes	**17** Tibia
4 Femur	**8** Hamstrings			

Left hip bone *lateral surface*

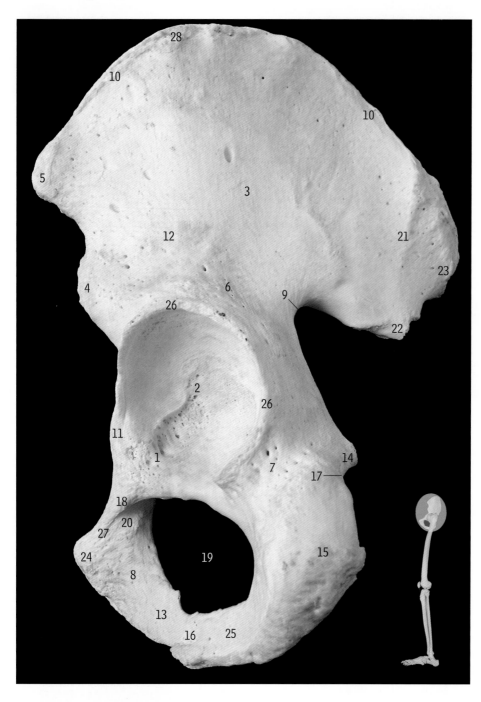

1 Acetabular notch
2 Acetabulum
3 Anterior gluteal line
4 Anterior inferior iliac spine
5 Anterior superior iliac spine
6 Body of ilium
7 Body of ischium
8 Body of pubis
9 Greater sciatic notch
10 Iliac crest
11 Iliopubic eminence
12 Inferior gluteal line
13 Inferior ramus of pubis
14 Ischial spine
15 Ischial tuberosity
16 Joint between 25 and 13
17 Lesser sciatic notch
18 Obturator crest
19 Obturator foramen
20 Obturator groove
21 Posterior gluteal line
22 Posterior inferior iliac spine
23 Posterior superior iliac spine
24 Pubic tubercle
25 Ramus of ischium
26 Rim of acetabulum
27 Superior ramus of pubis
28 Tubercle of iliac crest

The hip (innominate) bone is formed by the union of the ilium (6), ischium (7) and pubis (8).

The two hip bones articulate in the midline anteriorly at the pubic symphysis; posteriorly they are separated by the sacrum, forming the sacro-iliac joints. The two hip bones with the sacrum and coccyx constitute the pelvis (see page 92).

Left hip bone *attachments, lateral surface*

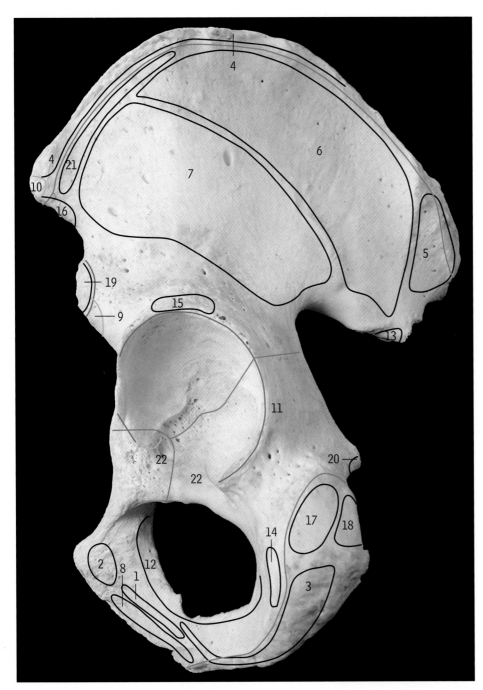

Blue lines, epiphysial lines
Green lines, capsular attachment
of hip joint
Pale green lines, ligament
attachments

1 Adductor brevis
2 Adductor longus
3 Adductor magnus
4 External oblique
5 Gluteus maximus
6 Gluteus medius
7 Gluteus minimus
8 Gracilis
9 Iliofemoral ligament
10 Inguinal ligament
11 Ischiofemoral ligament
12 Obturator externus
13 Piriformis
14 Quadratus femoris
15 Reflected head of rectus femoris
16 Sartorius
17 Semimembranosus
18 Semitendinosus and long head of
biceps femoris
19 Straight head of rectus femoris
20 Superior gemellus
21 Tensor fasciae latae
22 Transverse ligament

Left hip bone *medial surface*

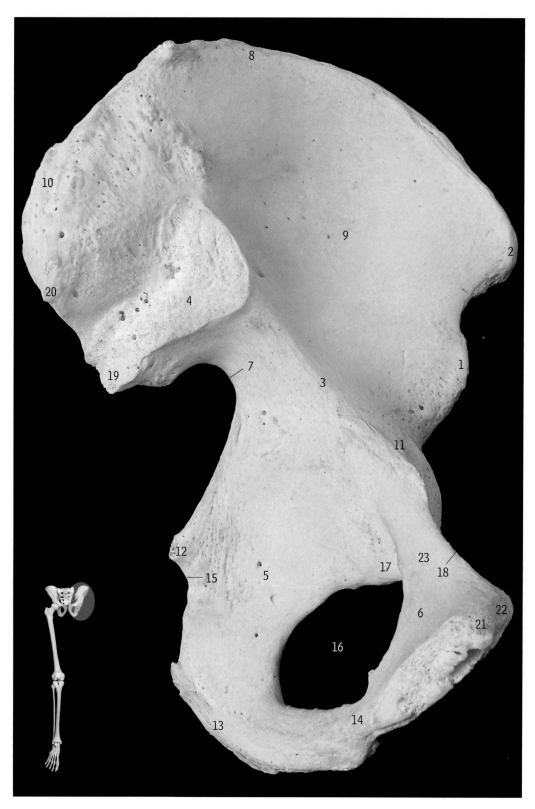

1 Anterior inferior iliac spine
2 Anterior superior iliac spine
3 Arcuate line
4 Auricular surface
5 Body of ischium
6 Body of pubis
7 Greater sciatic notch
8 Iliac crest
9 Iliac fossa
10 Iliac tuberosity
11 Iliopubic eminence
12 Ischial spine
13 Ischial tuberosity
14 Ischiopubic ramus
15 Lesser sciatic notch
16 Obturator foramen
17 Obturator groove
18 Pecten of pubis (pectineal line)
19 Posterior inferior iliac spine
20 Posterior superior iliac spine
21 Pubic crest
22 Pubic tubercle
23 Superior ramus of pubis

The auricular surface of the ilium (4) is the articular surface for the sacro-iliac joint.

The greater sciatic notch (7) is more hooked (J-shaped) in the male, whereas the female notch is more right-angled (L-shaped).

Left hip bone *attachments, medial surface*

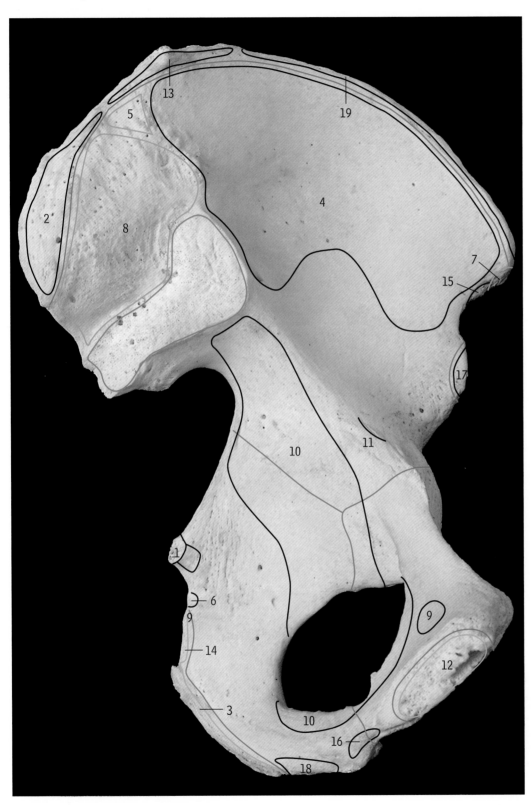

Blue lines, epiphysial lines
Green line, capsular attachment of sacro-iliac joint
Pale green lines, ligament attachments

1 Coccygeus and sacrospinous ligament
2 Erector spinae
3 Falciform process of sacrotuberous ligament
4 Iliacus
5 Iliolumbar ligament
6 Inferior gemellus
7 Inguinal ligament
8 Interosseous sacro-iliac ligament
9 Levator ani
10 Obturator internus
11 Psoas minor
12 Pubic symphysis
13 Quadratus lumborum
14 Sacrotuberous ligament
15 Sartorius
16 Sphincter urethrae
17 Straight head of rectus femoris
18 Superficial transverse perineal and ischiocavernosus
19 Transversus abdominis

Left hip bone *from above*

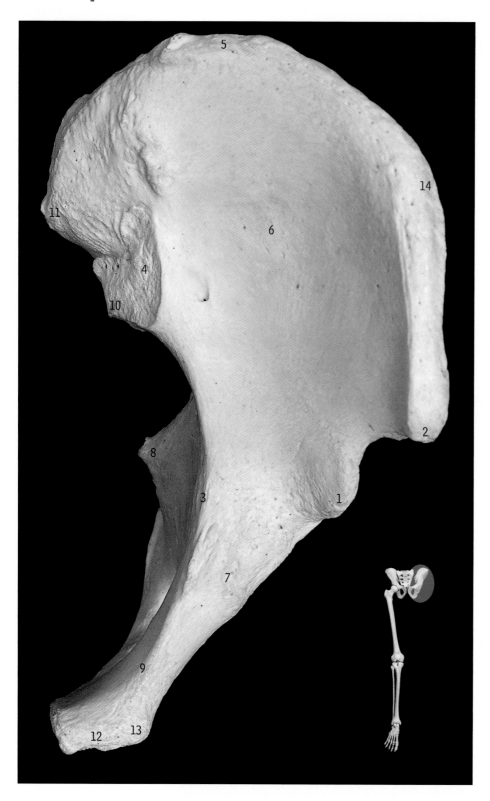

1 Anterior inferior iliac spine
2 Anterior superior iliac spine
3 Arcuate line
4 Auricular surface
5 Iliac crest
6 Iliac fossa
7 Iliopubic eminence
8 Ischial spine
9 Pecten of pubis (pectineal line)
10 Posterior inferior iliac spine
11 Posterior superior iliac spine
12 Pubic crest
13 Pubic tubercle
14 Tubercle of iliac crest

The arcuate line on the ilium (3) and the pecten and crest of the pubis (9 and 12) form part of the brim of the pelvis (the rest of the brim being formed by the promontory and upper surface of the lateral part of the sacrum – see pages 90 and 92).

The pecten of the pubis (9) is more commonly called the pectineal line.

Left hip bone *attachments, from above*

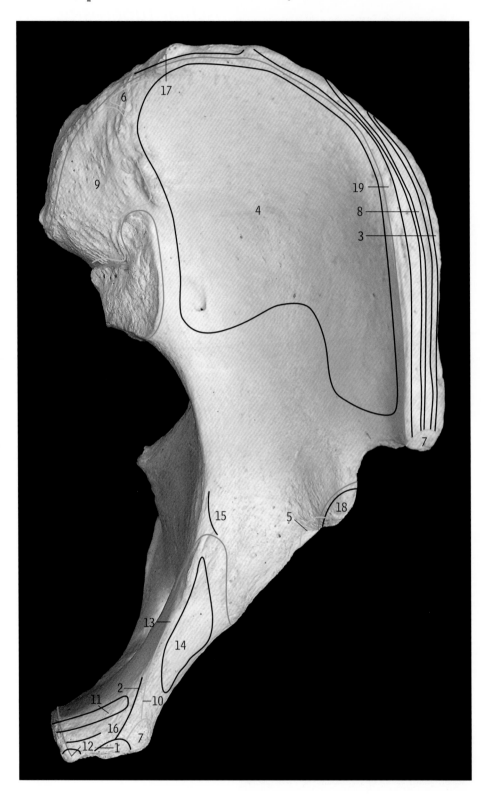

Blue lines, epiphysial lines
Green line, capsular attachment of sacro-iliac joint
Pale green lines, ligament attachments

1 Anterior wall of rectus sheath
2 Conjoint tendon
3 External oblique
4 Iliacus
5 Iliofemoral ligament
6 Iliolumbar ligament
7 Inguinal ligament
8 Internal oblique
9 Interosseous sacro-iliac ligament
10 Lacunar ligament
11 Lateral head of rectus abdominis
12 Medial head of rectus abdominis
13 Pectineal ligament
14 Pectineus
15 Psoas minor
16 Pyramidalis
17 Quadratus lumborum
18 Straight head of rectus femoris
19 Transversus abdominis

The inguinal ligament (7) is formed by the lower border of the aponeurosis of the external oblique muscle, and extends from the anterior superior iliac spine to the pubic tubercle.

The lacunar ligament (10, sometimes called the pectineal part of the inguinal ligament) is the part of the inguinal ligament that extends backwards from the medial end of the inguinal ligament to the pecten of the pubis.

The pectineal ligament (13) is the lateral extension of the lacunar ligament along the pecten. It is not classified as a part of the inguinal ligament, and must not be confused with the alternative name for the lacunar ligament, i.e. with the pectineal part of the inguinal ligament.

The conjoint tendon (2) is formed by the aponeuroses of the internal oblique and transversus muscles, and is attached to the pubic crest and the adjoining part of the pecten, blending medially with the anterior wall of the rectus sheath.

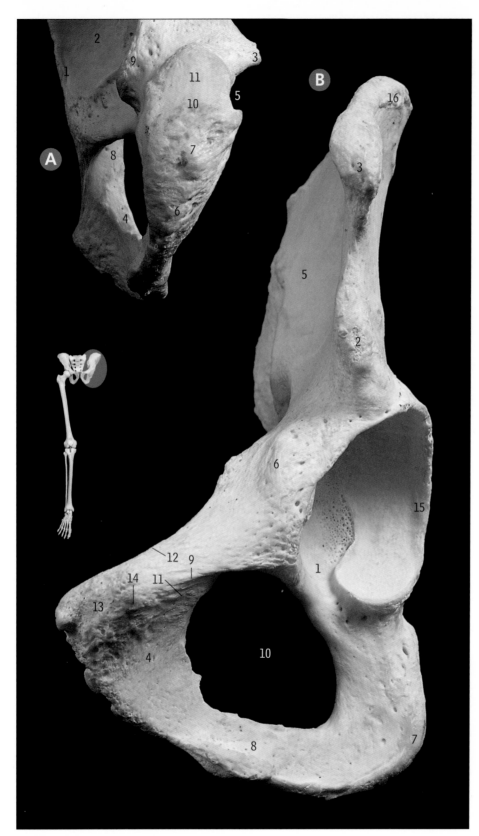

A Left hip bone
ischial tuberosity, from behind and below

1 Acetabular notch
2 Acetabulum
3 Ischial spine
4 Ischiopubic ramus
5 Lesser sciatic notch
6 Longitudinal ridge
7 Lower part of tuberosity
8 Obturator groove
9 Rim of acetabulum
10 Transverse ridge
11 Upper part of tuberosity

B Left hip bone
from the front

1 Acetabular notch
2 Anterior inferior iliac spine
3 Anterior superior iliac spine
4 Body of pubis
5 Iliac fossa
6 Iliopubic eminence
7 Ischial tuberosity
8 Ischiopubic ramus
9 Obturator crest
10 Obturator foramen
11 Obturator groove
12 Pecten of pubis (pectineal line)
13 Pubic crest
14 Pubic tubercle
15 Rim of acetabulum
16 Tubercle of iliac crest

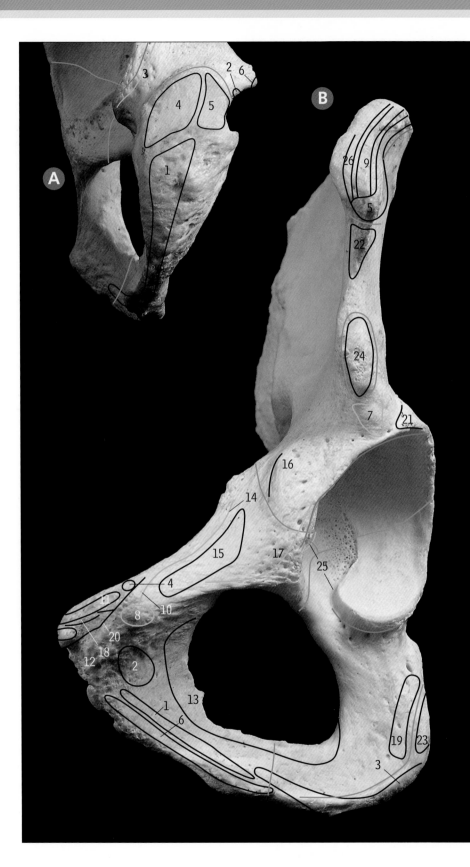

A Left hip bone attachments, ischial tuberosity, from behind and below

Blue lines, epiphysial lines
Green line, capsular attachment of hip joint
Pale green lines, ligament attachments

1 Adductor magnus
2 Inferior gemellus
3 Ischiofemoral ligament
4 Semimembranosus
5 Semitendinosus and long head of biceps femoris
6 Superior gemellus

The area on the ischial tuberosity medial to the adductor magnus attachment (1) is covered by fibrofatty tissue and the ischial bursa underlying gluteus maximus.

B Left hip bone attachments, from the front

Blue lines, epiphysial lines
Green line, capsular attachment of hip joint
Pale green lines, ligament attachments

1 Adductor brevis
2 Adductor longus
3 Adductor magnus
4 Conjoint tendon
5 External oblique and inguinal ligament
6 Gracilis
7 Iliofemoral ligament
8 Inguinal ligament
9 Internal oblique
10 Lacunar ligament
11 Lateral head of rectus abdominis
12 Medial head of rectus abdominis
13 Obturator externus
14 Pectineal ligament
15 Pectineus
16 Psoas minor
17 Pubofemoral ligament
18 Pyramidalis
19 Quadratus femoris
20 Rectus sheath
21 Reflected head of rectus femoris
22 Sartorius
23 Semimembranosus
24 Straight head of rectus femoris
25 Transverse ligament
26 Transversus abdominis

Left femur *proximal end*

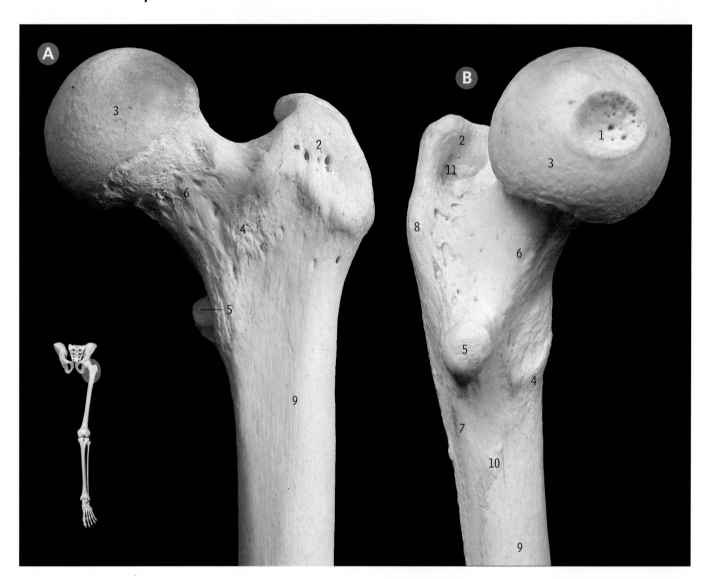

A from the front

B from the medial side

1	Fovea of head
2	Greater trochanter
3	Head
4	Intertrochanteric line
5	Lesser trochanter
6	Neck
7	Pectineal line
8	Quadrate tubercle on intertrochanteric crest
9	Shaft
10	Spiral line
11	Trochanteric fossa

The intertrochanteric *line* (4) is at the junction of the neck (6) and shaft (9) on the anterior surface; the intertrochanteric *crest* is in a similar position on the posterior surface (8, and page 296, A5).

The neck makes an angle with the shaft of about 125° in an adult.

The pectineal line of the femur (7) must not be confused with the pectineal line (pecten) of the pubis (9, page 290), nor with the spiral line of the femur (10) which is usually more prominent than the pectineal line.

Avulsion fractures, see pages 355–357.

Left femur *attachments, proximal end*

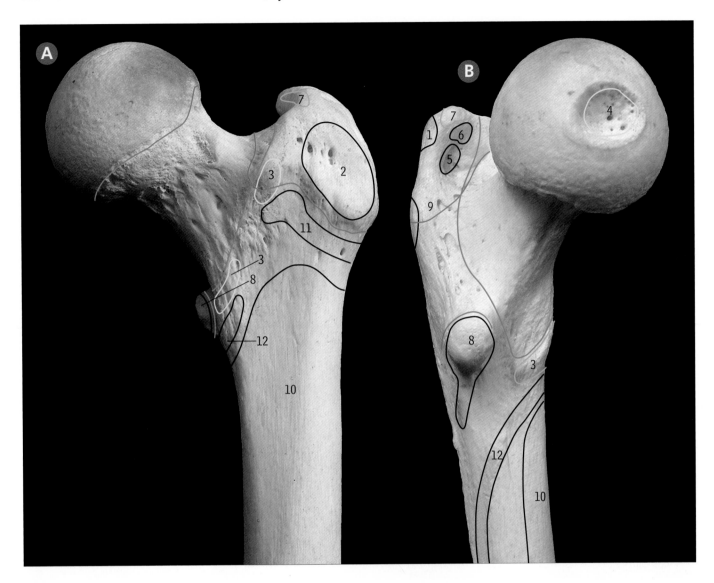

The iliofemoral ligament has the shape of an inverted V, with the stem attached to the anterior inferior iliac spine of the hip bone (page 293, B7), and the lateral and medial bands attached to the upper (lateral) and lower (medial) ends of the intertrochanteric line (page 296, 6), blending with the capsule of the hip joint.

The tendon of psoas major is attached to the lesser trochanter (page 296, 8); many of the muscle fibres of iliacus are inserted into the psoas tendon but some reach the femur below the trochanter.

A from the front

B from the medial side

Blue lines, epiphysial lines
Green line, capsular attachment of hip joint
Pale green lines, ligament attachments

1	Gluteus medius
2	Gluteus minimus
3	Iliofemoral ligament
4	Ligament of head of femur
5	Obturator externus
6	Obturator internus and gemelli
7	Piriformis
8	Psoas major and iliacus
9	Quadratus femoris
10	Vastus intermedius
11	Vastus lateralis
12	Vastus medialis

Intertrochanteric fracture–femur, slipped upper femoral epiphysis, see pages 355–357.

Left femur *proximal end*

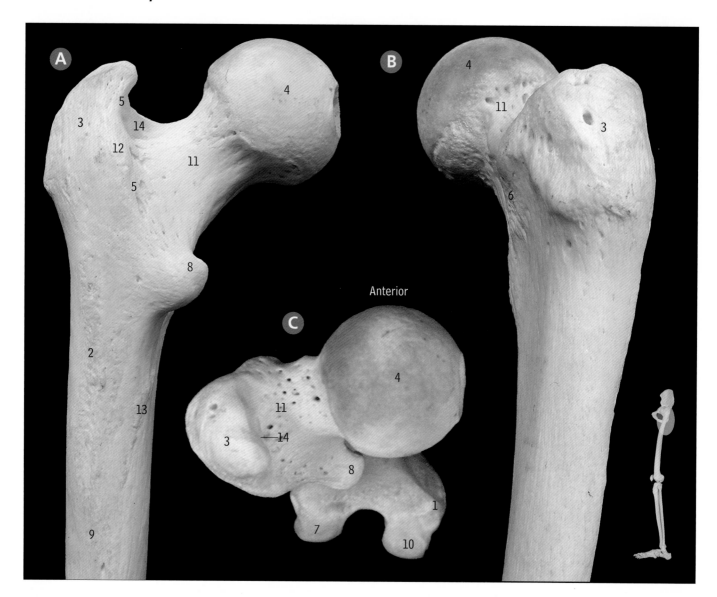

A from behind

B from the lateral side

C from above

1 Adductor tubercle at lower end
2 Gluteal tuberosity
3 Greater trochanter
4 Head
5 Intertrochanteric crest
6 Intertrochanteric line
7 Lateral condyle at lower end
8 Lesser trochanter
9 Linea aspera
10 Medial condyle at lower end
11 Neck
12 Quadrate tubercle
13 Spiral line
14 Trochanteric fossa

The neck of the femur passes forwards as well as upwards and medially (C11), making an angle of about 15° (in the adult) with the transverse axis of the lower end (the angle of femoral torsion or femoral anteversion).

The lesser trochanter (8) projects backwards and medially.

Fracture of the femoral neck, see pages 355–357.

Left femur *attachments, proximal end*

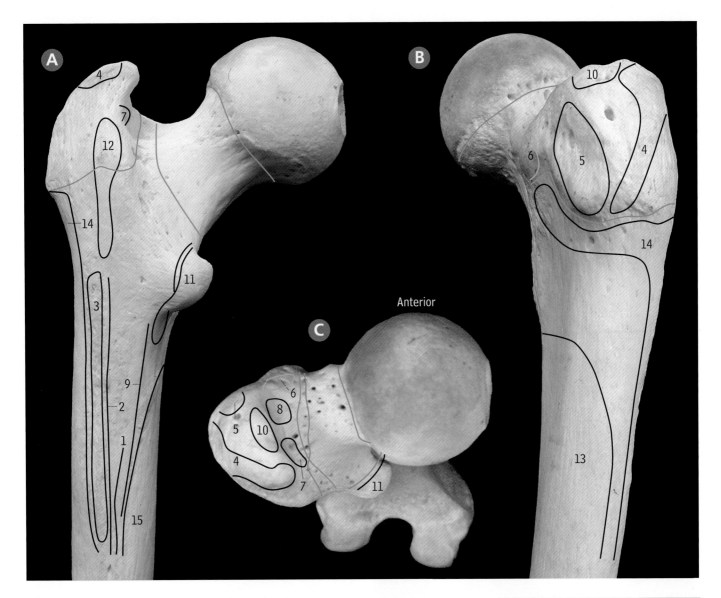

C Anterior

Exostoses femoral spurs, see pages 355–357.

A from behind

B from the lateral side

C from above

Blue lines, epiphysial lines
Green line, capsular attachment of hip joint
Pale green lines, ligament attachments

1 Adductor brevis
2 Adductor magnus
3 Gluteus maximus
4 Gluteus medius
5 Gluteus minimus
6 Iliofemoral ligament (lateral band)
7 Obturator externus
8 Obturator internus and gemelli
9 Pectineus
10 Piriformis
11 Psoas major and iliacus
12 Quadratus femoris
13 Vastus intermedius
14 Vastus lateralis
15 Vastus medialis

On the front of the femur (page 295) the capsule of the hip joint is attached to the intertrochanteric line, but at the back the capsule is attached to the neck of the femur and does not extend as far laterally as the intertrochanteric crest (page 296, A5).

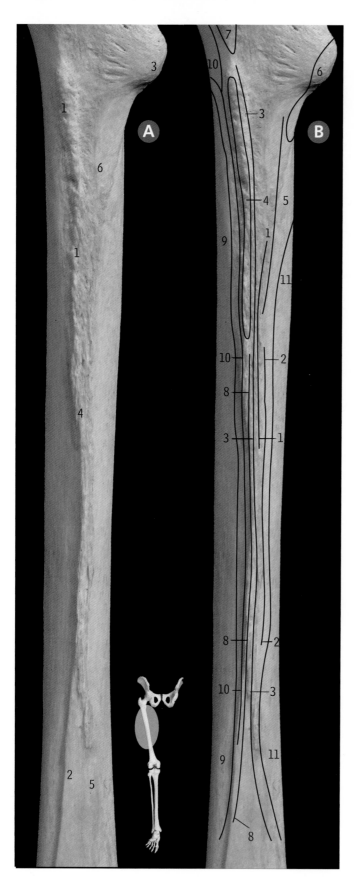

A Left femur *shaft, from behind*

1 Gluteal tuberosity   **4** Linea aspera
2 Lateral supracondylar line   **5** Medial supracondylar line
3 Lesser trochanter   **6** Pectineal line

> The rough linea aspera (4) often shows distinct medial and lateral lips; the lateral lip continues upwards as the gluteal tuberosity (1).

B Left femur
attachments, shaft, from behind

1 Adductor brevis   **7** Quadratus femoris
2 Adductor longus   **8** Short head of biceps femoris
3 Adductor magnus   **9** Vastus intermedius
4 Gluteus maximus   **10** Vastus lateralis
5 Pectineus   **11** Vastus medialis
6 Psoas major and iliacus

> For diagrammatic clarity, the muscle attachments to the linea aspera have been slightly separated.

C Left femur
upper end, from the front

This is the posterior half of a cleared and bisected specimen, to show the major groups of bone trabeculae.

1 Calcar femorale
2 From lateral surface of shaft to greater trochanter
3 From lateral surface of shaft to head
4 From medial surface of shaft to greater trochanter
5 From medial surface of shaft to head
6 Triangular area of few trabeculae

> The calcar femorale (1) is a dense concentration of trabeculae passing from the region of the lesser trochanter to the under-surface of the neck.

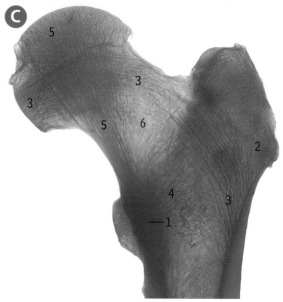

Fracture–femoral shaft, see pages 355–357.

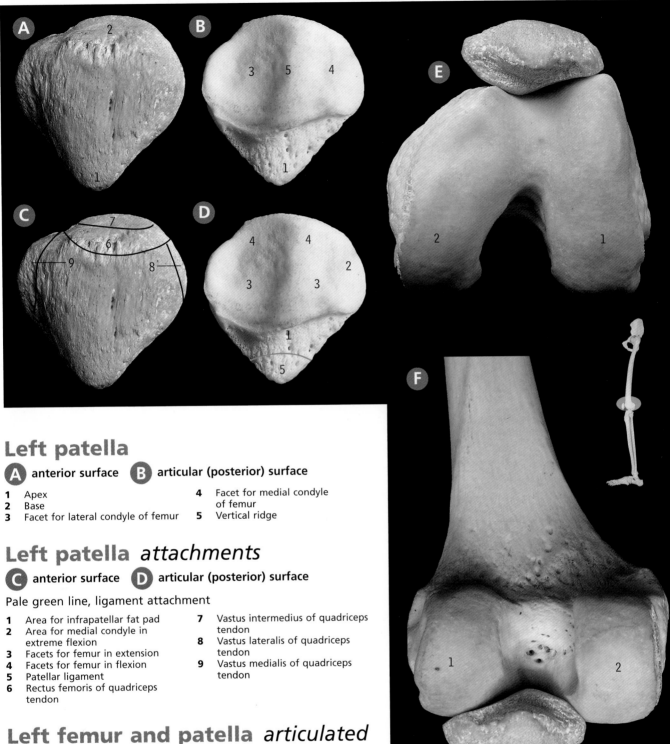

Left patella

A anterior surface **B** articular (posterior) surface

1 Apex
2 Base
3 Facet for lateral condyle of femur
4 Facet for medial condyle of femur
5 Vertical ridge

Left patella *attachments*

C anterior surface **D** articular (posterior) surface

Pale green line, ligament attachment

1 Area for infrapatellar fat pad
2 Area for medial condyle in extreme flexion
3 Facets for femur in extension
4 Facets for femur in flexion
5 Patellar ligament
6 Rectus femoris of quadriceps tendon
7 Vastus intermedius of quadriceps tendon
8 Vastus lateralis of quadriceps tendon
9 Vastus medialis of quadriceps tendon

Left femur and patella *articulated*

E from below with knee extended

F from below and behind with knee flexed

In flexion, note the increased area of contact between the medial condyle of the femur (2) and the patella.

1 Lateral condyle
2 Medial condyle

The most medial facet of the patella (D2) only comes into contact with the medial condyle in extreme flexion as in F.

Bipartite patella, dislocation of the patella, patellar fracture, see pages 355–357.

Left femur *distal end*

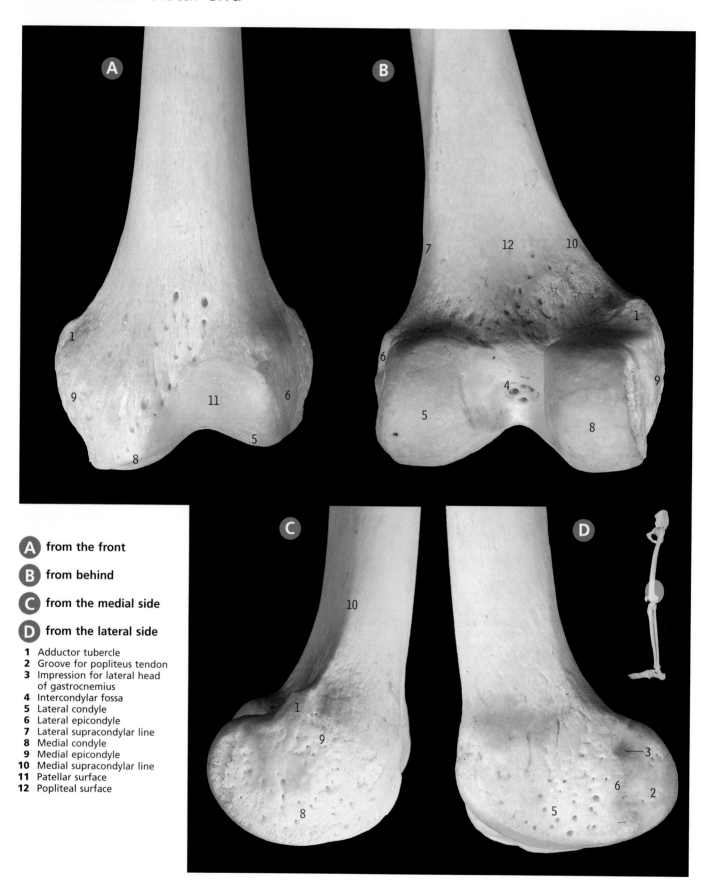

A from the front

B from behind

C from the medial side

D from the lateral side

1 Adductor tubercle
2 Groove for popliteus tendon
3 Impression for lateral head of gastrocnemius
4 Intercondylar fossa
5 Lateral condyle
6 Lateral epicondyle
7 Lateral supracondylar line
8 Medial condyle
9 Medial epicondyle
10 Medial supracondylar line
11 Patellar surface
12 Popliteal surface

Left femur *attachments, distal end*

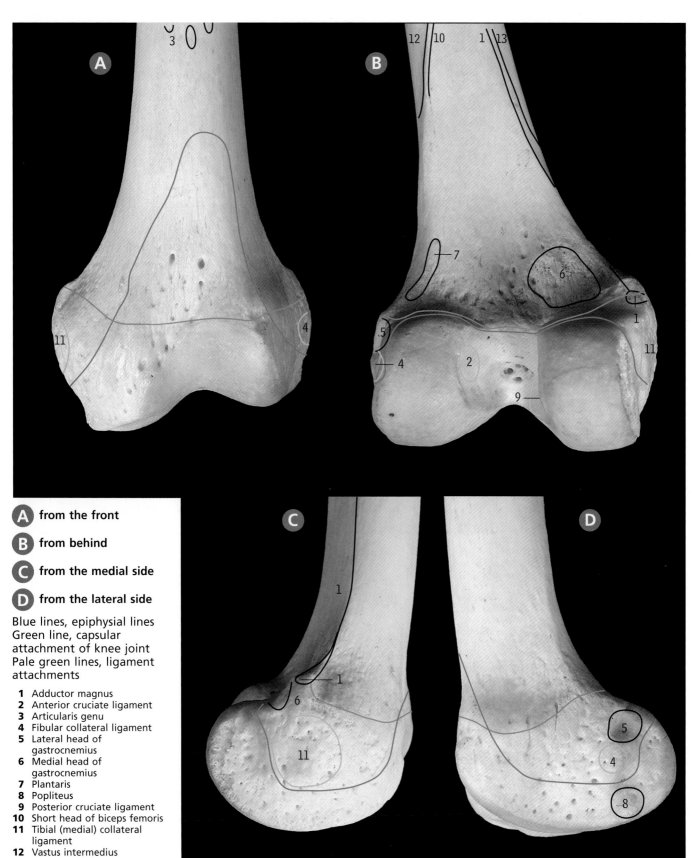

A from the front

B from behind

C from the medial side

D from the lateral side

Blue lines, epiphysial lines
Green line, capsular
attachment of knee joint
Pale green lines, ligament
attachments

1 Adductor magnus
2 Anterior cruciate ligament
3 Articularis genu
4 Fibular collateral ligament
5 Lateral head of
   gastrocnemius
6 Medial head of
   gastrocnemius
7 Plantaris
8 Popliteus
9 Posterior cruciate ligament
10 Short head of biceps femoris
11 Tibial (medial) collateral
   ligament
12 Vastus intermedius
13 Vastus medialis

Left tibia *proximal end*

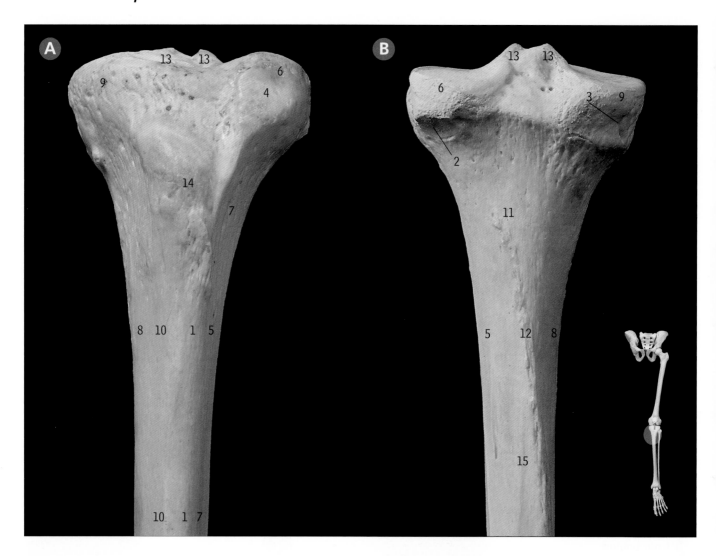

A from the front

B from behind

1 Anterior border
2 Articular facet for fibula
3 Groove for semimembranosus
4 Impression for iliotibial tract
5 Interosseous border
6 Lateral condyle
7 Lateral surface
8 Medial border
9 Medial condyle
10 Medial surface
11 Posterior surface
12 Soleal line
13 Tubercles of intercondylar eminence
14 Tuberosity
15 Vertical line

The shaft of the tibia has three borders: anterior (1), medial (8) and interosseous (5) – and three surfaces: medial (10), lateral (7) and posterior (11).

Much of the anterior border (1) forms a slightly curved crest commonly known as the shin. Most of the smooth medial surface (10) is subcutaneous. The posterior surface contains the soleal and vertical lines (12 and 15).

The tuberosity (14) is at the upper end of the anterior border.

Left tibia *attachments, proximal end*

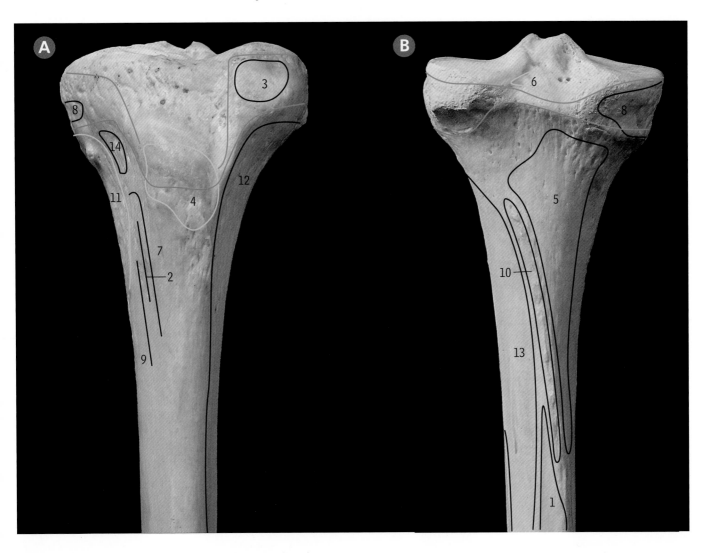

A from the front

B from behind

Blue lines, epiphysial lines
Green line, capsular
attachment of knee joint
Pale green lines, ligament
attachments

1 Flexor digitorum longus
2 Gracilis
3 Iliotibial tract
4 Patellar ligament
5 Popliteus
6 Posterior cruciate ligament
7 Sartorius
8 Semimembranosus

9 Semitendinosus
10 Soleus
11 Tibial (medial) collateral
  ligament
12 Tibialis anterior
13 Tibialis posterior
14 Vastus medialis

Left tibia *proximal end*

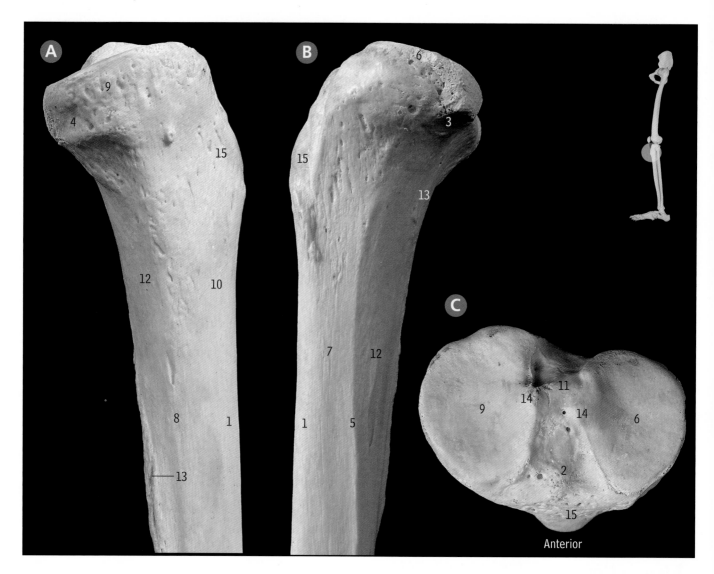

A **from the medial side**

B **from the lateral side**

C **from above (tibial plateau)**

1 Anterior border	**9** Medial condyle
2 Anterior intercondylar area	**10** Medial surface
3 Articular facet for fibula	**11** Posterior intercondylar area
4 Groove for semimembranosus	**12** Posterior surface
5 Interosseous border	**13** Soleal line
6 Lateral condyle	**14** Tubercles of intercondylar eminence
7 Lateral surface	**15** Tuberosity
8 Medial border	

The medial condyle (C9) is larger than the lateral condyle (C6).

The articular facet for the fibula is on the postero-inferior aspect of the lateral condyle (B3).

 Osgood–Schlatter's disease, see pages 355–357.

Left tibia *attachments, proximal end*

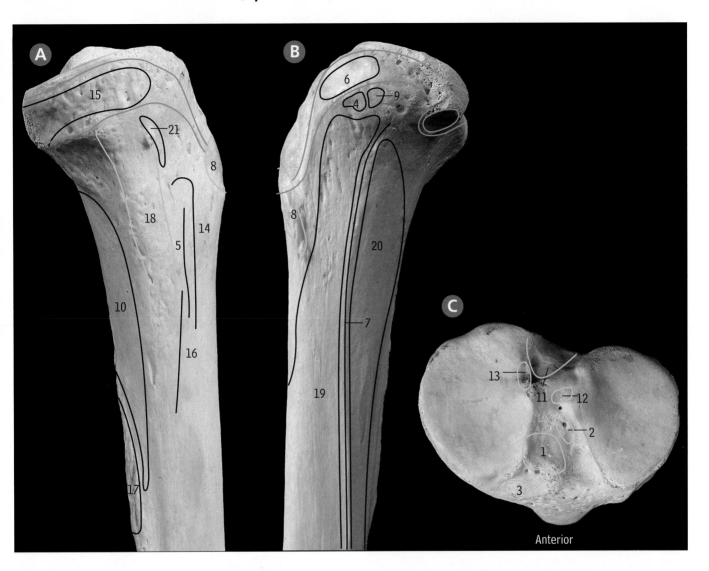

A from the medial side

B from the lateral side

C from above (tibial plateau)

Blue lines, epiphysial lines
Green lines, capsular attachments of knee joint and superior tibiofibular joint
Pale green lines, ligament attachments

1 Anterior cruciate ligament
2 Anterior horn of lateral meniscus
3 Anterior horn of medial meniscus
4 Extensor digitorum longus
5 Gracilis
6 Iliotibial tract
7 Interosseous membrane
8 Patellar ligament
9 Peroneus (fibularis) longus
10 Popliteus
11 Posterior cruciate ligament

12 Posterior horn of lateral meniscus
13 Posterior horn of medial meniscus
14 Sartorius
15 Semimembranosus
16 Semitendinosus
17 Soleus
18 Tibial (medial) collateral ligament
19 Tibialis anterior
20 Tibialis posterior
21 Vastus medialis

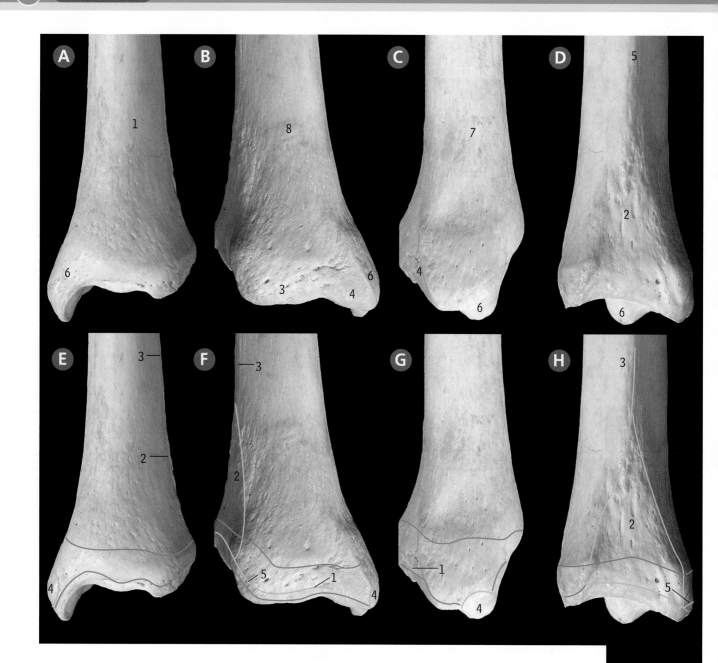

Left tibia *distal end*

A from the front

B from behind

C from the medial side

D from the lateral side

1 Anterior surface
2 Fibular notch
3 Groove for flexor hallucis longus
4 Groove for tibialis posterior
5 Interosseous border
6 Medial malleolus
7 Medial surface
8 Posterior surface

Left tibia *attachments, distal end*

E from the front

F from behind

G from the medial side

H from the lateral side

Blue line, epiphysial line
Green line, capsular attachment of ankle joint
Pale green lines, ligament attachment

1 Inferior transverse ligament
2 Interosseous ligament
3 Interosseous membrane
4 Medial collateral ligament
5 Posterior tibiofibular ligament

> The medial collateral ligament (G4) is commonly known as the deltoid ligament.

Tibial fractures, see pages 355–357.

Left tibia and fibula *articulated*

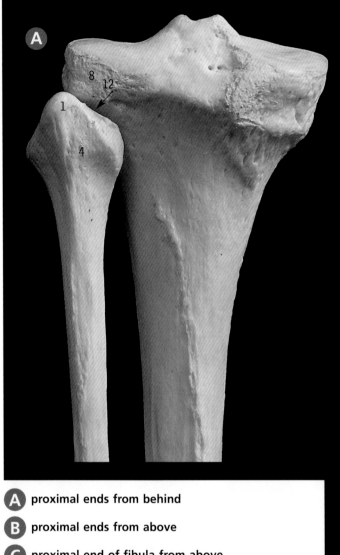

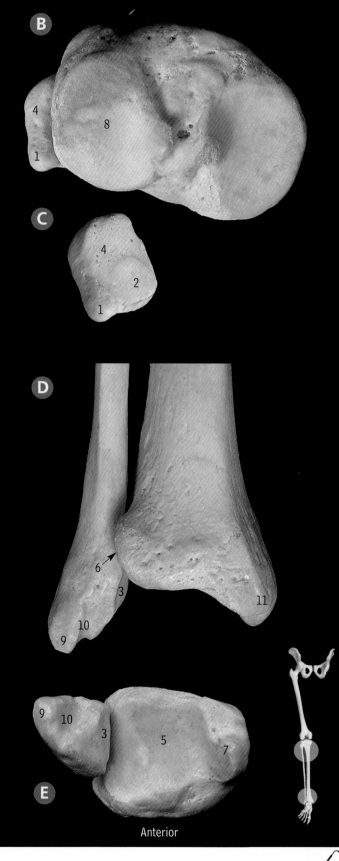

A proximal ends from behind

B proximal ends from above

C proximal end of fibula from above

D distal ends from behind

E distal ends from below

1 Apex of head (styloid process)
2 Articular facet (for superior tibiofibular joint)
3 Articular facet of lateral malleolus (for ankle joint)
4 Head of fibula
5 Inferior surface of tibia (for ankle joint)
6 Inferior tibiofibular joint
7 Lateral (articular) surface of medial malleolus (for ankle joint)
8 Lateral condyle of tibia
9 Lateral malleolus
10 Malleolar fossa
11 Medial malleolus
12 Superior tibiofibular joint

The superior tibiofibular joint (A12) is synovial.

The inferior tibiofibular joint (D6) is fibrous.

The lateral malleolus (D9) extends lower than the medial malleolus (D11).

Anterior

Tarsal dislocations, see pages 355–357.

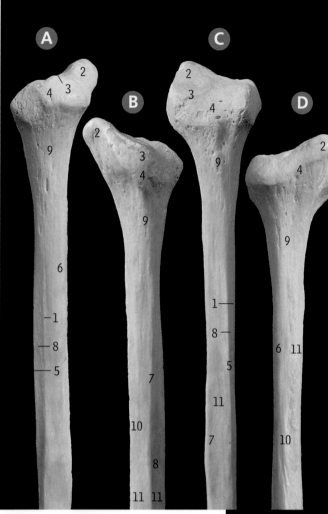

Left fibula *proximal end*

A from the front

B from behind

C from the medial side

D from the lateral side

1 Anterior border
2 Apex (styloid process)
3 Articular facet on upper surface
4 Head
5 Interosseous border
6 Lateral surface
7 Medial crest
8 Medial surface
9 Neck
10 Posterior border
11 Posterior surface

The fibula has three borders: anterior (A1), interosseous (A5) and posterior (B10) – and three surfaces: medial (A8), lateral (A6) and posterior (B11).

At first sight, much of the shaft appears to have four borders and four surfaces, but this is because the posterior surface (B11) is divided into two parts (medial and lateral) by the medial crest (B7).

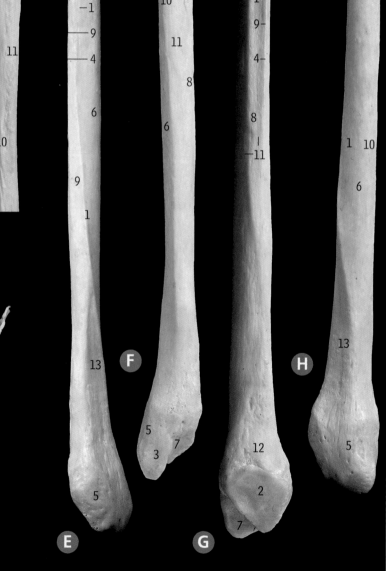

Left fibula *distal end*

E from the front

F from behind

G from the medial side

H from the lateral side

1 Anterior border
2 Articular surface of lateral malleolus
3 Groove for peroneus (fibularis) brevis
4 Interosseous border
5 Lateral malleolus
6 Lateral surface
7 Malleolar fossa
8 Medial crest
9 Medial surface
10 Posterior border
11 Posterior surface
12 Surface for interosseous ligament
13 Triangular subcutaneous area

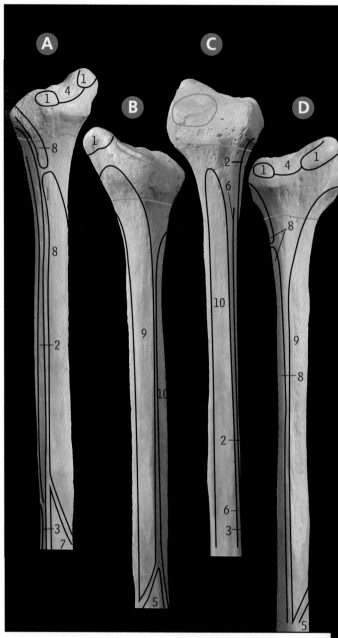

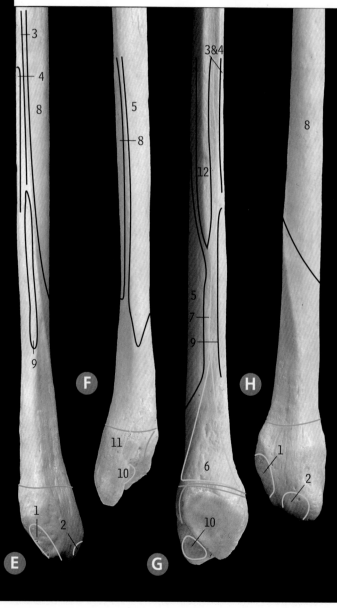

Left fibula
attachments, proximal end

A from the front   **C** from the medial side

B from behind   **D** from the lateral side

Blue line, epiphysial line
Green line, capsular attachment of superior tibiofibular joint
Pale green lines, ligament attachments

1 Biceps femoris
2 Extensor digitorum longus
3 Extensor hallucis longus
4 Fibular collateral ligament
5 Flexor hallucis longus
6 Interosseous membrane
7 Peroneus (fibularis) brevis
8 Peroneus (fibularis) longus
9 Soleus
10 Tibialis posterior

Left fibula
attachments, distal end

E from the front   **G** from the medial side

F from behind   **H** from the lateral side

Blue line, epiphysial line
Green line, capsular attachment of ankle joint
Pale green lines, ligament attachments

1 Anterior talofibular ligament
2 Calcaneofibular ligament
3 Extensor digitorum longus
4 Extensor hallucis longus
5 Flexor hallucis longus
6 Interosseous ligament
7 Interosseous membrane
8 Peroneus (fibularis) brevis
9 Peroneus (fibularis) tertius
10 Posterior talofibular ligament
11 Posterior tibiofibular ligament
12 Tibialis posterior

Bones of the left foot

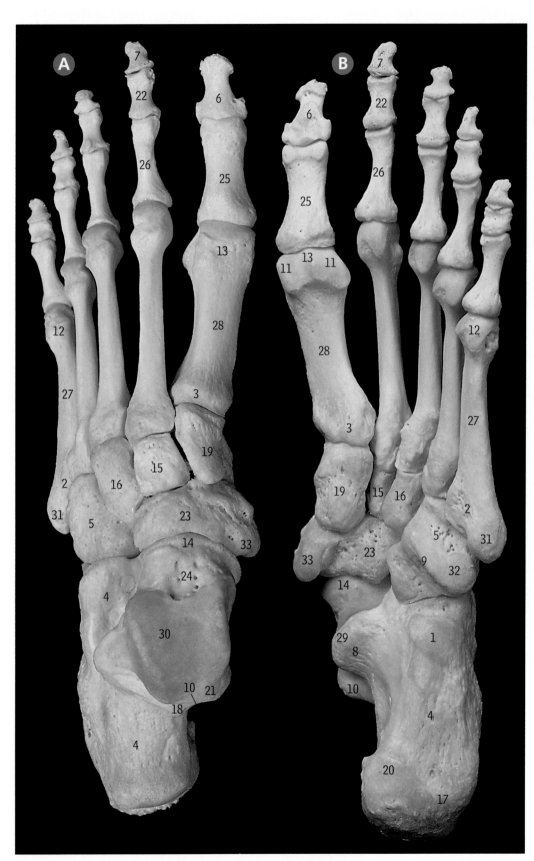

Dislocation of the toe, hallux valgus, see pages 355–357.

A from above (dorsum)

B from below (plantar surface)

1 Anterior tubercle of calcaneus
2 Base of fifth metatarsal
3 Base of first metatarsal
4 Calcaneus
5 Cuboid
6 Distal phalanx of great toe
7 Distal phalanx of second toe
8 Groove on calcaneus for flexor hallucis longus
9 Groove on cuboid for peroneus (fibularis) longus
10 Groove on talus for flexor hallucis longus
11 Grooves for sesamoid bones in flexor hallucis brevis
12 Head of fifth metatarsal
13 Head of first metatarsal
14 Head of talus
15 Intermediate cuneiform
16 Lateral cuneiform
17 Lateral process of calcaneus
18 Lateral tubercle of talus
19 Medial cuneiform
20 Medial process of calcaneus
21 Medial tubercle of talus
22 Middle phalanx of second toe
23 Navicular
24 Neck of talus
25 Proximal phalanx of great toe
26 Proximal phalanx of second toe
27 Shaft of fifth metatarsal
28 Shaft of first metatarsal
29 Sustentaculum tali of calcaneus
30 Trochlear surface of body of talus
31 Tuberosity of base of fifth metatarsal
32 Tuberosity of cuboid
33 Tuberosity of navicular

Bones of the left foot *attachments*

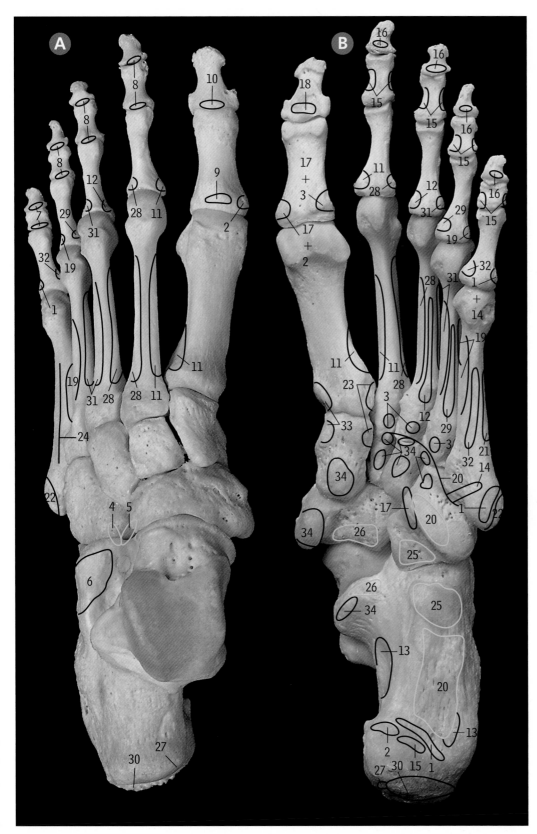

A from above

B from below

Joint capsules and minor ligaments have been omitted.

Pale green lines, ligament attachments

1 Abductor digiti minimi
2 Abductor hallucis
3 Adductor hallucis
4 Calcaneocuboid part of bifurcate ligament
5 Calcaneonavicular part of bifurcate ligament
6 Extensor digitorum brevis
7 Extensor digitorum longus
8 Extensor digitorum longus and brevis
9 Extensor hallucis brevis
10 Extensor hallucis longus
11 First dorsal interosseous
12 First plantar interosseous
13 Flexor accessorius
14 Flexor digiti minimi brevis
15 Flexor digitorum brevis
16 Flexor digitorum longus
17 Flexor hallucis brevis
18 Flexor hallucis longus
19 Fourth dorsal interosseous
20 Long plantar ligament
21 Opponens digiti minimi (part of 14)
22 Peroneus (fibularis) brevis
23 Peroneus (fibularis) longus
24 Peroneus (fibularis) tertius
25 Plantar calcaneocuboid (short plantar) ligament
26 Plantar calcaneonavicular (spring) ligament
27 Plantaris
28 Second dorsal interosseous
29 Second plantar interosseous
30 Tendo calcaneus (Achilles tendon)
31 Third dorsal interosseous
32 Third plantar interosseous
33 Tibialis anterior
34 Tibialis posterior

Hallux sesamoid fracture, metatarsal fractures, see pages 355–357.

Bones of the left foot

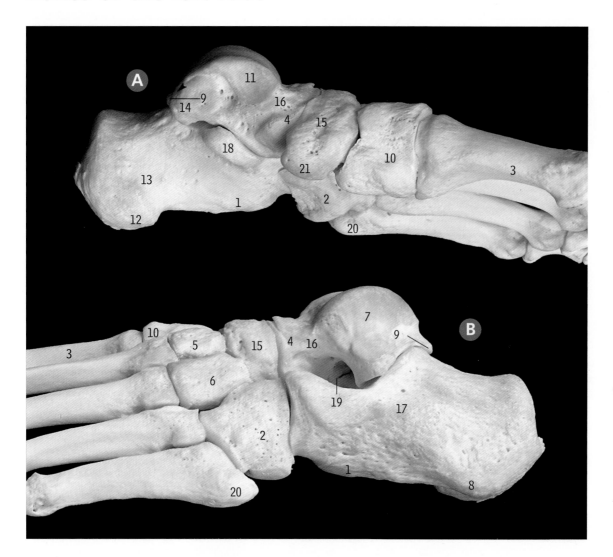

A from the medial side   **B** from the lateral side

1 Anterior tubercle of calcaneus	**9** Lateral tubercle of talus
2 Cuboid	**10** Medial cuneiform
3 First metatarsal	**11** Medial malleolar surface of talus
4 Head of talus	**12** Medial process of calcaneus
5 Intermediate cuneiform	**13** Medial surface of calcaneus
6 Lateral cuneiform	**14** Medial tubercle of talus
7 Lateral malleolar surface of talus	**15** Navicular
8 Lateral process of calcaneus	**16** Neck of talus

17 Peroneal (fibular) trochlea of calcaneus
18 Sustentaculum tali of calcaneus
19 Tarsal sinus
20 Tuberosity of base of fifth metatarsal
21 Tuberosity of navicular

Calcaneal fracture, hammer toe, os trigonum, see pages 355–357.

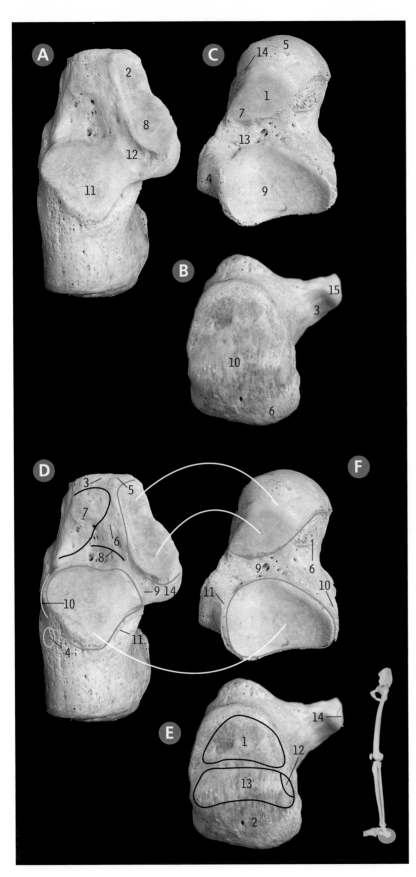

Bones of the left foot
Left calcaneus

A from above   **B** from behind

Left talus

C from below

1 Anterior calcanean articular surface of talus
2 Anterior talar articular surface of calcaneus
3 Groove of calcaneus for flexor hallucis longus
4 Groove of talus for flexor hallucis longus
5 Head of talus
6 Medial process of calcaneus
7 Middle calcanean articular surface of talus
8 Middle talar articular surface of calcaneus
9 Posterior calcanean articular surface of talus
10 Posterior surface of calcaneus
11 Posterior talar articular surface of calcaneus
12 Sulcus of calcaneus
13 Sulcus of talus
14 Surface of talus for plantar calcaneonavicular (spring) ligament
15 Sustentaculum tali of calcaneus

Left calcaneus, attachments

D from above   **E** from behind

Left talus, attachments

F from below

Curved lines indicate corresponding articular surfaces: green, capsular attachment of talocalcanean (subtalar) and talocalcaneonavicular joints; pale green lines, ligament attachments

1 Area for bursa
2 Area for fibrofatty tissue
3 Calcaneocuboid part of bifurcate ligament
4 Calcaneofibular ligament
5 Calcaneonavicular part of bifurcate ligament
6 Cervical ligament
7 Extensor digitorum brevis
8 Inferior extensor retinaculum
9 Interosseous talocalcanean (cervical) ligament
10 Lateral talocalcanean ligament
11 Medial talocalcanean ligament
12 Plantaris
13 Tendocalcaneus (Achilles tendon)
14 Tibiocalcanean part of deltoid ligament

The interosseous talocalcanean (cervical) ligament (9) is formed by thickening of the adjacent capsules of the talocalcanean and talocalcaneonavicular joints.

For different interpretations of the term 'subtalar joint' see the notes on page 348.

Left lower limb bones *secondary centres of ossification*

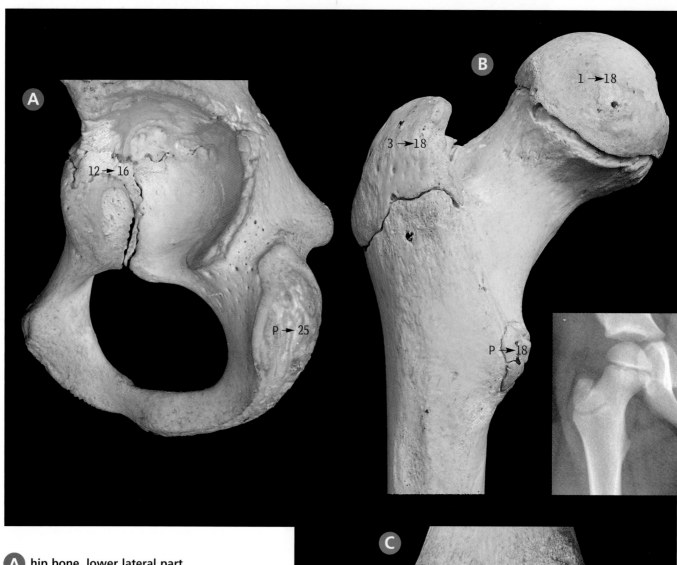

12 → 16

P → 25

1 → 18

3 → 18

P → 18

B → 20

A hip bone, lower lateral part

B **C** femur, proximal and distal ends

D **E** tibia, proximal and distal ends

F **G** fibula, proximal and distal ends

H calcaneus

I metatarsal and phalanges of second toe

J metatarsal and phalanges of great toe

Figures in years, commencement of ossification → fusion.
P, puberty, B, ninth intra-uterine month.
See introduction on page 125.

Slipped upper femoral epiphysis, see pages 355–357.

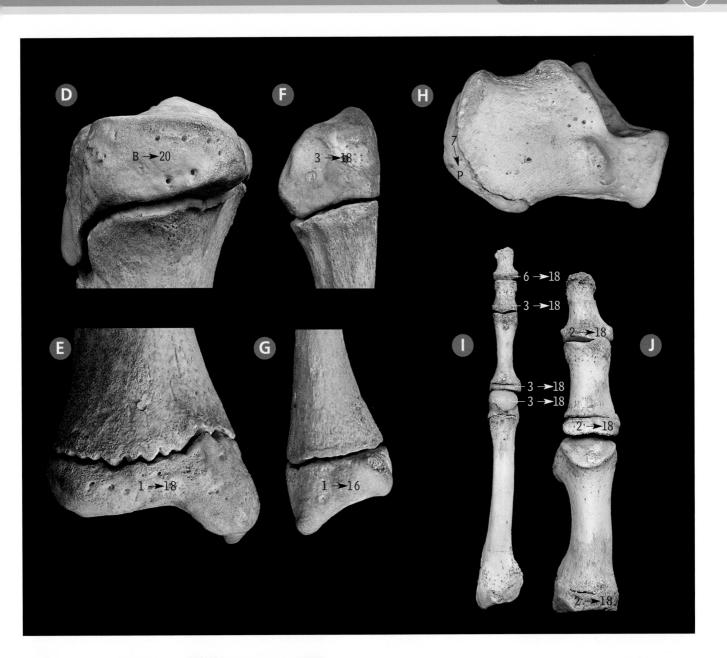

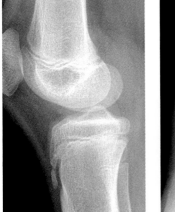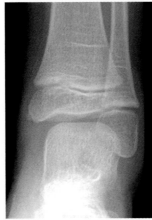

Note knee and ankle epiphyses as seen on plain x-rays

In the hip bone (A) one or more secondary centres appear in the Y-shaped cartilage between ilium, ischium and pubis. Other centres (not illustrated) are usually present for the iliac crest, anterior inferior iliac spine, and (possibly) the pubic tubercle and pubic crest (all P → 25).

The patella (not illustrated) begins to ossify from one or more centres between the third and sixth year.

All the phalanges, and the first metatarsal, have a secondary centre at their proximal ends; the other metatarsals have one at their distal ends.

Of the tarsal bones, the largest, the calcaneus, begins to ossify in the third intra-uterine month and the talus about three months later. The cuboid may begin to ossify either just before or just after birth, with the lateral cuneiform in the first year, medial cuneiform at two years and the intermediate cuneiform and navicular at three years.

The calcaneus (H) is the only tarsal bone to have a secondary centre.

A Gluteal region *surface features*

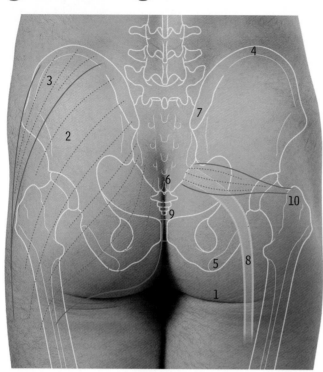

The iliac crest (4) with the posterior superior iliac spine (7), the tip of the coccyx (9), the ischial tuberosity (5) and the tip of the greater trochanter of the femur (10) are palpable landmarks. A line drawn from a point midway between the posterior superior iliac spine (7) and the tip of the coccyx (9) to the tip of the greater trochanter (10) marks the lower border of piriformis (illustrated on right buttock), which is a key feature of the gluteal region, where the most important structure is the sciatic nerve (indicated here in yellow, 8; see dissections and notes opposite).

1 Fold of buttock
2 Gluteus maximus
3 Gluteus medius
4 Iliac crest
5 Ischial tuberosity
6 Natal cleft
7 Posterior superior iliac spine
8 Sciatic nerve
9 Tip of coccyx
10 Tip of greater trochanter of femur

B Right gluteal region *superficial nerves*

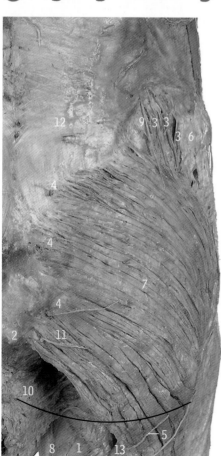

Skin and subcutaneous tissue have been removed, preserving cutaneous branches from the first three lumbar (3) and first three sacral (4) nerves, the cutaneous branches of the posterior femoral cutaneous nerve (5) and the perforating cutaneous nerve (11). The curved line near the bottom of the picture indicates the position of the gluteal fold (fold of the buttock). The muscle fibres of gluteus maximus (7) run downwards and laterally, and its lower border does not correspond to the gluteal fold.

1 Adductor magnus
2 Coccyx
3 Cutaneous branches of dorsal rami of first three lumbar nerves
4 Gluteal branches of dorsal rami of first three sacral nerves
5 Gluteal branches of the posterior femoral cutaneous nerve
6 Gluteal fascia overlying gluteus medius
7 Gluteus maximus
8 Gracilis
9 Iliac crest
10 Ischio-anal fossa and levator ani
11 Perforating cutaneous nerve
12 Posterior layer of lumbar fascia overlying erector spinae
13 Semitendinosus

The gluteal region or buttock is sometimes used as a site for intramuscular injections. The correct site is in the upper outer quadrant of the buttock, and for delineating this quadrant, it is essential to remember that the upper boundary of the buttock is the uppermost part of the iliac crest. The lower boundary is the fold of the buttock. Dividing the area between these two boundaries by a vertical line midway between the midline and the lateral side of the body indicates that the upper outer quadrant is well above and to the right of the label 7 in B, and this is the safe site for injection – well above and to the right of the sciatic nerve which is displayed in the dissections opposite.

Intramuscular injection–gluteal region, see pages 355–357.

Left gluteal region

A superficial dissection

B deeper dissection

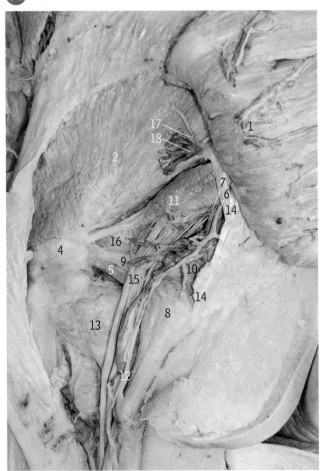

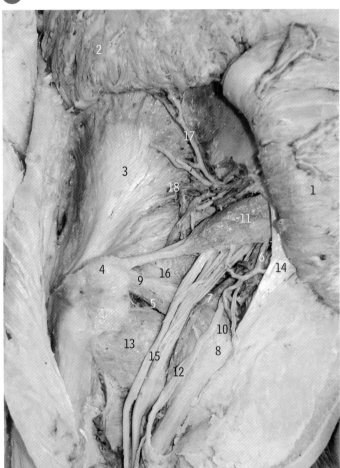

1 Gluteus maximus muscle, reflected	**10** Obturator internus muscle
2 Gluteus medius muscle, reflected	**11** Piriformis
3 Gluteus minimus muscle	**12** Posterior cutaneous nerve of thigh
4 Greater trochanter of femur	**13** Quadratus femoris muscle
5 Inferior gemellus muscle	**14** Sacrotuberous ligament
6 Inferior gluteal artery	**15** Sciatic nerve
7 Inferior gluteal vein	**16** Superior gemellus muscle
8 Ischial tuberosity	**17** Superior gluteal artery
9 Obturator internus tendon	**18** Superior gluteal vein

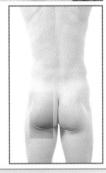

The two parts of the sciatic trunk (common peroneal [fibular] and tibial) usually divide from one another at the top of the popliteal fossa (page 330) but are sometimes separate as they emerge beneath piriformis, and the common peroneal (fibular) may even perforate piriformis.

Right thigh *posterior view*

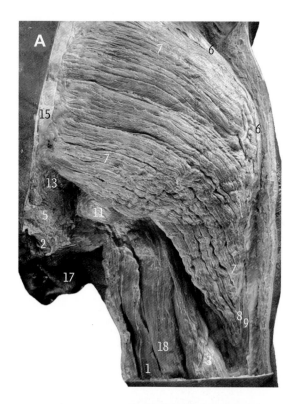

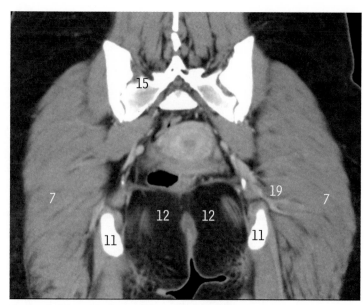

Coronal CT, posterior pelvic cavity, female

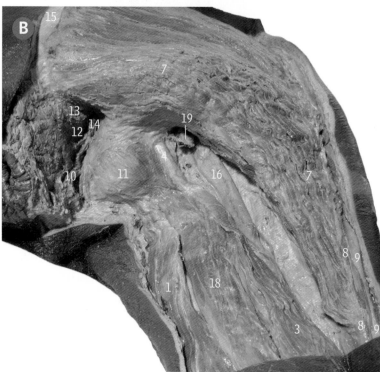

A Gluteal region and proximal hamstrings

B Deeper dissection revealing ischio-anal fossa

1 Adductor magnus, hamstring part
2 Anus
3 Biceps femoris
4 Biceps femoris, tendon of long head
5 External anal sphincter
6 Gluteal fascia
7 Gluteus maximus
8 Gluteus maximus, attachment to iliotibial tract
9 Iliotibial tract (thickened fascia lata)
10 Inferior rectal vessels
11 Ischial tuberosity
12 Ischio-anal fossa
13 Levator ani
14 Pudendal vessels and pudendal nerve
15 Sacrum, dorsal fascia
16 Sciatic nerve within fascial sheath
17 Scrotal skin
18 Semitendinosus
19 Superior gluteal vessels

Torn hamstrings, see pages 355–357.

C Right upper thigh *posterior view*

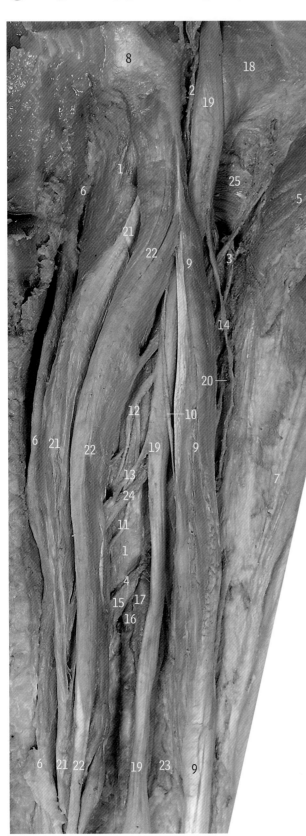

Gluteus maximus (5) has been reflected laterally and the gap between semitendinosus (22) and biceps femoris (9) has been opened up to show the sciatic trunk (19) and its muscular branches.

1 Adductor magnus
2 Anastomotic branch of inferior gluteal artery
3 First perforating artery
4 Fourth perforating artery
5 Gluteus maximus
6 Gracilis
7 Iliotibial tract overlying vastus lateralis
8 Ischial tuberosity
9 Long head of biceps femoris
10 Nerve to long head of biceps femoris
11 Nerve to semimembranosus
12 Nerve to semimembranosus and adductor magnus
13 Nerve to semitendinosus
14 Nerve to short head of biceps femoris
15 Opening in adductor magnus
16 Popliteal artery
17 Popliteal vein
18 Quadratus femoris
19 Sciatic trunk
20 Second perforating artery
21 Semimembranosus
22 Semitendinosus
23 Short head of biceps femoris
24 Third perforating artery
25 Upper part of adductor magnus ('adductor minimus')

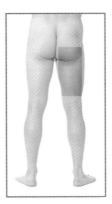

The only muscular branch to arise from the lateral side of the sciatic trunk (i.e. from the common peroneal (fibular) part of the nerve (19), uppermost 19, near the top of the picture), is the nerve to the short head of biceps (14). All the other muscular branches – to the long head of biceps femoris (10), semimembranosus (11), semimembranosus and adductor magnus (12) and semitendinosus (13) – arise from the medial side of the sciatic trunk (19, near the centre of the picture) (i.e. from the tibial part of the nerve).

D Femoral arteriogram

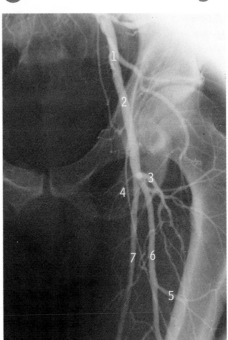

1 Catheter introduced into distal abdominal aorta via right common femoral artery
2 Common femoral artery
3 Lateral circumflex femoral artery
4 Medial circumflex femoral artery
5 Perforating artery
6 Profunda femoris artery
7 Superficial femoral artery

Anterior thigh and lower abdomen

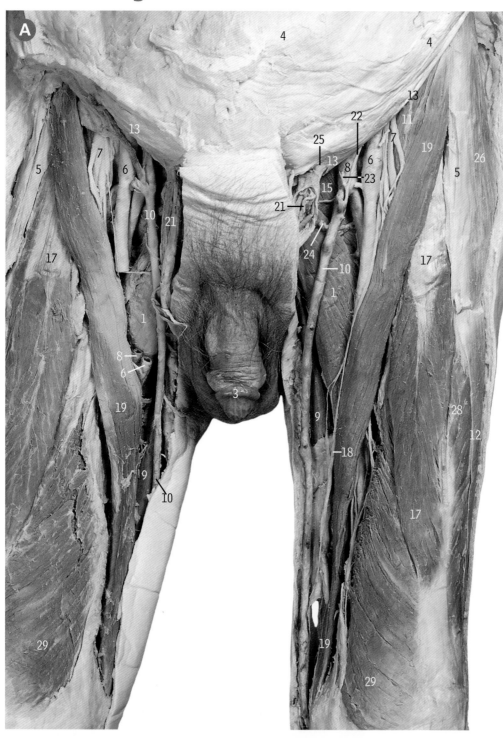

The boundaries of the femoral triangle are the inguinal ligament (13), the medial border of sartorius (19) and the medial border of adductor longus (1).

The femoral canal is the medial compartment of the femoral sheath (removed), which contains in its middle compartment the femoral vein (8), and in the lateral compartment the femoral artery (6). The femoral nerve (7) is lateral to the sheath, not within it.

Lumbar plexus block, varicella-zoster virus infection–lower limb, see pages 355–357.

Proximal anterior thigh *Sartorius retracted medially to show subsartorial canal*

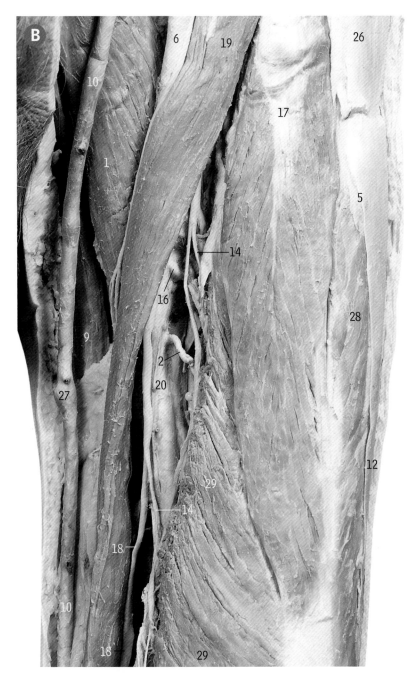

The boundaries of the femoral triangle are the inguinal ligament (13), the medial border of sartorius (19) and the medial border of adductor longus (1).

The femoral canal is the medial compartment of the femoral sheath (removed) which contains in its middle compartment the femoral vein (8), and in the lateral compartment the femoral artery (6). The femoral nerve (7) is lateral to the sheath, not within it.

 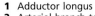

1 Adductor longus	**11** Iliopsoas	**21** Spermatic cord
2 Arterial branch to vastus medialis	**12** Iliotibial tract	**22** Superficial circumflex iliac vein
3 Corona of glans penis	**13** Inguinal ligament	**23** Superficial epigastric vein
4 External oblique aponeurosis	**14** Nerve to vastus medialis	**24** Superficial external pudendal vein
5 Fascia lata (cut edge)	**15** Pectineus	**25** Superficial inguinal ring
6 Femoral artery	**16** Perforating branch of profunda femoris artery	**26** Tensor fasciae latae deep to fascia lata
7 Femoral nerve	**17** Rectus femoris	**27** Valvular bulge in vein
8 Femoral vein	**18** Saphenous nerve	**28** Vastus lateralis
9 Gracilis	**19** Sartorius	**29** Vastus medialis
10 Great saphenous vein	**20** Subsartorial fascia (thickened aponeurosis)	

Femoral nerve paralysis, obturator nerve paralysis, see pages 355–357.

Ⓐ Right femoral artery

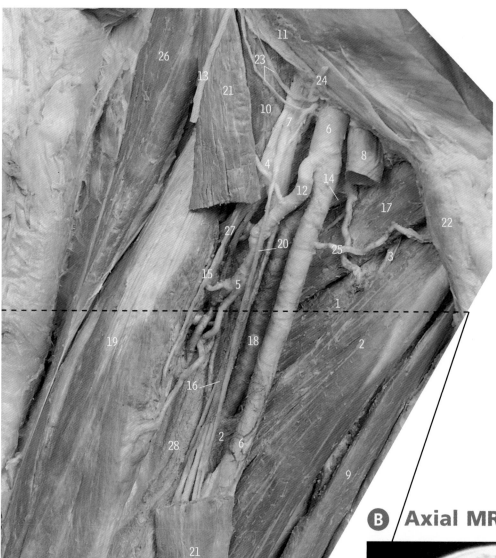

1 Adductor brevis
2 Adductor longus
3 Anterior branch of obturator nerve
4 Ascending branch of lateral circumflex femoral artery
5 Descending branch of lateral circumflex femoral artery
6 Femoral artery
7 Femoral nerve
8 Femoral vein
9 Gracilis
10 Iliacus
11 Inguinal ligament
12 Lateral circumflex femoral artery
13 Lateral femoral cutaneous nerve
14 Medial circumflex femoral artery
15 Nerve to rectus femoris
16 Nerve to vastus medialis
17 Pectineus
18 Profunda femoris artery
19 Rectus femoris
20 Saphenous nerve
21 Sartorius
22 Spermatic cord
23 Superficial circumflex iliac artery (double)
24 Superficial epigastric artery
25 Superficial external pudendal artery (low origin)
26 Tensor fasciae latae
27 Transverse branch of lateral circumflex femoral artery
28 Vastus intermedius
29 Vastus medialis

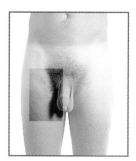

Ⓑ Axial MR image of thigh

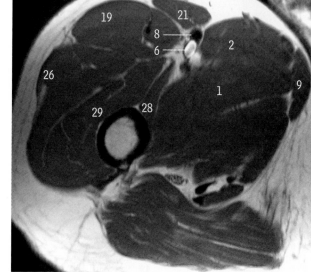

Femoral artery puncture, meralgia paraesthetica, see pages 355–357.

C Right distal thigh
from the front and medial side

The lower part of sartorius (13) has been displaced medially to open up the lower part of the adductor canal and expose the femoral artery (2) passing through the opening in adductor magnus (7) to enter the popliteal fossa behind the knee and become the popliteal artery (page 330).

1 Adductor magnus
2 Femoral artery
3 Gracilis
4 Iliotibial tract
5 Lowest (horizontal) fibres of vastus medialis
6 Medial patellar retinaculum
7 Opening in adductor magnus
8 Patella
9 Quadriceps tendon
10 Rectus femoris
11 Saphenous branch of descending genicular artery
12 Saphenous nerve
13 Sartorius
14 Vastus medialis and nerve

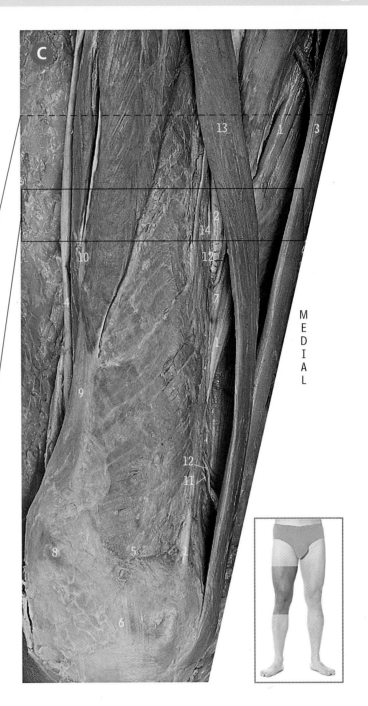

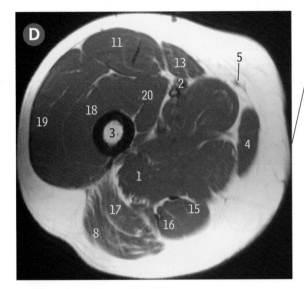

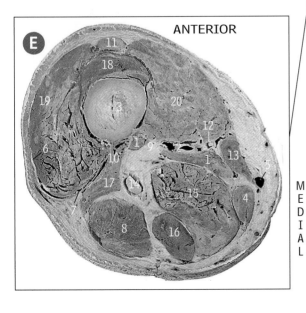

Right distal thigh

D axial MR image E cross-section

1 Adductor magnus
2 Femoral vessels
3 Femur
4 Gracilis
5 Great saphenous vein
6 Iliotibial tract
7 Lateral intermuscular septum
8 Long head of biceps femoris
9 Opening in adductor magnus
10 Profunda femoris vessels
11 Rectus femoris
12 Saphenous nerve
13 Sartorius
14 Sciatic nerve
15 Semimembranosus
16 Semitendinosus
17 Short head of biceps femoris
18 Vastus intermedius
19 Vastus lateralis
20 Vastus medialis

Femoropopliteal bypass, intermittent claudication, muscular transposition, rupture–quadriceps tendon, see pages 355–357.

Right hip joint

A *from the front and below* **B** *from the front and above*

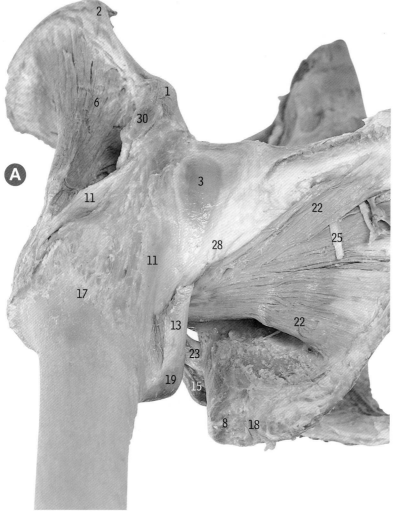

Some of the fibres of the ischiofemoral ligament help to form the zona orbicularis – circular fibres of the capsule that form a collar around the neck of the femur.

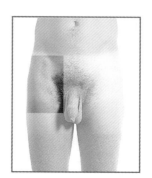

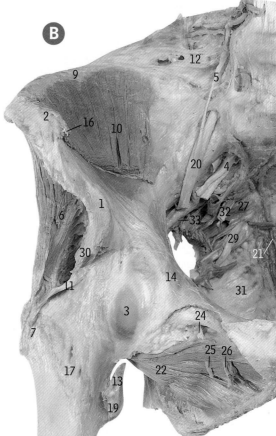

1 Anterior inferior iliac spine	**18** Ischial tuberosity
2 Anterior superior iliac spine	**19** Lesser trochanter
3 Bursa for psoas tendon	**20** Lumbosacral trunk
4 First sacral nerve root	**21** Median sacral artery
5 Fourth lumbar nerve root	**22** Obturator externus
6 Gluteus minimus muscle	**23** Obturator internus tendon
7 Greater trochanter	**24** Obturator nerve, anterior branch
8 Hamstring origin	**25** Obturator nerve, posterior branch
9 Iliac crest	**26** Obturator vessels
10 Iliacus muscle	**27** Piriformis muscle
11 Iliofemoral ligament	**28** Pubofemoral ligament
12 Iliolumbar ligament	**29** Pudendal nerve
13 Iliopsoas tendon	**30** Rectus femoris muscle
14 Iliopubic eminence	**31** Sacrospinous ligament
15 Inferior gemellus muscle	**32** Second sacral nerve root
16 Inguinal ligament	**33** Superior gluteal artery
17 Intertrochanteric line and capsule attachment	

Trendelenburg's sign, see pages 355–357.

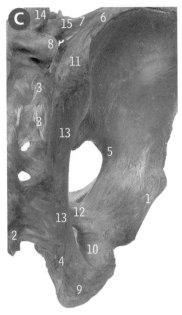

C Right vertebropelvic and sacro-iliac ligaments
from behind

1 Acetabular labrum
2 Coccyx
3 Dorsal sacro-iliac ligaments
4 Falciform process of sacrotuberous ligament
5 Greater sciatic notch
6 Iliac crest
7 Iliolumbar ligament
8 Inferior articular process of fifth lumbar vertebra
9 Ischial tuberosity
10 Lesser sciatic notch
11 Posterior superior iliac spine
12 Sacrospinous ligament and ischial spine
13 Sacrotuberous ligament
14 Superior articular process of fifth lumbar vertebra
15 Transverse process of fifth lumbar vertebra

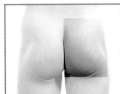

D Right hip joint with femur removed
from the right

The femur has been disarticulated from the acetabulum and removed, leaving the acetabular labrum, transverse ligament and the ligament teres. Refer to page 293, B, for bony attachments and musculature.

1 Acetabular fossa
2 Acetabular labrum
3 Adductor brevis muscle
4 Adductor longus muscle
5 Adductor magnus muscle
6 Articular surface
7 Gracilis muscle
8 Ligamentum teres femoris
9 Obturator externus muscle
10 Pectineus muscle
11 Quadratus femoris muscle
12 Reflected head of rectus femoris muscle
13 Straight head of rectus femoris muscle
14 Transverse ligament

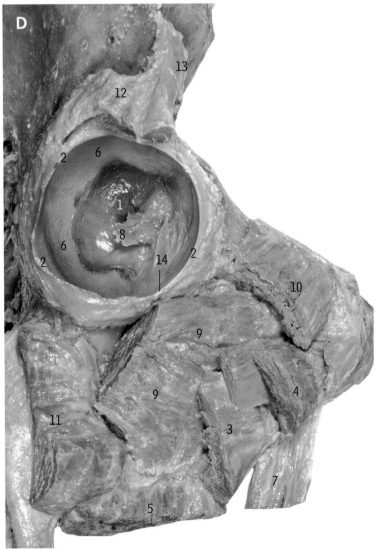

Avascular necrosis of the head of the femur, see pages 355–357.

Left hip joint Ⓐ *coronal section, from the front*

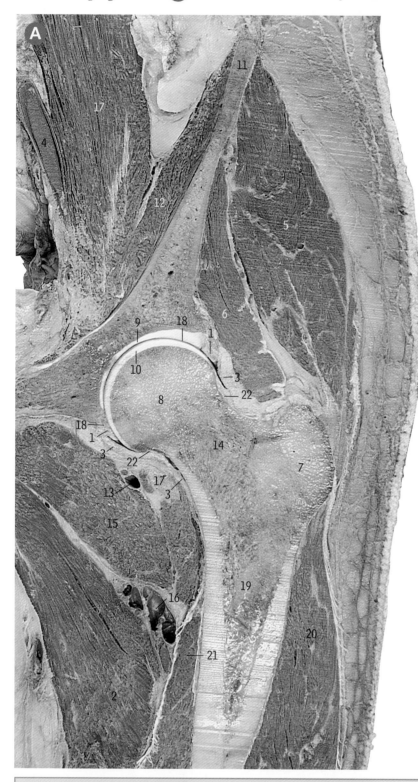

The section has almost passed through the centre of the head (8) of the femur and the centre of the greater trochanter (7). Above the neck of the femur (14), gluteus minimus (6) with gluteus medius (5) above it run down to their attachments to the greater trochanter (7), while below the neck the tendon of psoas major (17) and muscle fibres of iliacus (12) pass backwards towards the lesser trochanter. The circular fibres of the zona orbicularis (22) constrict the capsule (3) around the intracapsular part of the neck of the femur.

1 Acetabular labrum
2 Adductor longus
3 Capsule of hip joint
4 External iliac artery
5 Gluteus medius
6 Gluteus minimus
7 Greater trochanter
8 Head of femur
9 Hyaline cartilage of acetabulum
10 Hyaline cartilage of head
11 Iliac crest
12 Iliacus
13 Medial circumflex femoral vessels
14 Neck of femur
15 Pectineus
16 Profunda femoris vessels
17 Psoas major
18 Rim of acetabulum
19 Shaft of femur
20 Vastus lateralis
21 Vastus medialis
22 Zona orbicularis of capsule

*Contrast outlines the joint cavity
** Ligamentum teres

Ⓑ *coronal MR, arthrogram*

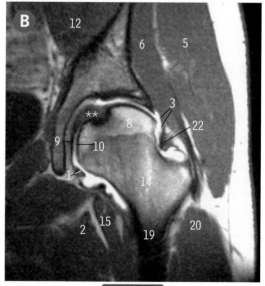

The convergence of gluteus medius and minimus (5 and 6) on to the greater trochanter is well displayed in this section. These muscles are classified as abductors of the femur at the hip joint, but their more important action is in walking, where they act to prevent adduction – preventing the pelvis from tilting to the opposite side when the opposite limb is off the ground (see Trendelenburg's sign, page 357).

Total hip replacement surgery, see pages 355–357.

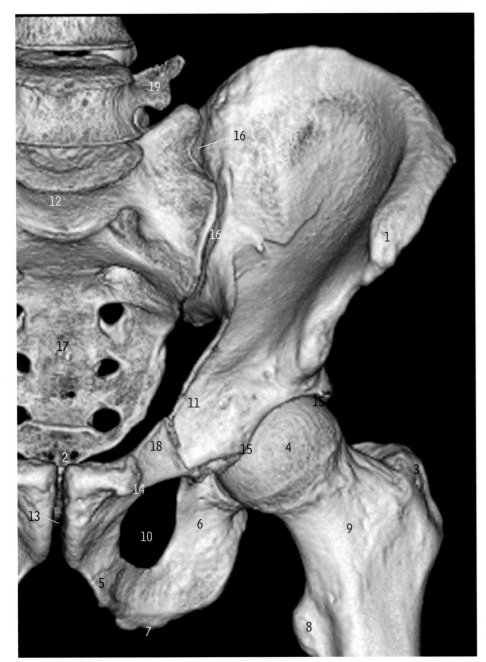

C Left hip and sacro-iliac joint

3D surface rendered 64 slice CT

1 Anterior superior iliac spine
2 First coccygeal vertebra
3 Greater trochanter of femur
4 Head of femur
5 Inferior pubic ramus
6 Ischium
7 Ischial tuberosity
8 Lesser trochanter of femur
9 Neck of femur
10 Obturator foramen
11 Pectineal line
12 Promontory of sacrum
13 Pubic symphysis
14 Pubic tubercle
15 Rim of acetabulum
16 Sacro-iliac joint
17 Sacrum
18 Superior pubic ramus
19 Transverse process of fifth lumbar vertebra

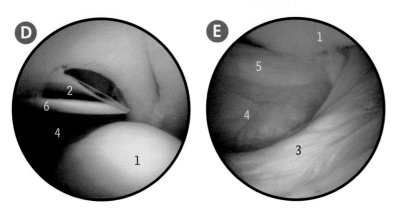

Hip joint

D E arthroscopic views

1 Femoral head
2 Irrigation needle
3 Ligamentum teres
4 Synovium
5 Transverse ligament
6 Zona orbicularis

Posterior hip dislocation, see pages 355–357.

Right knee
partially flexed

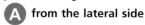

A from the lateral side

B from the medial side

1 Biceps femoris
2 Common peroneal (fibular) nerve
3 Head of fibula
4 Iliotibial tract
5 Lateral head of gastrocnemius
6 Margin of condyle of femur
7 Margin of condyle of tibia
8 Patella
9 Patellar ligament
10 Popliteal fossa
11 Semimembranosus
12 Semitendinosus
13 Tuberosity of tibia
14 Vastus medialis

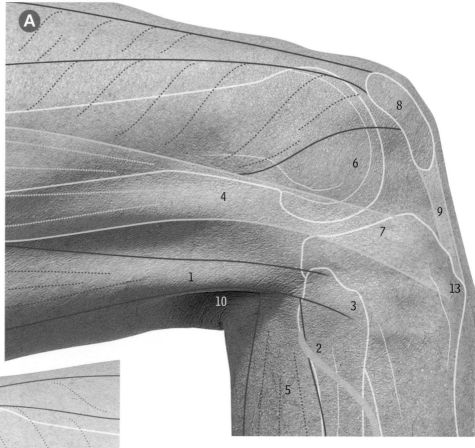

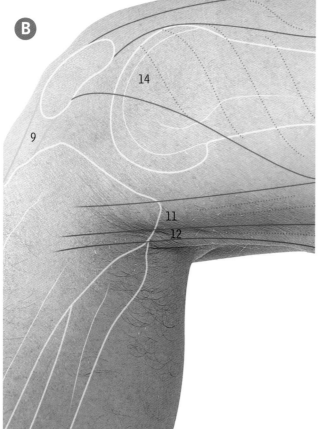

Behind the knee on the lateral side, the rounded tendon of biceps femoris (1) can be felt easily, with the broad strap-like iliotibial tract (4) in front of it, with a furrow between them. On the medial side, two tendons can be felt – the narrow rounded semitendinosus (12) just behind the broader semimembranosus (11). At the front, the patellar ligament (9) keeps the patella (8) at a constant distance from the tibial tuberosity (13), while at the side the adjacent margins of the femoral and tibial condyles (6 and 7) can be palpated.

Genu valgum, genu varum patellar tendon reflex, see pages 355–357.

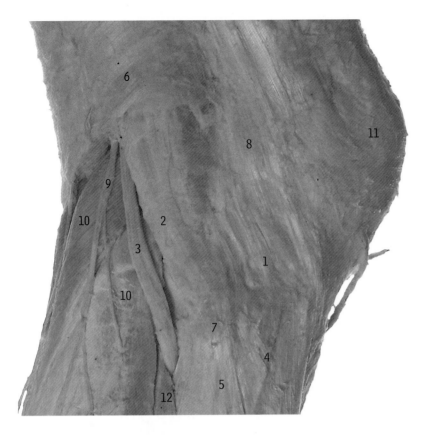

C Right knee
superficial dissection, from the lateral side

The fascia behind biceps femoris (2) has been removed to show the common peroneal (fibular) nerve (3) passing downwards immediately behind the tendon, and then running between the adjacent borders of soleus (12) and peroneus (fibularis) longus (5), under cover of which it lies against the neck of the fibula. Minor superficial vessels and nerves have been removed.

1 Attachment of iliotibial tract to tibia
2 Biceps femoris
3 Common peroneal (fibular) nerve
4 Deep fascia overlying extensor muscles
5 Deep fascia overlying peroneus (fibularis) longus
6 Fascia lata
7 Head of fibula
8 Iliotibial tract
9 Lateral cutaneous nerve of calf
10 Lateral head of gastrocnemius
11 Patella
12 Soleus

The iliotibial tract (8) is the thickened lateral part of the fascia lata (6). At its upper part, the tensor fasciae latae and most of gluteus maximus are inserted into it.

Its subcutaneous position and contact with the neck of the fibula make the common peroneal (fibular) nerve (3) the most commonly injured nerve in the lower limb.

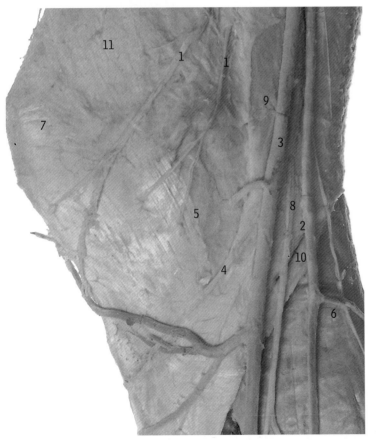

D Right knee
superficial dissection, from the medial side

The great saphenous vein (3) runs upwards about a hand's breadth behind the medial border of the patella (7). The saphenous nerve (8) becomes superficial between the tendons of sartorius (9) and gracilis (2), and its infrapatellar branch (4) curls forwards a little below the upper margin of the tibial condyle.

1 Branches of medial femoral cutaneous nerve
2 Gracilis
3 Great saphenous vein
4 Infrapatellar branch of saphenous nerve
5 Level of margin of medial condyle of tibia
6 Medial head of gastrocnemius
7 Patella
8 Saphenous nerve
9 Sartorius
10 Semitendinosus
11 Vastus medialis

Right popliteal fossa *superficial dissections*

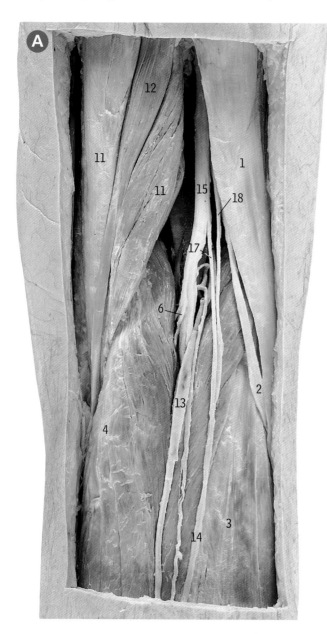

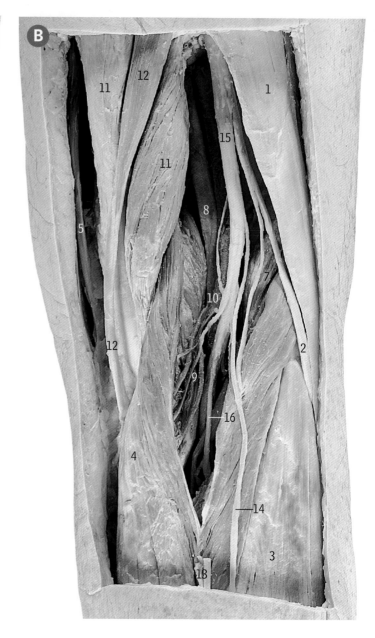

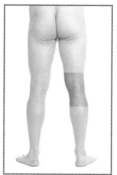

A Skin and fascia forming the roof of the diamond-shaped popliteal fossa and the fat within it have been removed but the small saphenous vein which pierces the fascia has been preserved. A high (proximal) union of the lateral and medial sural cutaneous nerves places the sural nerve in this field.

B Heads of gastrocnemius have been separated to show deeper structures.

1 Biceps femoris
2 Common peroneal (fibular) nerve
3 Gastrocnemius, lateral head
4 Gastrocnemius, medial head
5 Gracilis
6 Nerve to medial head of gastrocnemius
7 Plantaris
8 Popliteal artery
9 Popliteal vascular branches to gastrocnemius
10 Popliteal vein
11 Semimembranosus
12 Semitendinosus
13 Small saphenous vein
14 Sural nerve
15 Tibial nerve
16 Tibial nerve, muscular branches
17 Sural nerve, branch from tibial
18 Sural nerve, branch from common peroneal (fibular)

Popliteal fossa *progressive dissections*

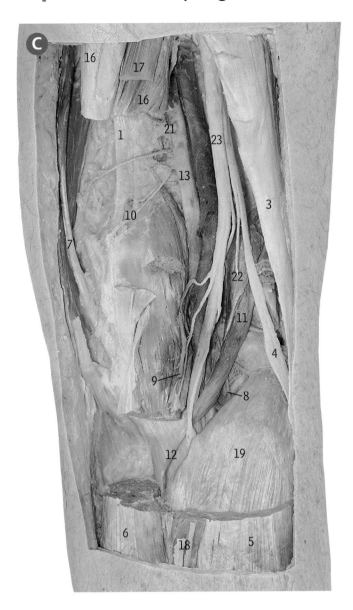

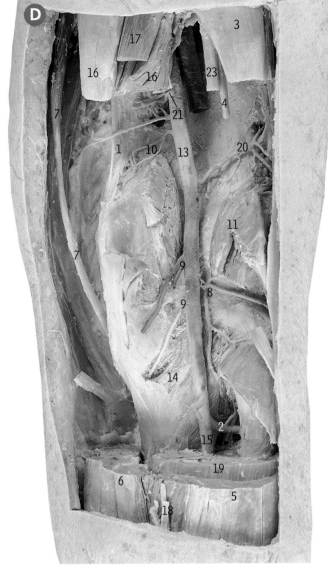

 C Removal of semitendinosus, semimembranosus and most of the origins of the gastrocnemius reveals plantaris and branches of the deeply situated popliteal artery and soleus.

D Removal of the muscular boundaries of the popliteal fossa shows the popliteal artery, its genicular anastomoses and its terminal branches, the anterior and posterior tibial arteries.

1 Adductor magnus	**13** Popliteal artery
2 Anterior tibial artery	**14** Popliteus
3 Biceps femoris	**15** Posterior tibial artery
4 Common peroneal (fibular) nerve	**16** Semimembranosus
5 Gastrocnemius, lateral head	**17** Semitendinosus
6 Gastrocnemius, medial head	**18** Short saphenous vein
7 Gracilis	**19** Soleus
8 Inferior lateral genicular artery	**20** Superior lateral genicular artery
9 Inferior medial genicular artery	**21** Superior medial genicular artery
10 Middle genicular artery	**22** Sural nerve
11 Plantaris muscle	**23** Tibial nerve
12 Plantaris tendon	

Popliteal (Baker's) cyst, popliteal artery aneurysm, sural nerve graft, see pages 355–357.

Left knee joint *ligaments*

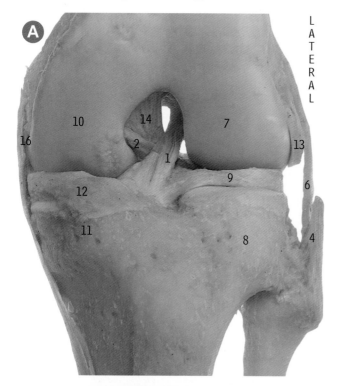

L A T E R A L

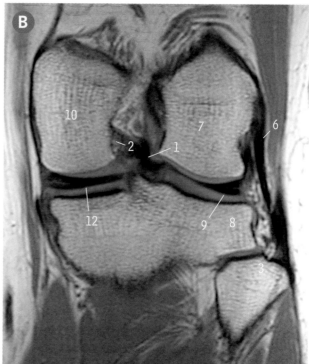

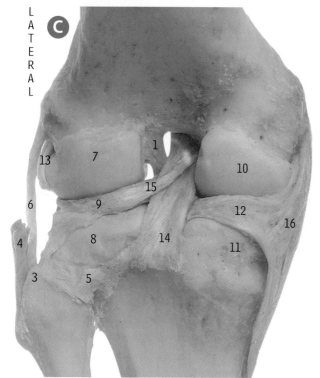

L A T E R A L

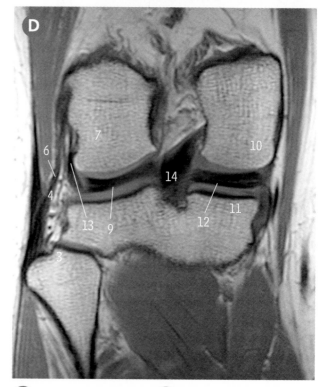

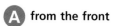
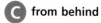

A from the front   **C** from behind

The capsule of the knee joint and all surrounding tissues have been removed, leaving only the ligaments of the joint, which is partially flexed.

B coronal MR image   **D** coronal MR image

1 Anterior cruciate ligament
2 Anterior meniscofemoral ligament
3 Apex of head of fibula
4 Biceps femoris tendon
5 Capsule of superior tibiofibular joint
6 Fibular (lateral) collateral ligament
7 Lateral condyle of femur
8 Lateral condyle of tibia

9 Lateral meniscus
10 Medial condyle of femur
11 Medial condyle of tibia
12 Medial meniscus
13 Popliteus tendon
14 Posterior cruciate ligament
15 Posterior meniscofemoral ligament
16 Tibial (medial) collateral ligament

The fibular collateral (lateral) ligament (A6) is a rounded cord about 5 cm long, passing from the lateral epicondyle of the femur to the head of the fibula just in front of its apex (C3), largely under cover of the tendon of biceps femoris (C4).

The medial meniscus is attached to the deep part of the tibial (medial) collateral ligament. This helps to anchor the meniscus but makes it liable to become trapped and torn by rotatory movements between the tibia and femur.

The lateral meniscus (A9) is not attached to the fibular (lateral) collateral ligament (A6), but is attached posteriorly to the popliteus muscle.

The tibial collateral (medial) ligament is a broad flat band about 12 cm long, passing from the medial epicondyle of the femur to the medial condyle of the tibia and an extensive area of the medial surface of the tibia below the condyle.

The cruciate ligaments are named from their attachments to the tibia.

The anterior cruciate ligament (A1) passes upwards, backwards and laterally to be attached to the medial side of the lateral condyle of the femur (C7).

The posterior cruciate ligament (C14) passes upwards, forwards and medially to be attached to the lateral surface of the medial condyle of the femur (A10).

Left knee tibial plateau *from above*

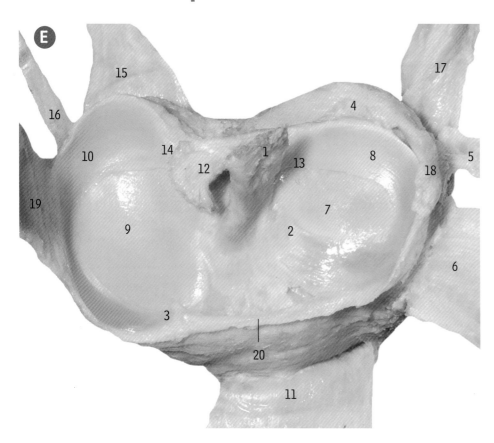

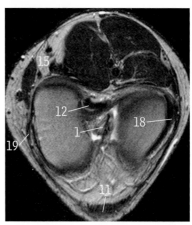

Axial MR, knee

1 Anterior cruciate ligament	**5** Fibular collateral ligament	**12** Posterior cruciate ligament	**17** Tendon of biceps femoris muscle
2 Anterior horn of lateral meniscus	**6** Iliotibial tract	**13** Posterior horn of lateral meniscus	**18** Tendon of popliteus muscle
3 Anterior horn of medial meniscus	**7** Lateral condyle of tibia	**14** Posterior horn of medial meniscus	**19** Tibial collateral ligament attachment to medial meniscus
4 Attachment of lateral meniscus to popliteus muscle	**8** Lateral meniscus	**15** Semimembranosus (tendon)	**20** Transverse ligament
	9 Medial condyle of tibia	**16** Semitendinosus (tendon)	
	10 Medial meniscus		
	11 Patellar ligament (tendon)		

Meniscal tears, rupture–anterior cruciate ligament, see pages 355–357.

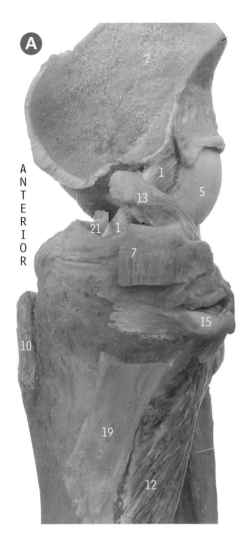

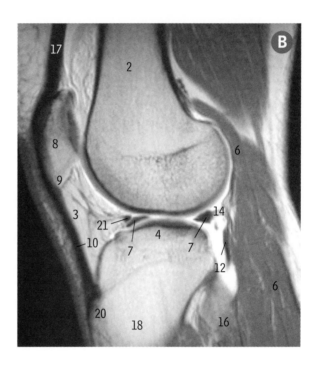

Right knee joint

A from the medial side with the medial femoral condyle removed

B sagittal MR image

Removal of the medial half of the lower end of the femur enables the X-shaped crossover of the cruciate ligaments to be seen; the anterior cruciate (1) is passing backwards and laterally, while the posterior cruciate (13) passes forwards and medially. The MR image in B shows the infrapatellar fat pad (3).

1 Anterior cruciate ligament	**8** Patella	**15** Semimembranosus
2 Femur	**9** Patellar apex	**16** Soleus
3 Infrapatellar fat pad (Hoffa)	**10** Patellar ligament (tendon)	**17** Tendon of quadriceps
4 Intercondylar notch	**11** Popliteal artery and vein	**18** Tibia
5 Lateral condyle of femur	**12** Popliteus	**19** Tibial (medial) collateral ligament
6 Lateral head of gastrocnemius muscle	**13** Posterior cruciate ligament	**20** Tibial tubercle
7 Lateral meniscus	**14** Posterior meniscofemoral ligament	**21** Transverse (intermeniscal) ligament

Left knee *arthroscopic views*

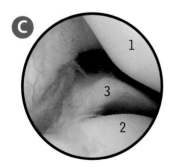

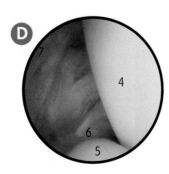

C anterolateral approach

D posteromedial approach

1 Lateral condyle of femur	**5** Medial meniscus
2 Lateral condyle of tibia	**6** Posterior cruciate ligament
3 Lateral meniscus	**7** Posterior part of capsule
4 Medial condyle of femur	

Rupture–posterior cruciate ligament, suprapatellar bursitis, see pages 355–357.

E

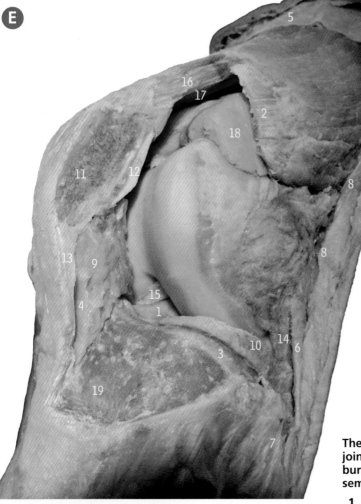

E Left knee joint
opened from the lateral side to reveal internal structures

1 Anterior cruciate ligament
2 Aponeurosis of vastus lateralis (cut edge)
3 Articular cartilage, tibial plateau
4 Deep infrapatellar bursa
5 Fascia lata (deep fascia)
6 Fibular collateral ligament
7 Head of fibula
8 Iliotibial tract (cut edge)
9 Infrapatellar fat pad (Hoffa)
10 Lateral meniscus
11 Patella
12 Patellar articular cartilage
13 Patellar ligament (tendon)
14 Popliteus tendon, attachment to lateral tibial epicondyle
15 Posterior cruciate ligament
16 Quadriceps tendon
17 Suprapatellar bursa
18 Suprapatellar fat pad
19 Tibial tuberosity

F Left knee joint
from the medial side, with synovial and bursal cavities injected

The resin injection has distended the synovial cavity of the joint (3) and extends into the suprapatellar bursa (10), the bursa round the popliteus tendon (2) and the semimembranosus bursa (9).

1 Articularis genu
2 Bursa of popliteus tendon
3 Capsule
4 Medial meniscus
5 Patella
6 Patellar ligament
7 Quadriceps tendon
8 Semimembranosus
9 Semimembranosus bursa
10 Suprapatellar bursa
11 Tibial (medial) collateral ligament

The suprapatellar bursa (F10) always communicates with the joint cavity. The bursa around the popliteus tendon (F2) usually does so. The semimembranosus bursa (F9) may do so.

F

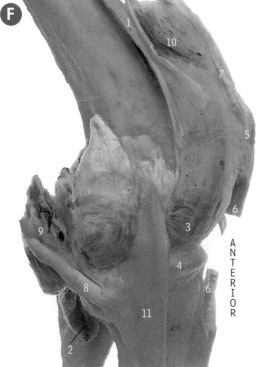

G Anterior cruciate ligament
anterior arthroscopic view

G

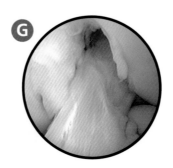

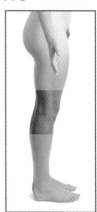

Knee joint aspiration and injection, lower limb bursitis, prepatellar bursitis, see pages 355–357.

Knee *radiographs and arthroscopic views*

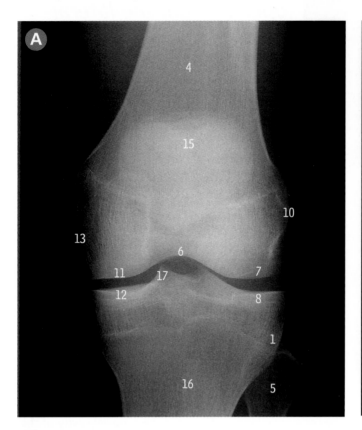

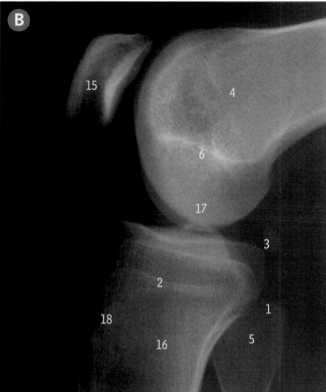

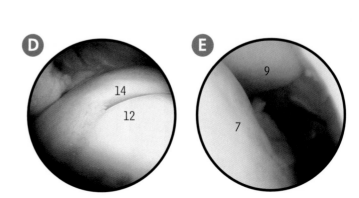

A from the front

B from the lateral side in partial flexion

C skyline view projection

D anterolateral approach

E lateral view of patella

In A, the shadow of the patella (15) is superimposed on that of the femur. The regular space between the condyles of the femur and tibia (7 and 8, 11 and 12) is due to the thickness of the hyaline cartilage on the articulating surface, with the menisci at the periphery. In C, with the knee flexed, the view should be compared with the bones seen on page 299, E, and the lateral edge of the patella (9) is seen in the arthroscopic view in E.

1	Apex (styloid process) of fibula	**10**	Lateral epicondyle of femur
2	Epiphysial line	**11**	Medial condyle of femur
3	Fabella	**12**	Medial condyle of tibia
4	Femur	**13**	Medial epicondyle of femur
5	Head of fibula	**14**	Medial meniscus
6	Intercondylar fossa	**15**	Patella
7	Lateral condyle of femur	**16**	Tibia
8	Lateral condyle of tibia	**17**	Tubercles of intercondylar eminence
9	Lateral edge of patella	**18**	Tuberosity of tibia

Knee joint replacement surgeries, see pages 355–357.

Ⓐ Left leg *from the front and lateral side*

1 Anterior tibial artery overlying interosseous membrane
2 Branch of deep peroneal (fibular) nerve to tibialis anterior
3 Deep peroneal (fibular) nerve
4 Extensor digitorum longus
5 Extensor hallucis longus
6 Head of fibula
7 Lateral branch of superficial peroneal (fibular) nerve

8 Medial branch of superficial peroneal (fibular) nerve
9 Peroneus (fibularis) longus
10 Recurrent branch of common peroneal (fibular) nerve
11 Superficial peroneal (fibular) nerve
12 Tibialis anterior and overlying fascia
13 Tuberosity of tibia and patellar ligament

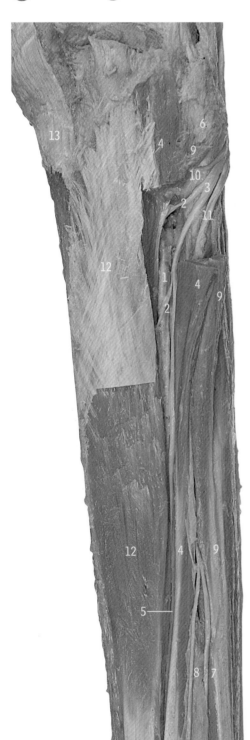

Ⓑ Left knee *from the lateral side to show common peroneal (fibular) nerve and articular branches*

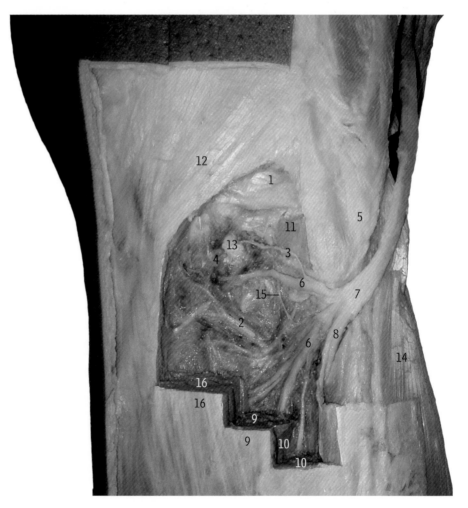

1 Anterior ligament of fibular head
2 Anterior tibial recurrent artery and vein
3 Articular branch from deep common peroneal (fibular) nerve
4 Articular vessels
5 Biceps femoris tendon
6 Common peroneal (fibular) nerve, deep branches
7 Common peroneal (fibular) nerve, overlying neck of fibula
8 Common peroneal (fibular) nerve, superficial branch

9 Extensor digitorum longus
10 Peroneus (fibularis) longus
11 Head of fibula
12 Iliotibial tract
13 Interosseous membrane
14 Lateral head, gastrocnemius muscle
15 Recurrent branch of deep peroneal (fibular) nerve
16 Tibialis anterior

Common peroneal (fibular) nerve paralysis, see pages 355–357.

Left knee and leg

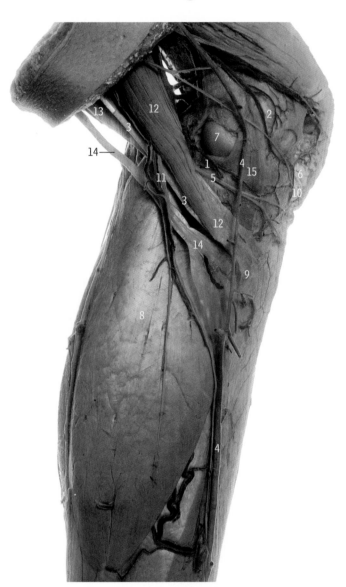

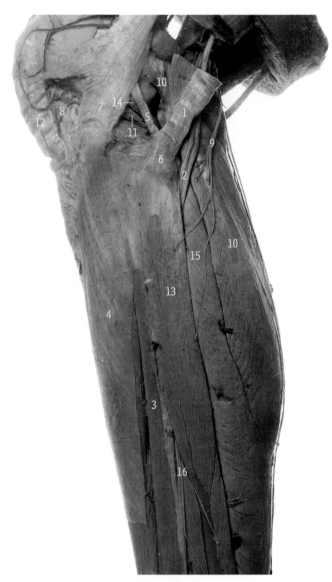

Left knee and leg Ⓐ *from the medial side and behind*

A small window has been cut in the capsule of the knee joint to show part of the medial condyle of the femur (7) and the medial meniscus (1).

1 Branch of saphenous artery overlying medial meniscus
2 Branches of superior medial genicular artery
3 Gracilis
4 Great saphenous vein
5 Infrapatellar branch of saphenous nerve
6 Infrapatellar fat pad
7 Medial condyle of femur (part of capsule removed)
8 Medial head of gastrocnemius
9 Medial surface of tibia
10 Patellar ligament
11 Saphenous nerve and artery
12 Sartorius
13 Semimembranosus
14 Semitendinosus
15 Tibial (medial) collateral ligament

Ⓑ *from the lateral side*

A small window has been cut in the capsule of the knee joint to show the tendon of popliteus (14) passing deep to the fibular (lateral) collateral ligament (5). The common peroneal (fibular) nerve (2) runs down behind biceps femoris (1) to pass through the gap between peroneus (fibularis) longus (13) and soleus (15). The superficial peroneal (fibular) nerve becomes superficial between peroneus (fibularis) longus (13) and extensor digitorum longus (3).

1 Biceps femoris
2 Common peroneal (fibular) nerve
3 Extensor digitorum longus
4 Fascia overlying tibialis anterior
5 Fibular (lateral) collateral ligament
6 Head of fibula
7 Iliotibial tract
8 Infrapatellar fat pad
9 Lateral cutaneous nerve of calf
10 Lateral head of gastrocnemius
11 Lateral meniscus
12 Patellar ligament
13 Peroneus (fibularis) longus
14 Popliteus
15 Soleus
16 Superficial peroneal (fibular) nerve

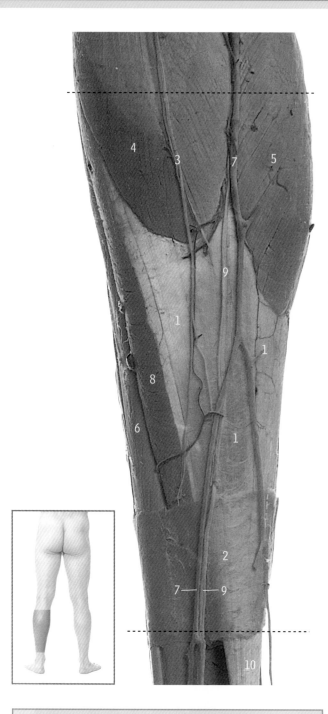

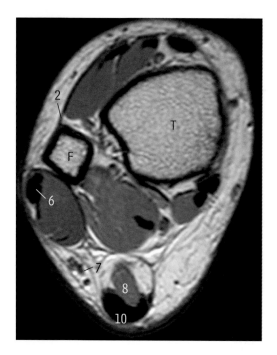

Axial T1w MR, calf

Axial T1w MR, lower leg

Below knee level, the great saphenous vein (A4) is accompanied by the saphenous nerve (A11).

In the calf, the small saphenous vein (C7) is accompanied by the sural nerve (C9).

Ⓒ Left calf
superficial dissection, from behind

1 Aponeurosis of gastrocnemius	**7** Small saphenous vein
2 Deep fascia	**8** Soleus
3 Lateral cutaneous nerve of calf	**9** Sural nerve
4 Lateral head of gastrocnemius	**10** Tendocalcaneus (Achilles
5 Medial head of gastrocnemius	tendon)
6 Peroneus (fibularis) longus	

Vein harvest for coronary artery bypass grafting (CABG), see pages 355–357.

Ⓐ Right leg *posterior view*

Ⓑ Right calf *including muscles, nerves and veins*

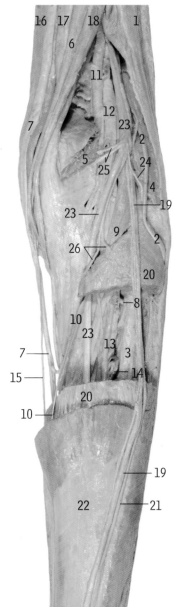

1. Biceps femoris muscle
2. Common peroneal (fibular) nerve
3. Fibula, posterior surface
4. Gastrocnemius muscle, lateral head
5. Gastrocnemius muscle, medial head
6. Gracilis muscle
7. Great saphenous vein
8. Peroneal (fibular) vein
9. Plantaris muscle
10. Plantaris tendon
11. Popliteal artery
12. Popliteal vein
13. Posterior tibial artery and vein
14. Posterior tibial artery and vein, soleal branches
15. Saphenous nerve
16. Sartorius muscle
17. Semimembranosus muscle
18. Semitendinosus muscle
19. Small saphenous veins, displaced laterally
20. Soleus muscle
21. Sural nerve, displaced laterally
22. Tendocalcaneus (formation)
23. Tibial nerve
24. Tibial nerve, muscular branches of lateral head of gastrocnemius
25. Tibial nerve, muscular branches of medial head of gastrocnemius
26. Tibial nerve, muscular branches of soleus

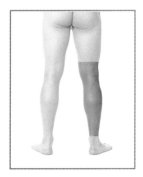

1. Biceps femoris muscle
2. Common peroneal (fibular) nerve
3. Gastrocnemius muscle, lateral head
4. Gastrocnemius muscle, medial head
5. Gracilis muscle
6. Gracilis tendon
7. Great saphenous vein
8. Lateral sural cutaneous nerve
9. Medial sural cutaneous nerve
10. Popliteal vein
11. Sartorius muscle
12. Semimembranosus muscle
13. Semitendinosus muscle
14. Small saphenous vein
15. Soleus muscle
16. Tendocalcaneus (Achilles)
17. Tendocalcaneus (formation)
18. Tibial nerve
19. Venous network, formation of small saphenous vein

Compartment syndrome, see pages 355–357.

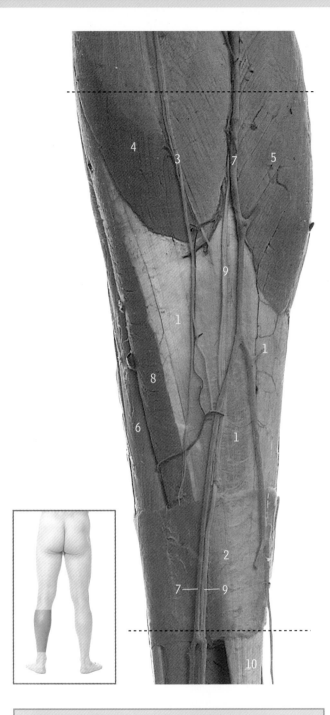

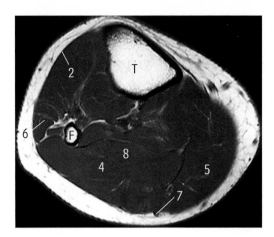

Axial T1w MR, calf

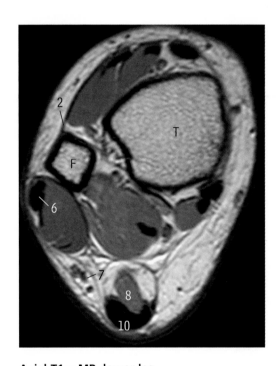

Axial T1w MR, lower leg

Below knee level, the great saphenous vein (A4) is accompanied by the saphenous nerve (A11).

In the calf, the small saphenous vein (C7) is accompanied by the sural nerve (C9).

C Left calf
superficial dissection, from behind

1 Aponeurosis of gastrocnemius
2 Deep fascia
3 Lateral cutaneous nerve of calf
4 Lateral head of gastrocnemius
5 Medial head of gastrocnemius
6 Peroneus (fibularis) longus
7 Small saphenous vein
8 Soleus
9 Sural nerve
10 Tendocalcaneus (Achilles tendon)

Vein harvest for coronary artery bypass grafting (CABG), see pages 355–357.

Left leg and ankle *superficial veins and nerves*

A *from the medial side* **B** *from behind*

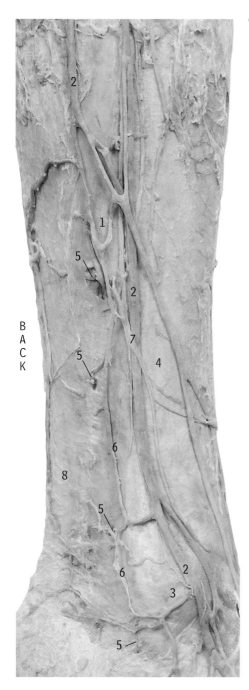

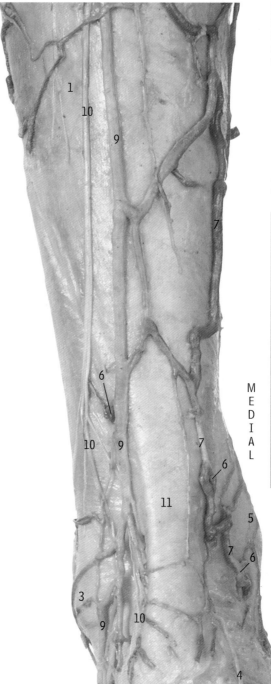

In B (a different specimen from that in A), the posterior arch vein (7) on the medial side is large and becoming varicose.

1 Deep fascia
2 Fibrofatty tissue of heel
3 Lateral malleolus
4 Medial calcanean nerve
5 Medial malleolus
6 Perforating vein
7 Posterior arch vein
8 Posterior surface of calcaneus
9 Small saphenous vein
10 Sural nerve
11 Tendocalcaneus (under fascia)

The perforating veins are communications between the superficial veins (outside the deep fascia) and the deep veins (inside the fascia). The commonest sites for them are just behind the tibia, behind the fibula and in the adductor canal. These communicating vessels possess valves which direct the blood flow from superficial to deep; venous return from the limb is then brought about by the pumping action of the deep muscles (which are all below the deep fascia). If the valves become incompetent or the deep veins blocked, pressure in the superficial veins increases and they become varicose (dilated and tortuous) (see page 357).

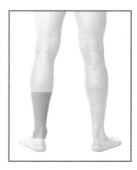

1 Deep fascia over soleus
2 Great saphenous vein
3 Medial malleolus
4 Medial (subcutaneous) surface of tibia
5 Perforating veins
6 Posterior arch vein
7 Saphenous nerve
8 Tendocalcaneus (Achilles tendon)

 Ankle ulceration from varicose veins, deep vein thrombosis (DVT), see pages 355–357.

Ⓐ Left popliteal fossa and proximal calf   Ⓑ Left distal calf and ankle

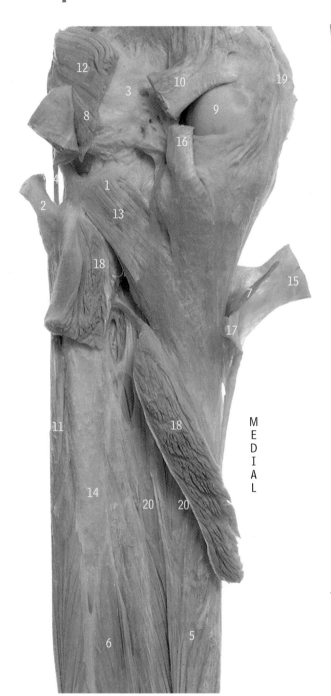

1 Fascia overlying tibialis posterior
2 Flexor digitorum longus
3 Flexor hallucis longus
4 Lateral malleolus
5 Medial malleolus
6 Part of flexor retinaculum
7 Peroneus (fibularis) brevis
8 Peroneus (fibularis) longus
9 Position of posterior tibial vessels and tibial nerve
10 Posterior talofibular ligament
11 Superior peroneal (fibular) retinaculum
12 Tendocalcaneus (Achilles tendon)
13 Tibialis posterior

Axial MR, just above ankle joint

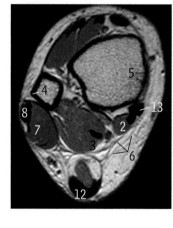

1 Attachment of popliteus to lateral meniscus
2 Biceps femoris
3 Capsule of knee joint
4 Fibular (lateral) collateral ligament
5 Flexor digitorum longus
6 Flexor hallucis longus
7 Gracilis
8 Lateral head of gastrocnemius
9 Medial condyle of femur
10 Medial head of gastrocnemius

11 Peroneus (fibularis) longus
12 Plantaris
13 Popliteus
14 Posterior surface of fibula (soleus removed)
15 Sartorius
16 Semimembranosus
17 Semitendinosus
18 Soleus
19 Tibial (medial) collateral ligament
20 Tibialis posterior

Tibialis posterior tendonitis, see pages 355–357.

A Right leg *posterior view*

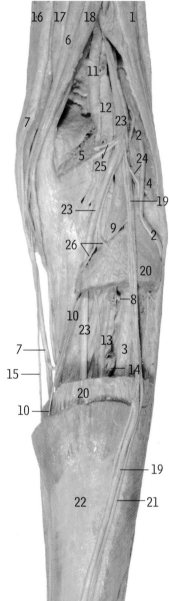

B Right calf *including muscles, nerves and veins*

1	Biceps femoris muscle
2	Common peroneal (fibular) nerve
3	Fibula, posterior surface
4	Gastrocnemius muscle, lateral head
5	Gastrocnemius muscle, medial head
6	Gracilis muscle
7	Great saphenous vein
8	Peroneal (fibular) vein
9	Plantaris muscle
10	Plantaris tendon
11	Popliteal artery
12	Popliteal vein
13	Posterior tibial artery and vein
14	Posterior tibial artery and vein, soleal branches
15	Saphenous nerve
16	Sartorius muscle
17	Semimembranosus muscle
18	Semitendinosus muscle
19	Small saphenous veins, displaced laterally
20	Soleus muscle
21	Sural nerve, displaced laterally
22	Tendocalcaneus (formation)
23	Tibial nerve
24	Tibial nerve, muscular branches of lateral head of gastrocnemius
25	Tibial nerve, muscular branches of medial head of gastrocnemius
26	Tibial nerve, muscular branches of soleus

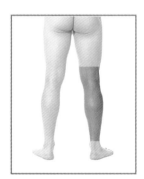

1	Biceps femoris muscle	**10**	Popliteal vein
2	Common peroneal (fibular) nerve	**11**	Sartorius muscle
		12	Semimembranosus muscle
3	Gastrocnemius muscle, lateral head	**13**	Semitendinosus muscle
		14	Small saphenous vein
4	Gastrocnemius muscle, medial head	**15**	Soleus muscle
		16	Tendocalcaneus (Achilles)
5	Gracilis muscle	**17**	Tendocalcaneus (formation)
6	Gracilis tendon	**18**	Tibial nerve
7	Great saphenous vein	**19**	Venous network, formation of small saphenous vein
8	Lateral sural cutaneous nerve		
9	Medial sural cutaneous nerve		

Compartment syndrome, see pages 355–357.

C Right lower leg
deep dissection

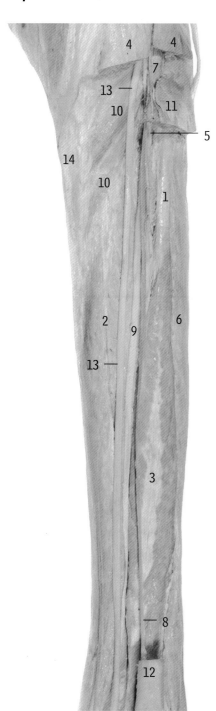

D Popliteal angiogram

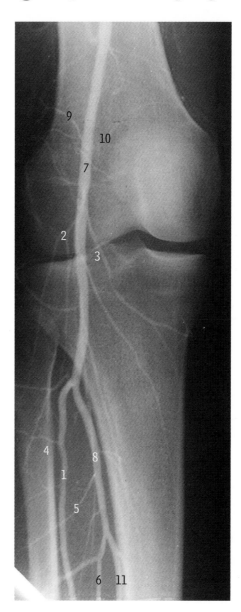

1 Anterior tibial artery
2 Inferior lateral genicular artery
3 Inferior medial genicular artery
4 Muscular branches of anterior tibial artery
5 Muscular branches of tibioperoneal trunk
6 Peroneal (fibular) artery
7 Popliteal artery
8 Tibioperoneal trunk
9 Superior lateral genicular artery
10 Superior medial genicular artery
11 Posterior tibial artery

1 Fibula (posterior surface)
2 Flexor digitorum longus muscle
3 Flexor hallucis longus muscle
4 Gastrocnemius muscle
5 Peroneal (fibular) artery
6 Peroneus (fibularis) longus
7 Plantaris muscle
8 Plantaris tendon
9 Posterior tibial artery
10 Popliteus muscle
11 Soleus muscle
12 Tendocalcaneus (Achilles)
13 Tibial nerve
14 Tibia, posterior surface

Ⓐ Right ankle and foot

from the lateral side

1 Extensor digitorum brevis
2 Lateral malleolus
3 Peroneus (fibularis) longus and brevis
4 Small saphenous vein
5 Tendocalcaneus (Achilles tendon)
6 Tibialis anterior
7 Tuberosity of base of fifth metatarsal

The great saphenous vein (B7) runs upwards in front of the medial malleolus (B9).

The small saphenous vein (A4) runs upwards behind the lateral malleolus (A2).

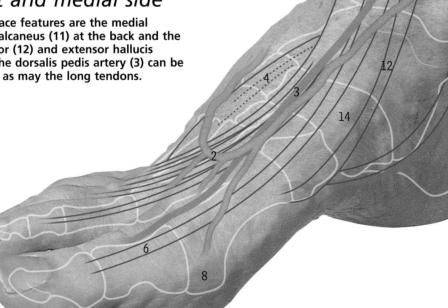

Ⓑ Right ankle and foot

from the front and medial side

The most prominent surface features are the medial malleolus (9), the tendocalcaneus (11) at the back and the tendons of tibialis anterior (12) and extensor hallucis longus (6) at the front. The dorsalis pedis artery (3) can be palpated where labelled, as may the long tendons.

1 Calcaneus
2 Dorsal venous arch
3 Dorsalis pedis artery
4 Extensor digitorum brevis
5 Extensor digitorum longus
6 Extensor hallucis longus
7 Great saphenous vein
8 Head of first metatarsal
9 Medial malleolus
10 Posterior tibial artery
11 Tendocalcaneus (Achilles tendon)
12 Tibialis anterior
13 Tibialis posterior
14 Tuberosity of navicular

Achilles tendon tendocalcaneus reflex (ankle jerk), rupture – Achilles tendon, talipes equinovarus (club foot), venous cutdown, see pages 355–357.

C Right ankle and foot *from the lateral side*

Fascia has been removed but the thickenings that form the superior and inferior extensor retinacula (16 and 6) and the superior and inferior peroneal (fibular) retinacula (17 and 7) have been preserved. The synovial sheaths of tendons have been emphasised by blue tissue.

1 Abductor digiti minimi
2 Dorsal digital expansion
3 Extensor digitorum brevis
4 Extensor digitorum longus
5 Extensor hallucis longus
6 Inferior extensor retinaculum
7 Inferior peroneal (fibular) retinaculum
8 Lateral malleolus
9 Lateral surface of calcaneus
10 Medial and lateral branches of superficial peroneal (fibular) nerve

11 Peroneus (fibularis) brevis
12 Peroneus (fibularis) longus
13 Peroneus (fibularis) tertius
14 Soleus
15 Subcutaneous area of fibula
16 Superior extensor retinaculum
17 Superior peroneal (fibular) retinaculum
18 Sural nerve
19 Tendocalcaneus (Achilles tendon)
20 Tibialis anterior

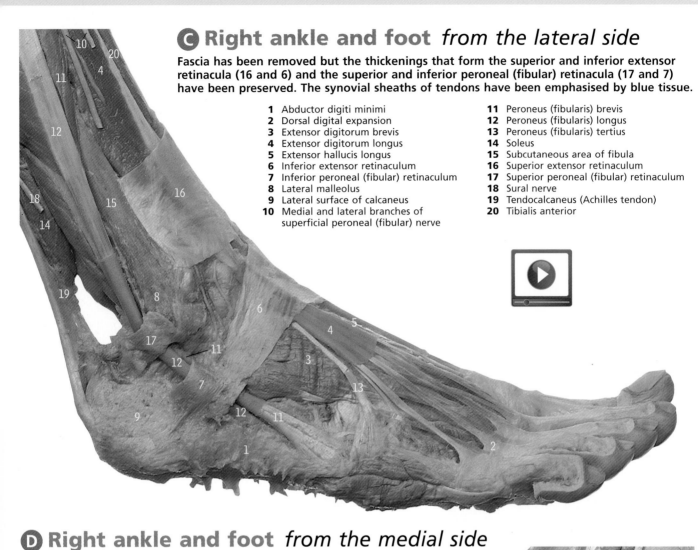

D Right ankle and foot *from the medial side*

1 Abductor hallucis
2 Extensor hallucis longus
3 Flexor digitorum longus
4 Flexor hallucis longus
5 Flexor retinaculum
6 Inferior extensor retinaculum (lower band)
7 Inferior extensor retinaculum (upper band)
8 Medial calcanean nerve
9 Medial malleolus

10 Medial surface of tibia
11 Plantaris tendon
12 Posterior surface of calcaneus
13 Posterior tibial artery and venae comitantes
14 Soleus
15 Tendocalcaneus (Achilles tendon)
16 Tibial nerve
17 Tibialis anterior
18 Tibialis posterior

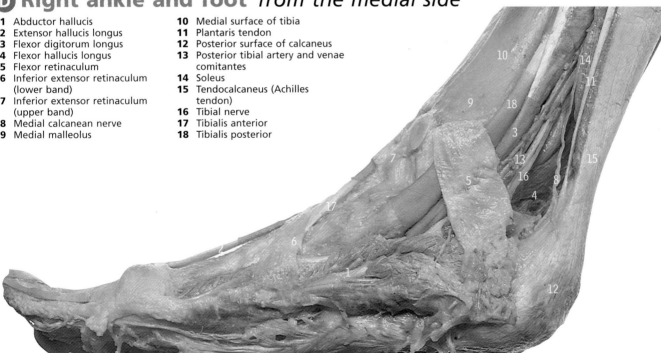

Ankle arthroscopy, digital abnormalities, see pages 355–357.

A Right lower leg and ankle
from the medial side and behind

B Right ankle
from the medial side

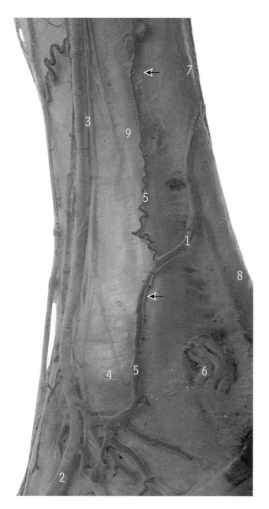

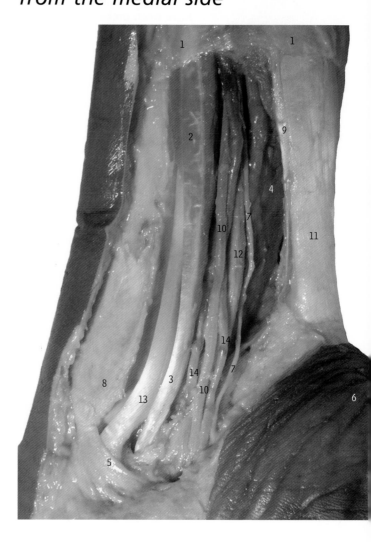

The deep fascia remains intact apart from a small window cut to show the position of the posterior tibial vessels and tibial nerve (6). The great saphenous vein (3) runs upwards in front of the medial malleolus (4) with the posterior arch vein (5) behind it. The arrows indicate common levels for perforating veins (page 340, A5 and B6).

1 Communication with small saphenous vein
2 Dorsal venous arch
3 Great saphenous vein and saphenous nerve
4 Medial malleolus
5 Posterior arch vein
6 Posterior tibial vessels and tibial nerve
7 Small saphenous vein
8 Tendocalcaneus (Achilles tendon)
9 Tibialis posterior and flexor digitorum longus underlying deep fascia

1 Deep fascia of calf
2 Flexor digitorum longus
3 Flexor digitorum longus, tendon
4 Flexor hallucis longus
5 Flexor retinaculum
6 Heel
7 Medial calcanean nerve
8 Medial malleolus, tibia
9 Plantaris tendon
10 Posterior tibial artery
11 Tendocalcaneus (Achilles tendon)
12 Tibial nerve
13 Tibialis posterior tendon
14 Venae comitantes of posterior tibial artery

The deep veins of the calf, deep to and within soleus, are sites for potentially dangerous venous thrombosis (see page 355).

 Ulceration of the foot, varicose veins, see pages 355–357.

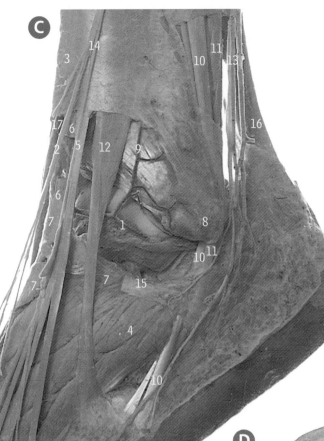

C Left ankle and foot
from the front and lateral side

The foot is plantar flexed and part of the capsule of the ankle joint has been removed to show the talus (1). The tendons of peroneus (fibularis) tertius (12) and extensor digitorum longus (5) lie superficial to extensor digitorum brevis (4). The sural nerve and small saphenous vein (13) pass behind the lateral malleolus (8).

1 Anterior lateral malleolar artery overlying talus (ankle joint capsule removed)
2 Anterior tibial vessels and deep peroneal (fibular) nerve
3 Deep fascia forming superior extensor retinaculum
4 Extensor digitorum brevis
5 Extensor digitorum longus
6 Extensor hallucis longus
7 Inferior extensor retinaculum (partly removed)
8 Lateral malleolus
9 Perforating branch of peroneal (fibular) artery
10 Peroneus (fibularis) brevis
11 Peroneus (fibularis) longus
12 Peroneus (fibularis) tertius
13 Small saphenous vein and sural nerve
14 Superficial peroneal (fibular) nerve
15 Tarsal sinus
16 Tendocalcaneus (Achilles tendon)
17 Tibialis anterior

Left ankle

D cross-section
E axial MR image

This section, looking down from above, emphasises the positions of tendons, vessels and nerves in the ankle region. The talus (18) is in the centre, with the medial malleolus (9) on the left of the picture and the lateral malleolus (8) on the right. The great saphenous vein (7) and saphenous nerve (15) are in front of the medial malleolus, with the tendon of tibialis posterior (22) immediately behind it. The small saphenous vein (16) and the sural nerve (17) are behind the lateral malleolus, with the tendons of peroneus (fibularis) longus (11) and peroneus (fibularis) brevis (10) intervening. At the front of the ankle, the dorsalis pedis vessels (2) and deep peroneal (fibular) nerve (1) are between the tendons of extensor hallucis longus (4) and extensor digitorum longus (3). Behind the medial malleolus (9) and tibialis posterior (22), the posterior tibial vessels (14) and tibial nerve (20) are between the tendons of flexor digitorum longus (5) and flexor hallucis longus (6).

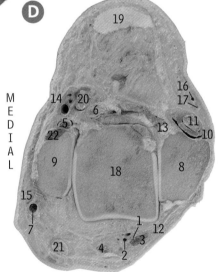

1 Deep peroneal (fibular) nerve
2 Dorsalis pedis artery and venae comitantes
3 Extensor digitorum longus
4 Extensor hallucis longus
5 Flexor digitorum longus
6 Flexor hallucis longus
7 Great saphenous vein
8 Lateral malleolus of fibula
9 Medial malleolus of tibia
10 Peroneus (fibularis) brevis
11 Peroneus (fibularis) longus
12 Peroneus (fibularis) tertius
13 Posterior talofibular ligament
14 Posterior tibial artery and venae comitantes
15 Saphenous nerve
16 Small saphenous vein
17 Sural nerve
18 Talus
19 Tendocalcaneus (Achilles tendon)
20 Tibial nerve
21 Tibialis anterior
22 Tibialis posterior

Charcot foot, see pages 355–357.

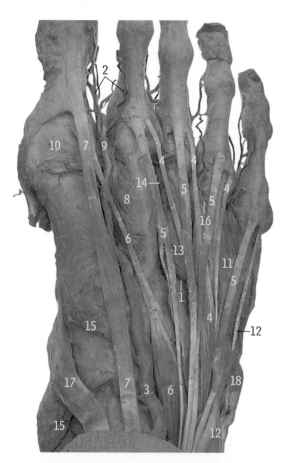

Ⓐ Dorsum of the right foot

1	Arcuate artery	**11**	Fourth dorsal interosseous
2	Digital arteries	**12**	Peroneus (fibularis) tertius
3	Dorsalis pedis artery	**13**	Second dorsal interosseous
4	Extensor digitorum brevis	**14**	Second dorsal metatarsal artery
5	Extensor digitorum longus	**15**	Tarsal arteries
6	Extensor hallucis brevis	**16**	Third dorsal interosseous
7	Extensor hallucis longus	**17**	Tibialis anterior
8	First dorsal interosseous	**18**	Tuberosity of base of fifth
9	First dorsal metatarsal artery		metatarsal and peroneus (fibularis)
10	First metatarsophalangeal joint		brevis

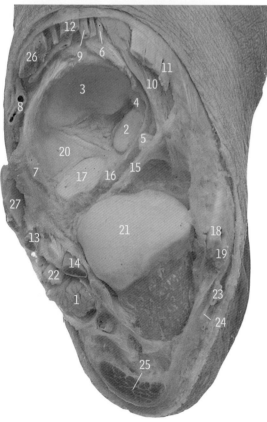

Ⓑ Right talocalcanean and talocalcaneonavicular joints

The talus has been removed to show the articular surfaces of the calcaneus (21, 17 and 2), navicular (3) and plantar calcaneonavicular (spring) ligament (20).

1	Abductor hallucis	**15**	Inferior extensor retinaculum
2	Anterior articular surface on calcaneus for talus	**16**	Interosseous talocalcanean ligament
3	Articular surface on navicular for talus	**17**	Middle articular surface on calcaneus for talus
4	Calcaneonavicular part of bifurcate ligament	**18**	Peroneus (fibularis) brevis
5	Cervical ligament	**19**	Peroneus (fibularis) longus
6	Deep peroneal (fibular) nerve	**20**	Plantar calcaneonavicular (spring) ligament
7	Deltoid ligament	**21**	Posterior articular surface on calcaneus for talus
8	Dorsal venous arch	**22**	Posterior tibial vessels and medial and lateral plantar nerves
9	Dorsalis pedis artery and vena comitans	**23**	Small saphenous vein
10	Extensor digitorum brevis	**24**	Sural nerve
11	Extensor digitorum longus	**25**	Tendocalcaneus (Achilles tendon)
12	Extensor hallucis longus	**26**	Tibialis anterior
13	Flexor digitorum longus	**27**	Tibialis posterior
14	Flexor hallucis longus		

Clinicians sometimes use the term subtalar joint as a combined name for both the talocalcanean joint and the talocalcanean part of the talocalcaneonavicular joint, because it is at both these joints beneath the talus that most of the movements of inversion and eversion of the foot occur, on the axis of the cervical ligament.

Ankle block, malignant melanoma, tarsal tunnel syndrome, see pages 355–357.

Left ankle and foot *ligaments*

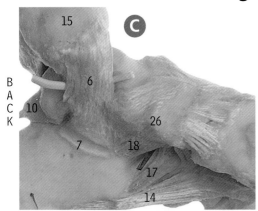

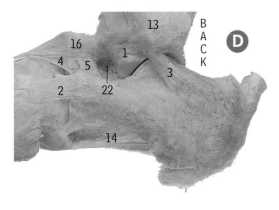

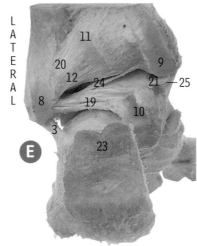

C from the medial side

D from the lateral side

E from behind

In C, the marker below the medial malleolus (15) passes between the superficial and deep parts of the deltoid ligament (6). The marker below the tuberosity of the navicular (26) passes between the plantar calcaneonavicular (spring) and calcaneocuboid (short plantar) ligaments (18 and 17).

1 Anterior talofibular ligament
2 Calcaneocuboid part of bifurcate ligament
3 Calcaneofibular ligament
4 Calcaneonavicular part of bifurcate ligament
5 Cervical ligament
6 Deltoid ligament
7 Groove below sustentaculum tali for flexor hallucis longus
8 Groove on lateral malleolus for peroneus (fibularis) brevis
9 Groove on medial malleolus for tibialis posterior
10 Groove on talus for flexor hallucis longus
11 Groove on tibia for flexor hallucis longus
12 Inferior transverse ligament
13 Lateral malleolus
14 Long plantar ligament
15 Medial malleolus
16 Neck of talus
17 Plantar calcaneocuboid (short plantar) ligament
18 Plantar calcaneonavicular (spring) ligament
19 Posterior talofibular ligament
20 Posterior tibiofibular ligament
21 Posterior tibiotalar part of deltoid ligament
22 Tarsal sinus
23 Tendocalcaneus (Achilles tendon)
24 Tibial slip of posterior talofibular ligament
25 Tibiocalcanean part of deltoid ligament
26 Tuberosity of navicular

F Left foot *sagittal section, from the right*

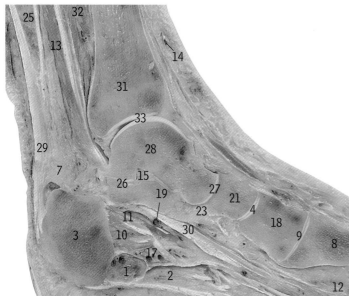

1 Abductor digiti minimi
2 Abductor hallucis
3 Calcaneus
4 Cuneonavicular joint
5 Distal phalanx
6 Extensor hallucis longus
7 Fat pad
8 First metatarsal
9 First tarsometatarsal (cuneometatarsal) joint
10 Flexor accessorius
11 Flexor digitorum brevis
12 Flexor hallucis brevis
13 Flexor hallucis longus
14 Great saphenous vein
15 Interosseous talocalcanean ligament
16 Interphalangeal joint
17 Lateral plantar nerve and vessels
18 Medial cuneiform
19 Medial plantar artery
20 Metatarsophalangeal joint of great toe
21 Navicular
22 Plantar aponeurosis
23 Plantar calcaneonavicular (spring) ligament
24 Proximal phalanx
25 Soleus muscle
26 Talocalcanean (subtalar) joint
27 Talonavicular part of talocalcaneonavicular joint
28 Talus
29 Tendocalcaneus (Achilles tendon)
30 Tendon of flexor hallucis
31 Tibia
32 Tibialis posterior muscle
33 Tibiotalar part of ankle joint

Sprained ankle, see pages 355–357.

Sole of the left foot

A *plantar aponeurosis* **B** *superficial neuromuscular layer*

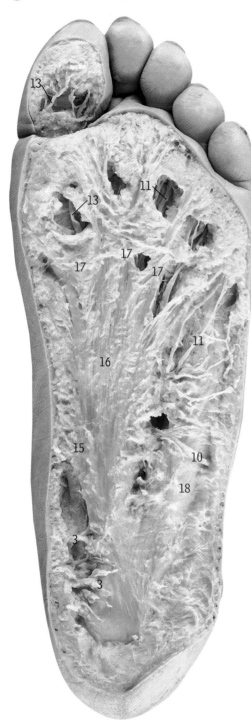

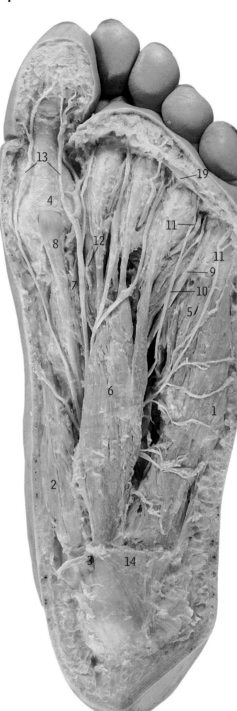

1	Abductor digiti minimi
2	Abductor hallucis
3	Calcaneal neurovascular bundle
4	Fibrous flexor sheath
5	Flexor digiti minimi brevis
6	Flexor digitorum brevis
7	Flexor hallucis brevis
8	Flexor hallucis longus
9	Lateral plantar artery
10	Lateral plantar nerve
11	Lateral plantar nerve, digital branches
12	Lumbrical
13	Medial plantar nerve, digital branches
14	Plantar aponeurosis
15	Plantar aponeurosis, overlying abductor hallucis
16	Plantar aponeurosis, overlying flexor digitorum brevis
17	Plantar aponeurosis, digital slips
18	Plantar aponeurosis, overlying abductor digiti minimi
19	Superficial transverse metatarsal ligament

Removal of the plantar skin reveals the plantar aponeurosis with thick central and digital slips and thin lateral and medial parts.

Deep to the plantar aponeurosis lie the superficial plantar nerves, arteries and muscles.

Flat foot (pes planus), plantar fasciitis, see pages 355–357.

Sole of the left foot

C *after removal of flexor digitorum brevis*
D *after removal of flexor digitorum longus*

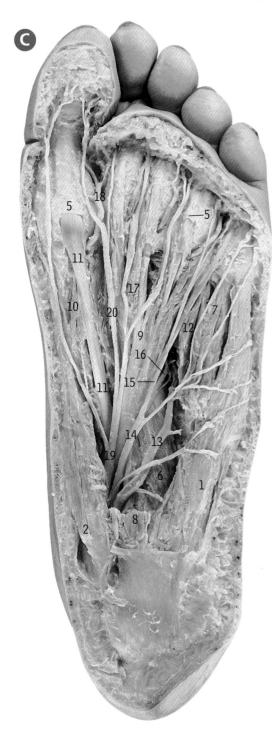

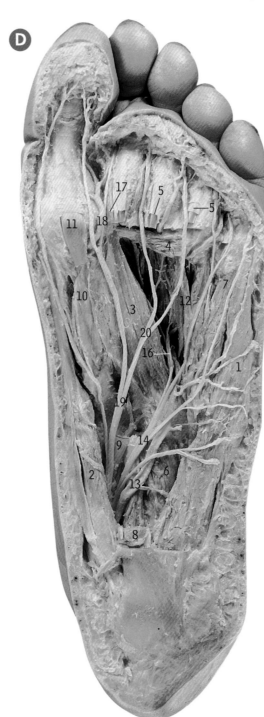

1 Abductor digiti minimi
2 Abductor hallucis
3 Adductor hallucis, oblique head
4 Adductor hallucis, transverse head
5 Fibrous sheath, flexors
6 Flexor accessorius (quadratus plantae)
7 Flexor digiti minimi brevis
8 Flexor digitorum brevis (cut)
9 Flexor digitorum longus
10 Flexor hallucis brevis
11 Flexor hallucis longus
12 Interossei
13 Lateral plantar artery
14 Lateral plantar nerve
15 Lateral plantar nerve, common digital branch
16 Lateral plantar nerve, deep branch
17 Lumbrical
18 Medial plantar artery
19 Medial plantar nerve
20 Medial plantar nerve, common digital branch

Extensor plantar response–Babinski sign, see pages 355–357.

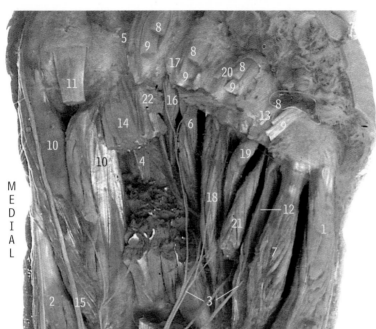

Ⓐ Sole of the left foot

deep muscles, interossei

1 Abductor digiti minimi
2 Abductor hallucis
3 Branches of deep branch of lateral plantar nerve
4 First dorsal interosseous
5 First lumbrical
6 First plantar interosseous
7 Flexor digiti minimi brevis
8 Flexor digitorum brevis
9 Flexor digitorum longus
10 Flexor hallucis brevis
11 Flexor hallucis longus
12 Fourth dorsal interosseous
13 Fourth lumbrical

14 Oblique head of adductor hallucis
15 Plantar digital nerve of great toe
16 Second dorsal interosseous
17 Second lumbrical
18 Second plantar interosseous
19 Third dorsal interosseous
20 Third lumbrical
21 Third plantar interosseous
22 Transverse head of adductor hallucis

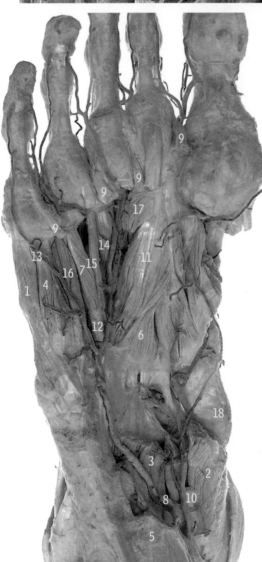

Ⓑ Sole of the right foot

plantar arch

Most of the flexor muscles and tendons have been removed to show the lateral plantar artery (8) crossing flexor accessorius (quadratus plantae) (3) to become the plantar arch (12) which would lie deep to the flexor tendons.

1 Abductor digiti minimi
2 Abductor hallucis
3 Flexor accessorius (quadratus plantae)
4 Flexor digiti minimi brevis
5 Flexor digitorum brevis
6 Flexor hallucis brevis
7 Fourth dorsal interosseous
8 Lateral plantar artery
9 Lumbrical

10 Medial plantar artery and nerve
11 Oblique head of adductor hallucis
12 Plantar arch
13 Plantar digital artery
14 Plantar metatarsal artery
15 Second plantar interosseous
16 Third plantar interosseous
17 Transverse head of adductor hallucis
18 Tuberosity of navicular

Sole of the left foot **C** *ligaments and tendons* **D** *ligaments*

C

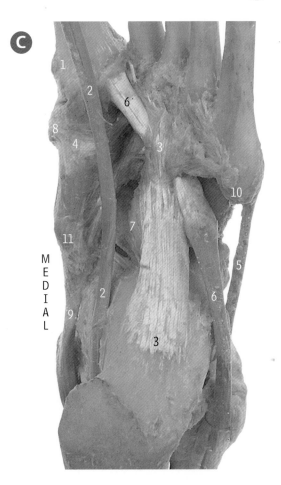

M
E
D
I
A
L

D

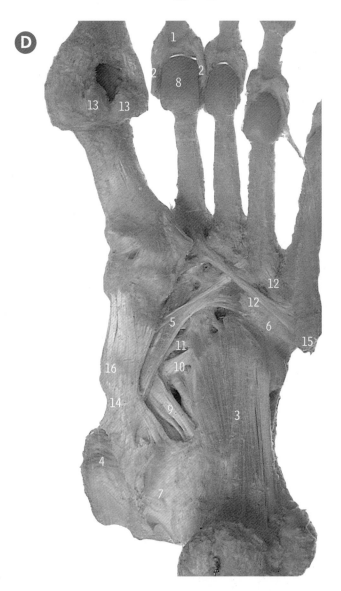

The anterior end of the long plantar ligament (3) forms with the groove of the cuboid (D6) a tunnel for the peroneus (fibularis) longus tendon (6) which runs to the medial cuneiform (4) and the base of the first metatarsal (1).

1 Base of first metatarsal
2 Flexor hallucis longus
3 Long plantar ligament
4 Medial cuneiform
5 Peroneus (fibularis) brevis
6 Peroneus (fibularis) longus
7 Plantar calcaneocuboid (short plantar) ligament
8 Tibialis anterior
9 Tibialis posterior
10 Tuberosity of base of fifth metatarsal
11 Tuberosity of navicular

The plantar calcaneonavicular ligament (D9), commonly called the spring ligament, is one of the most important in the foot. It stretches between the sustentaculum tali (D7) and the tuberosity of the navicular (D16), blending on its medial side with the deltoid ligament of the ankle joint and supporting the upper surface part of the head of the talus.

The anterior end of the long plantar ligament (3) has been removed to show the groove for peroneus (fibularis) longus on the cuboid (6).

1 Base of proximal phalanx
2 Collateral ligament of metatarsophalangeal joint
3 Deep fibres of long plantar ligament
4 Deltoid ligament
5 Fibrous slip from tibialis posterior
6 Groove on cuboid for peroneus (fibularis) longus
7 Groove on sustentaculum tali for flexor hallucis longus
8 Head of second metatarsal
9 Plantar calcaneonavicular (spring) ligament
10 Plantar cuboideonavicular ligament
11 Plantar cuneonavicular ligament
12 Plantar metatarsal ligament
13 Sesamoid bone
14 Tibialis posterior
15 Tuberosity of base of fifth metatarsal
16 Tuberosity of navicular

Ankle A *anteroposterior projection* B *lateral projection*

1 Calcaneus
2 Cuboid
3 Fibula
4 Head of talus
5 Lateral cuneiform
6 Lateral malleolus of fibula
7 Posterior talar process
8 Medial malleolus of tibia
9 Medial tubercle of talus
10 Navicular
11 Region of inferior tibiofibular joint
12 Sustentaculum tali of calcaneus
13 Talus
14 Tibia
15 Tuberosity of base of fifth metatarsal

* The side view in B shows a small calcaneal spur.

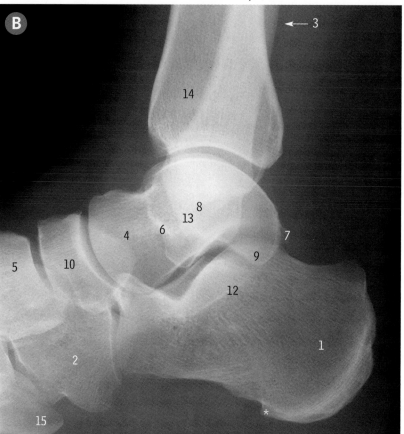

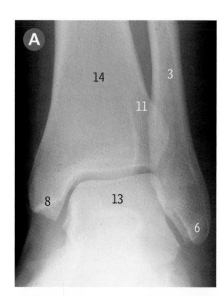

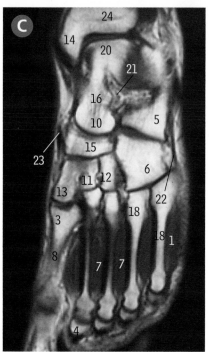

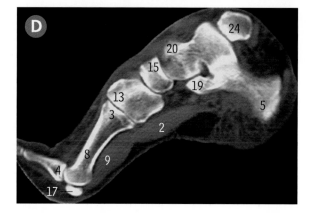

Foot

C *long axis MR image*

D *sagittal CT through hallux*

1 Abductor digiti minimi
2 Abductor hallucis
3 Base of metatarsal
4 Base of proximal phalanx
5 Calcaneus
6 Cuboid
7 Dorsal interossei muscle
8 First metatarsal
9 Flexor digitorum brevis
10 Head of talus
11 Intermediate cuneiform
12 Lateral cuneiform
13 Medial cuneiform

14 Medial malleolus
15 Navicular
16 Neck of talus
17 Sesamoid bone in flexor hallucis brevis
18 Shaft of metatarsal
19 Sustentaculum tali of calcaneus
20 Talus
21 Tarsal sinus (talocalcaneal cervical ligament)
22 Tendon of peroneus (fibularis) brevis muscle
23 Tendon of tibialis anterior
24 Tibia

Pott's and other fractures of the ankle, see pages 355–357.

Lower limb

Clinical thumbnails, see website for details and further clinical images to download into your own notes.

Achilles tendon tendocalcaneus reflex (ankle jerk)

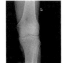
Ankle arthroscopy

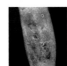
Ankle block

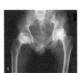
Ankle ulceration from varicose veins

Avascular necrosis of the head of the femur

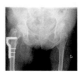
Avulsion fractures

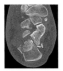
Bipartite patella

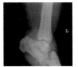
Calcaneal fracture

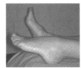
Charcot foot

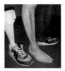
Common peroneal (fibular) nerve paralysis

Compartment syndrome

Deep vein thrombosis (DVT)

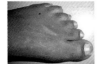
Digital abnormalities

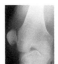
Dislocation of the patella

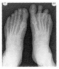
Dislocation of the toe

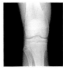
Exostoses femoral spurs

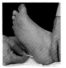
Extensor plantar response – Babinski sign

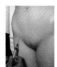
Femoral artery puncture

Femoral nerve paralysis

Femoropopliteal bypass

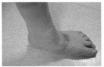
Flat foot (pes planus)

Fracture – femoral neck

Fracture – femoral shaft

Genu valgum, genu varum

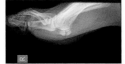
Hallux sesamoid fracture

Hallux valgus

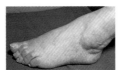
Hammer toe

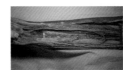
Intermittent claudication

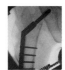
Intertrochanteric fracture – femur

Intramuscular injection – gluteal region

Knee joint aspiration and injection

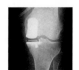
Knee joint replacement surgeries

Lower limb bursitis

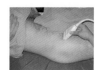
Lumbar plexus block

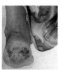
Malignant melanoma

Meniscal tears

Meralgia paraesthetica

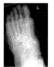
Metatarsal fractures

Muscular transposition

Obturator nerve paralysis

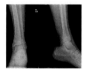
Os trigonum

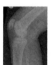
Osgood–Schlatter's disease

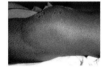
Patellar fracture

Patellar tendon reflex

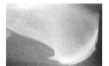
Plantar fasciitis

Popliteal artery aneurysm

Popliteal (Baker's) cyst

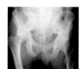
Posterior hip dislocation

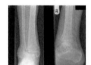
Pott's and other fractures of the ankle

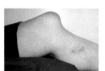
Prepatellar bursitis

Rupture – Achilles tendon

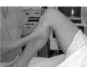
Rupture – anterior cruciate ligament

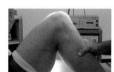
Rupture – posterior cruciate ligament

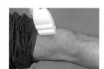
Rupture – quadriceps tendon

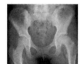
Slipped upper femoral epiphysis

Sprained ankle

Suprapatellar bursitis

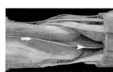
Sural nerve graft

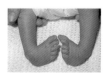
Talipes equinovarus (club foot)

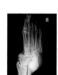
Tarsal dislocations

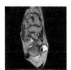

Tarsal
tunnel
syndrome

Tibial
fractures

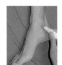

Tibialis
posterior
tendonitis

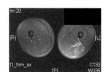

Torn hamstrings

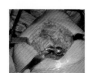

Total hip
replacement
surgery

Trendelenburg's
sign

Ulceration of
the leg

Varicella-zoster
virus infection –
lower limb

Varicose
veins

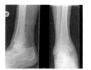

Vein harvest for
coronary artery
bypass grafting
(CABG)

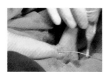

Venous
cutdown

Lymphatics

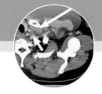
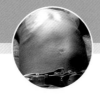

Lymphatic system

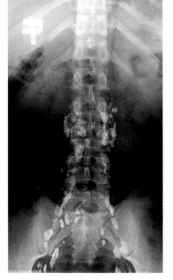

Lumbar spine - AP phase 2

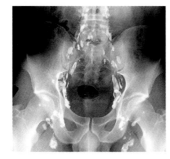

Pelvis - AP phase 2, NB nodes

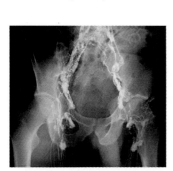

Pelvis - AP phase 1, NB vessels

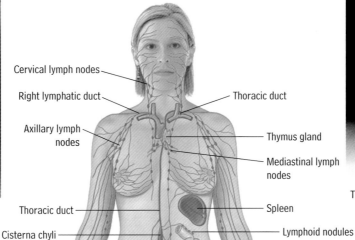

Cervical lymph nodes

Right lymphatic duct

Axillary lymph nodes

Thoracic duct

Cisterna chyli

Inguinal lymph nodes

Thoracic duct

Thymus gland

Mediastinal lymph nodes

Spleen

Lymphoid nodules of intestine

Lumbar lymph nodes

Iliac lymph nodes

Bone marrow

Thoracic duct termination in neck

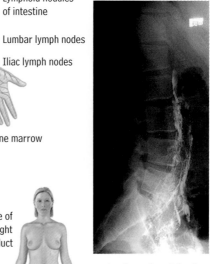

Lumbar spine - lateral phase 1, NB vessels

Drainage of the right lymphatic duct

Drainage of the thoracic duct

The lymphangiograms shown on this page are rarely performed clinically due to advances in CT scanning; however they do illustrate perfectly the detailed anatomy. Phase 1 images are taken on day one and best show the vessels whereas phase 2 are taken at about 48 hours and best image the lymph nodes.

Lymphatic system–methylene blue test, see page 369.

Ⓐ Thymus

lying in the superior and anterior mediastinum as seen through a split-sternal approach

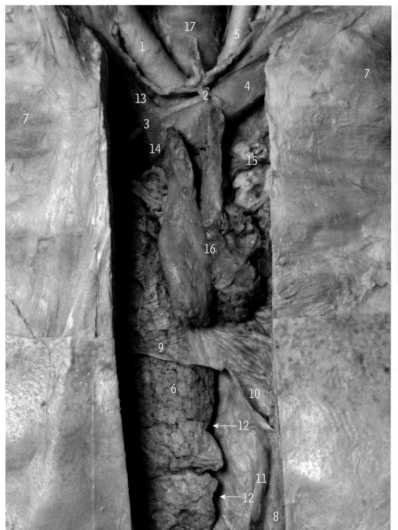

Ⓑ Chest radiograph of a child

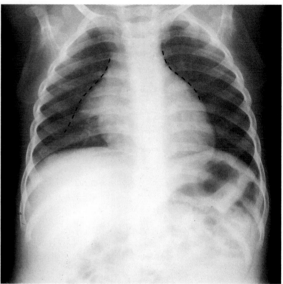

Child's thymus can normally be seen under the age of 2 on a plain chest radiograph, appearing as a spinnaker sail (sail sign), as outlined by the interrupted line.

Ⓒ Palatine tonsils

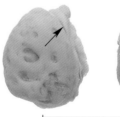

2 cm

The palatine tonsils (commonly referred to as 'the tonsils') are masses of lymphoid tissue that are frequently enlarged in childhood but become much reduced in size in later life. Together with the lymphoid tissue in the posterior part of the tongue (lingual tonsil) and in the posterior wall of the nasopharynx (pharyngeal tonsil) and the tubal tonsil they form a protective 'ring' of lymphoid tissue (Waldeyer's ring) at the upper end of the respiratory and alimentary tracts.

The pits on the medial surfaces of these operation specimens from a child aged 14 years are the openings of the tonsillar crypts. The arrows indicate the intratonsillar clefts (the remains of the embryonic second pharyngeal pouch).

1 Brachiocephalic trunk (artery)	**5** Left common carotid artery	**10** Pleura (cut edge of left sac)	**15** Thymic vein draining into internal thoracic vein
2 Inferior thyroid vein	**6** Lung, upper lobe right	**11** Pleura (cut edge of right sac)	**16** Thymus gland (bilobed)
3 Internal thoracic vein, right	**7** Pectoralis major	**12** Pleural cavity	**17** Trachea
4 Left brachiocephalic vein	**8** Pericardium, fibrous	**13** Right brachiocephalic vein	
	9 Pleura	**14** Superior vena cava	

Thymus, tonsillitis, see page 369.

A Neck dissection *termination of the thoracic duct into the left subclavian vein in the root of neck – as seen from left side*

SUPERIOR

RIGHT/ANTERIOR

LEFT/POSTERIOR

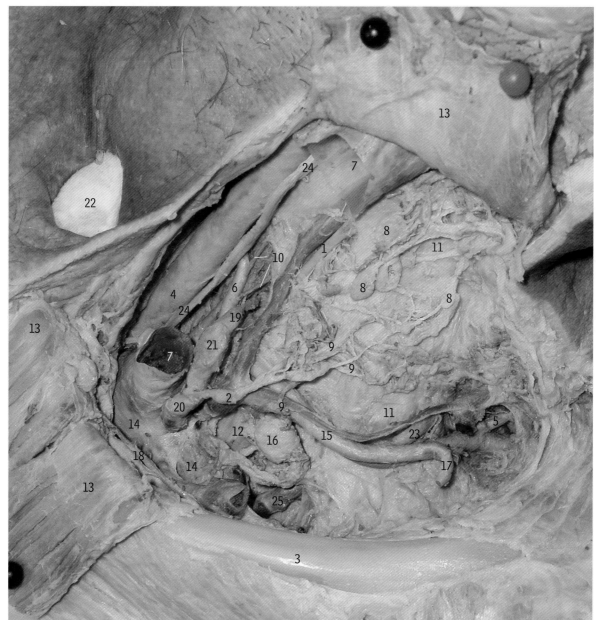

INFERIOR

1 Ascending cervical artery and vein	**10** Muscular arterial branches to longus colli	**18** Thoraco-acromial artery, clavicular branch
2 Cervical lymphatic trunk	**11** Prevertebral fascia	**19** Thoracic duct
3 Clavicle (left)	**12** Scalenus anterior	**20** Thoracic duct, termination
4 Common carotid artery	**13** Sternocleidomastoid (reflected and pinned)	**21** Thoracic duct, ampulla
5 Dorsal scapular artery		**22** Tracheostomy site (midline)
6 Inferior thyroid artery	**14** Subclavian vein	**23** Transverse cervical artery and vein
7 Internal jugular vein	**15** Superficial cervical artery	**24** Vagus nerve
8 Lymph nodes, deep cervical chain	**16** Supraclavicular node (Virchow – enlarged)	**25** Vertebral vein
9 Lymph vessel from node to cervical trunk	**17** Suprascapular artery	

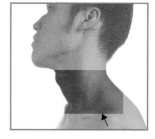

A Thoracic duct
cervical part

B First day lymphangiogram

C Lymphangio-gram of thorax

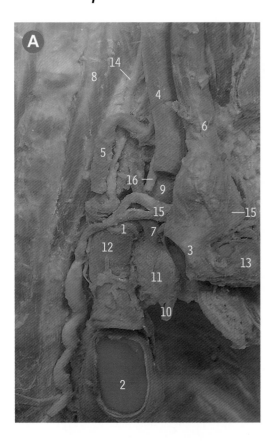

In this deep dissection of the left side of the root of the neck and upper thorax, the internal jugular vein (6) joins the subclavian vein (13) to form the left brachiocephalic vein (3). The thoracic duct (15) is double for a short distance just before passing in front of the vertebral artery (9) and behind the common carotid artery (4), whose lower end has been cut away to show the duct). The duct then runs behind the internal jugular vein (6) before draining into the junction of that vein with the subclavian vein (13).

1 Ansa subclavia
2 Arch of aorta
3 Brachiocephalic vein
4 Common carotid artery
5 Inferior thyroid artery
6 Internal jugular vein
7 Internal thoracic artery
8 Longus colli
9 Origin of vertebral artery
10 Phrenic nerve
11 Pleura
12 Subclavian artery
13 Subclavian vein
14 Sympathetic trunk
15 Thoracic duct
16 Vagus nerve

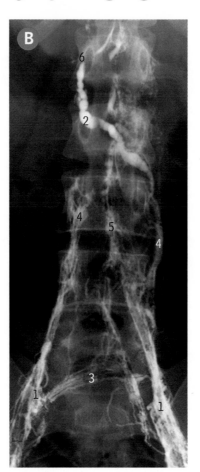

1 Common iliac vessels
2 Cisterna chyli
3 Lumbar crossover
4 Para-aortic vessels
5 Pre-aortic vessels
6 Thoracic duct

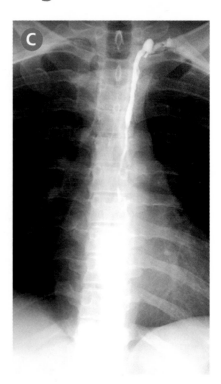

Thoracic duct termination in neck
(Here seen superiorly at venous confluence of left internal jugular vein and subclavian vein.)

Virchow's node, see page 369.

Right axilla with moderate lymphadenopathy

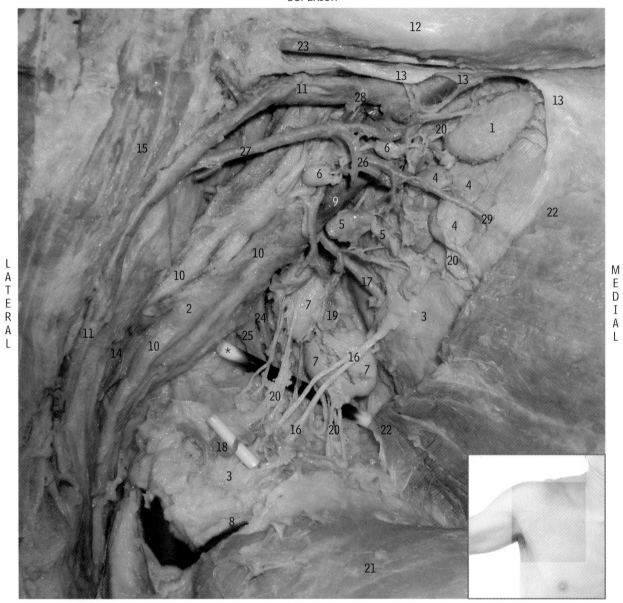

SUPERIOR

LATERAL

MEDIAL

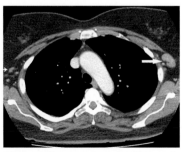

1	Apical node (infraclavicular – enlarged)	**16**	Intercostobrachial nerve
2	Axillary fascial sheath	**17**	Lateral thoracic artery
3	Axillary fat	**18**	Lateral thoracic, axillary skin and sweat gland branches
4	Axillary nodes, anterior or pectoral group		
5	Axillary nodes, central group	**19**	Lateral thoracic, nodal arterial branch
6	Axillary nodes, lateral group (normal)	**20**	Lymphatic vessels
7	Axillary nodes, posterior group (enlarged)	**21**	Pectoralis major (reflected)
8	Axillary skin	**22**	Pectoralis minor
9	Axillary vein	**23**	Subclavius
10	Brachial plexus within axillary sheath	**24**	Subscapular artery
11	Cephalic vein	**25**	Subscapular vein
12	Clavicle	**26**	Thoraco-acromial artery
13	Clavipectoral fascia (cut)	**27**	Thoraco-acromial artery, deltoid branch
14	Coracobrachialis	**28**	Thoraco-acromial artery, clavicular branch
15	Deltoid	**29**	Thoraco-acromial artery, pectoral branch

* Quill placed to lift vessels and nerves

Axial CT, axilla*

*Arrow points to enlarged axillary node

Axillary lymph node (sentinel node) dissection for breast cancer, lymphangitis, lymphoedema, see page 369.

A Right axilla and lymph nodes *from the front*

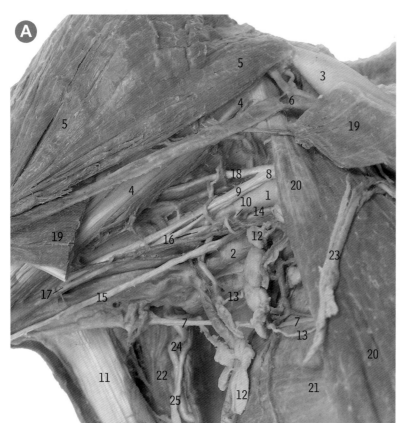

Pectoralis major (19) has been reflected and the clavipectoral fascia removed, together with the axillary sheath which surrounded the axillary artery and brachial plexus.

1 Axillary artery
2 Axillary vein
3 Clavicle
4 Coracobrachialis
5 Deltoid
6 Entry of cephalic vein into deltoid vein
7 Intercostobrachial nerve
8 Lateral cord of brachial plexus
9 Lateral root of median nerve
10 Lateral thoracic artery
11 Latissimus dorsi
12 Lymph nodes
13 Lymph vessels
14 Medial cord of the brachial plexus
15 Medial cutaneous nerve of arm
16 Medial root of median nerve
17 Median nerve
18 Musculocutaneous nerve
19 Pectoralis major
20 Pectoralis minor
21 Serratus anterior
22 Subscapularis
23 Thoracoacromial vessels and lateral pectoral nerve
24 Thoracodorsal artery
25 Thoracodorsal nerve

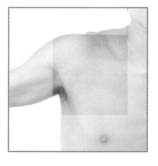

Coronal CT*

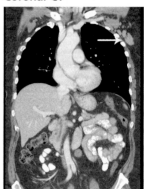

B Right cubital fossa *lymph nodes*

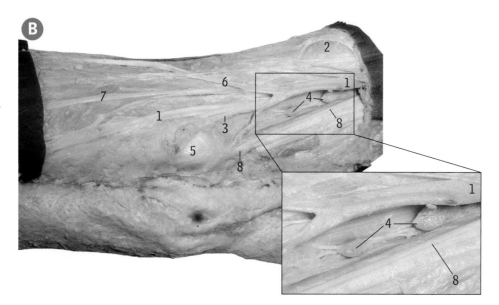

1 Basilic vein
2 Biceps brachii
3 Branches of medial cutaneous nerve of forearm
4 Cubital lymph nodes
5 Medial epicondyle of humerus
6 Median cubital vein
7 Median forearm vein
8 Ulnar nerve

Parasagittal CT*

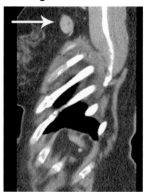

*Arrows indicate axillary lymphadenopathy

Cisterna chyli in posterior upper abdominal wall

Note split right crus

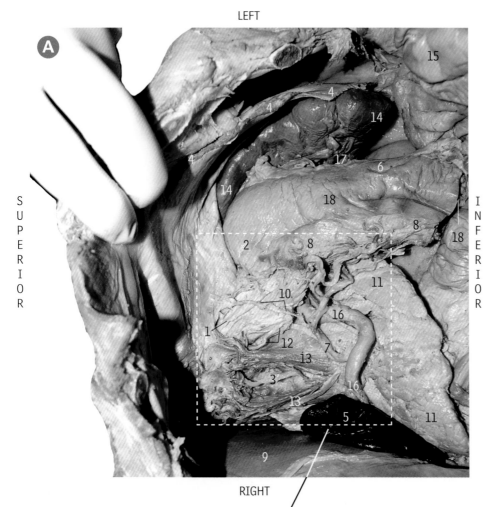

LEFT

A

SUPERIOR

INFERIOR

RIGHT

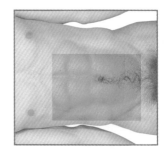

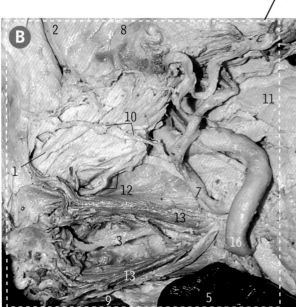

B

1	Anterior vagal trunk
2	Cardia of stomach
3	Cisterna chyli
4	Diaphragm
5	Gall bladder
6	Greater curvature of stomach
7	Left gastric artery
8	Lesser curvature of stomach
9	Liver
10	Oesophageal artery
11	Pancreas
12	Posterior vagal trunk
13	Right crus of the diaphragm (split)
14	Spleen
15	Splenic flexure
16	Splenic artery
17	Splenic hilum with splenic artery and vein
18	Stomach (cut)

Female pelvis *left half of midline sagittal section with lymphadenopathy*

Retroverted uterus – a normal variant

SUPERIOR

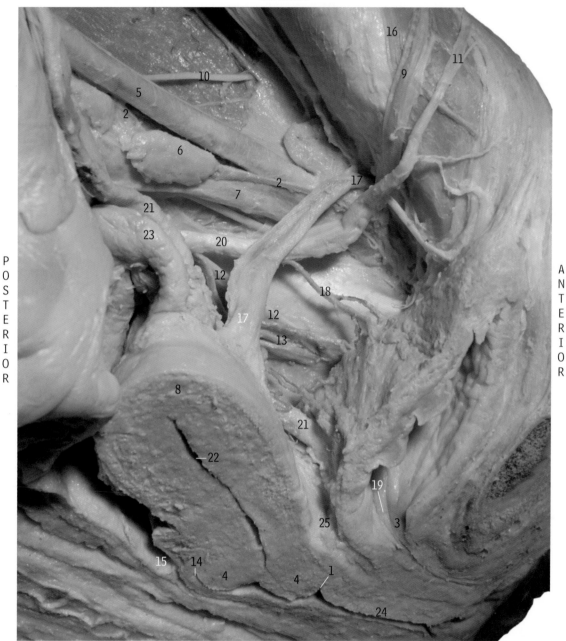

POSTERIOR

ANTERIOR

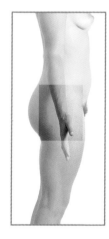

INFERIOR

1 Anterior vaginal fornix	**10** Lateral cutaneous nerve of thigh	**19** Trigone of bladder
2 Arterial supply to lymph node	**11** Medial umbilical ligament	**20** Umbilical artery (remnant)
3 Bladder neck	**12** Obturator nerve	**21** Ureter
4 Cervix	**13** Obturator vessels	**22** Uterine cavity
5 External iliac artery	**14** Posterior vaginal fornix	**23** Uterine tube (Fallopian)
6 External iliac lymph node (enlarged)	**15** Rectouterine peritoneal pouch (Douglas)	**24** Vagina
7 External iliac vein	**16** Rectus abdominis	**25** Vesicouterine peritoneal pouch
8 Fundus of uterus	**17** Round ligament of uterus	
9 Inferior epigastric vessels	**18** Superior vesical artery	

Gross lymphadenopathy of the pelvis *relationship of nodal groups*

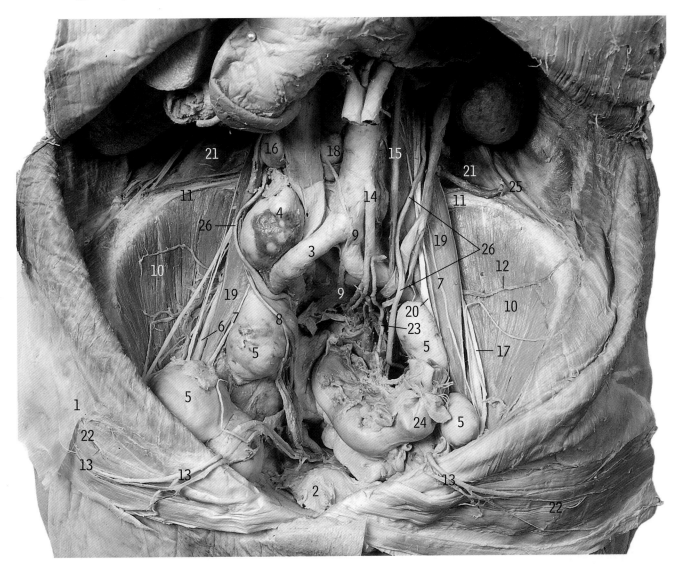

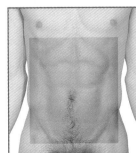

1 Arcuate line of posterior rectus sheath
2 Bladder
3 Common iliac artery
4 Common iliac node (grossly enlarged)
5 External iliac node (grossly enlarged)
6 Femoral nerve
7 Genitofemoral nerve
8 Gonadal vein
9 Hypogastric plexus, superior
10 Iliacus
11 Iliolumbar ligament
12 Iliolumbar vein
13 Inferior epigastric vessels
14 Inferior mesenteric artery
15 Inferior mesenteric vein
16 Lateral aortic (right chain) node (enlarged)
17 Lateral cutaneous nerve of thigh
18 Pre-aortic (aortocaval) node (enlarged)
19 Psoas major
20 Psoas minor
21 Quadratus lumborum
22 Rectus abdominis
23 Sigmoid branches of left colic artery
24 Sigmoid colon
25 Subcostal nerve
26 Ureter

Lymphadenopathy, lymphoma and splenomegaly, see page 369.

Lymphatics of thigh and superficial inguinal lymph nodes

A *minor lymphadenopathy*

B *moderate lymphadenopathy*

* Marker quill is in the right anterior superior iliac spine

LATERAL

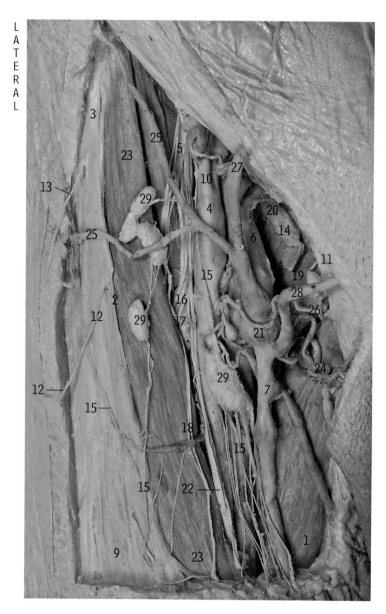

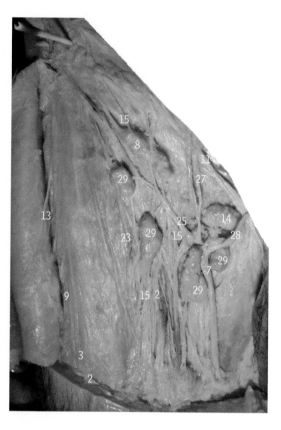

1 Adductor longus
2 Fascia lata, cut edge
3 Fascia lata overlying tensor fasciae latae
4 Femoral artery
5 Femoral nerve
6 Femoral vein
7 Great saphenous vein
8 Horizontal chain of superficial inguinal nodes
9 Iliotibial tract overlying vastus lateralis
10 Inferior epigastric vessels
11 Inguinal ligament
12 Intermediate cutaneous nerve of thigh
13 Lateral cutaneous nerve of thigh
14 Lymph node (Cloquet)
15 Lymph vessels
16 Muscular branches of femoral nerve overlying lateral circumflex femoral vessels
17 Nerve to sartorius
18 Nerve to vastus lateralis
19 Pectineus
20 Position of femoral canal
21 Saphena varix
22 Saphenous nerve
23 Sartorius
24 Scrotal veins
25 Superficial circumflex iliac vein
26 Superficial external pudendal artery
27 Superficial epigastric vein
28 Superficial external pudendal vein
29 Vertical chain of superficial inguinal lymph nodes

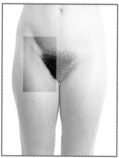

The boundaries of the femoral triangle are the inguinal ligament (11), the medial border of sartorius (23) and the medial border of adductor longus (1).

The femoral canal (20) is the medial compartment of the femoral sheath (removed) which contains in its middle compartment the femoral vein (6) and in the lateral compartment the femoral artery (4). The femoral nerve (5) is lateral to the sheath, not within it.

Milroy's disease, lymphangioma circumscriptum, lymphogranuloma venereum (LGV), elephantiasis, see page 369.

Lymphatics

Clinical thumbnails, see website for details and further clinical images to download into your own notes.

Axillary lymph node
(sentinel node)
dissection for breast
cancer

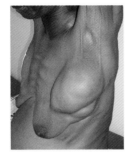

Axillary node
enlargement

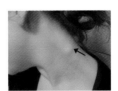

Elephantiasis

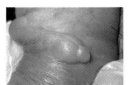

Lymphadenopathy

Lymphangioma
circumscriptum

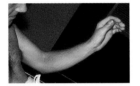

Lymphangitis

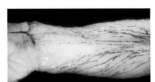

Lymphatic system –
methylene blue test

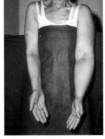

Lymphoedema

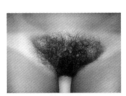

Lymphogranuloma
venereum (LGV)

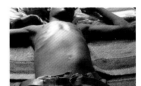

Lymphoma and
splenomegaly

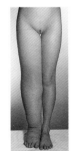

Milroy's disease

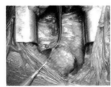

Thymus

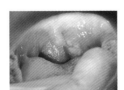

Tonsillitis

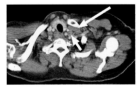

Virchow's node

Index

Page numbers followed by "f" indicate figures, "t" indicate tables, and "b" indicate boxes. Page numbers preceded by "e" indicate online material.